Hair and Scalp Disorders

Hair and Scalp Disorders
Common Presenting Signs, Differential Diagnosis and Treatment

Second Edition

Rodney PR Dawber MA MB ChB FRCP
Senior Clinical Lecturer in Dermatology
University of Oxford

Consultant Dermatologist
Oxford Hospitals

Chairman Oxford Hair Foundation

Churchill Hospital
Old Road
Headington
Oxford
OX3 7LJ
UK

Dominique Van Neste MD PhD
Managing Director
Skinterface sprl
9 rue du Sondart
7500 Tournai
Belgium
info@skinterface.be
www.skinterface.be

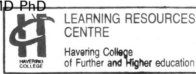
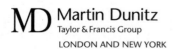
Martin Dunitz
Taylor & Francis Group
LONDON AND NEW YORK

© 1995, 2004 Martin Dunitz, an imprint of the Taylor & Francis Group plc

First published in the United Kingdom in 1995 by
Martin Dunitz, an imprint of the Taylor & Francis Group plc, 11 New Fetter Lane,
London EC4P 4EE

Tel.:   +44 (0) 20 7583 9855
Fax.:   +44 (0) 20 7842 2298
E-mail: info@dunitz.co.uk
Website: http://www.dunitz.co.uk

Although every effort has been made to ensure that all owners of copyright material
have been acknowledged in this publication, we would be glad to acknowledge in
subsequent reprints or editions any omissions brought to our attention.

A CIP record for this book is available from the British Library.

ISBN 1 84184 193 5

Distributed in North and South America by

Taylor & Francis
2000 NW Corporate Blvd
Boca Raton, FL 33431, USA

Within Continental USA
Tel.:   800 272 7737; Fax.:   800 374 3401
Outside Continental USA
Tel.:   561 994 0555; Fax.:   561 361 6018
E-mail: orders@crcpress.com

Distributed in the rest of the world by

Thomson Publishing Services
Cheriton House
North Way
Andover, Hampshire SP10 5BE, UK
Tel.:   +44 (0)1264 332424
E-mail: salesorder.tandf@thomsonpublishingservices.co.uk

Composition by EXPO Holdings, Malaysia
Printed and bound in Spain by Grafos SA

Contents

Preface

In the first edition of the book we aimed to provide a succinct volume to complement the greater detail of the major textbooks in the field – a guide to clinicians in primary care – and in dermatology, trichology and associated specialities. We were reassured that it has been sufficiently successful to merit a further edition, despite the massive increase in hair literature and books. We have again concentrated mainly on ordering the various sections based on presenting symptoms and signs, differential diagnosis and pragmatic therapeutics. Most changes in recent years have been in the scientific basis of hair and scalp disorders; the 'measurement' of hair loss, and the pathogenesis of diseases and syndromes such as female pattern hair loss (FPHL), androgenetic alopecia (AGA) and chronic telogen effluvium (CTE). Because of these advances, the management of diffuse hair loss, particularly in women, and alopecia areata has improved enormously, and this is reflected in the descriptions in the relevant sections. We hope that the book will provide practitioners with the knowledge and confidence to manage the 'core' of hair and scalp disorders.

1 Hair science

ANATOMY AND PHYSIOLOGY

Introduction

In contrast with other sections dedicated to scalp hair, this section also contains much information on human hair from other body sites and on animal hair. Indeed, there has been much to learn from scientists working in other fields such as animal biology, the wool industry and even cosmetic sciences. They have generated important information that applies in some cases to human scalp hair. Hair has no vital function in humans, yet its psychological importance is immeasurable. If the inevitability of scalp baldness makes it tolerable to genetically disposed men, in women, loss of hair from the scalp is no less distressing than growth of body or facial hair in excess of the culturally acceptable amount; subtle loss in women may be a much greater clinical problem than the overt loss in men. Sudden changes of hair appearance, even though reversible, as in chemotherapy-associated hair loss or scalp shaving before brain surgery, are clearly the first psychological obstacles that the patient has to accept before proceeding with the proposed treatment.

The evolutionary history of hair is no less of an enigma (Figure 1.1). Whatever its origin, it is clear that the warm-blooded mammals owe much of their evolutionary success to the properties of the hairy covering as a heat insulator. Paradoxically, the movement of humans from their ancestral forest home to populate the globe is linked

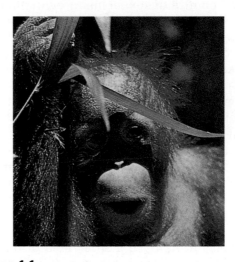

Figure 1.1
The coat in monkeys and apes is an important heat insulator. Many of these primates also develop androgenetic alopecia!

with a reversion to relative nudity and an ability to keep cool.

Hair serves many other purposes; in particular, it is concerned with sexual and social communication by constructing adornments such as the mane of the lion or the beard of the human male, or assisting in the dispersal of scents secreted by complexes of sebaceous or apocrine glands. From the anthropological standpoint, we have the magnificent display of scalp hair by many women, with cosmetic assistance.

For these evolutionary reasons, hair follicles are not all under identical control mechanisms. To match the animal pelage to seasonal changes in ambient temperature or environmental background requires moulting and replacement of the hairs. The process appears to involve an inherent follicular rhythm, modified by circulating hormones such as steroids or thyroxine, whose secretion is, in turn, geared to environmental cues through the hypothalamus and hypophysis. In a subtle way, these control mechanisms may still be important in *Homo sapiens*.

The control of sexual hair growth must be clearly differentiated from that of the moult cycle. The development of pubic, axillary and other body hair is delayed until puberty because it is dependent upon androgens in both sexes. The serum level and the local transformation of such hormones play a crucial role in the sexual hair phenotype. That 'male' hormones (present and functioning in both sexes!) are also a prerequisite for the manifestation of pattern baldness still defies adequate explanation.

Hair grows from follicles (Figures 1.2, 1.3), which are stocking-like invaginations of the superficial epithelium, each of which encloses at its base a small area of dermis known as the dermal papilla (Figures 1.3, 1.4). The cylinder of hair may be regarded as a holocrine secretion arising by division of cells surrounding the papilla, in a region known as the bulb. The follicles are sloped, not vertical, in the dermis, the longer ones extending into the subcutaneous fat layer. An oblique muscle, the arrector pili, runs from the mid-region of the follicle wall to the dermoepidermal junction. Above the muscle one or more sebaceous glands, and also in some regions of the body an apocrine gland, open into the follicle. At the level of attachment of the arrector pili muscle to the follicle is the 'bulge zone' of the root sheaths. This is considered to be the stem cell site from which the 'new' matrix cells generate as a new hair cycle is initiated. Indeed, in all mammals, including humans, but with the possible exception of the merino sheep, hair follicles show intermittent activity. Thus, each hair grows to a maximum length, is retained for a time without further growth, and is eventually shed and replaced. In humans, the hair cycle occurs a sufficient number of times to maintain hair on most body sites and at least on some areas of the scalp.

> **Though hair is not a requirement for physical existence in humans, it is extremely important to one's social and psychological equilibrium – a very delicate interplay between important perception of self by self and others**

Development and distribution of hair follicles

The 'nucleus' of hair follicles appears first in the regions of the eyebrows, upper lip and chin at about 9 weeks of embryonic development, and in other regions in the fourth month; by 22 weeks, the full complement of follicles is established. The diffusion of this phenomenon is a complex

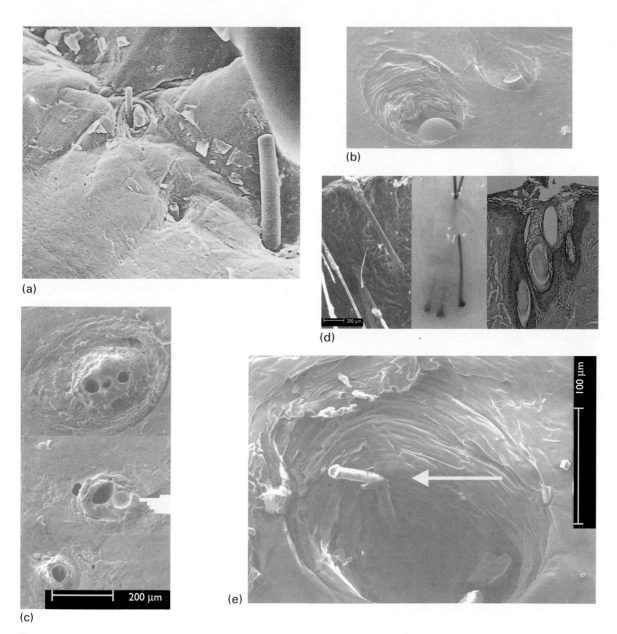

Figure 1.2
Hairs emerging at the skin surface: scanning electron micrograph (SEM) of surface replicas. On some body sites, thin hair may rise almost at right angles from the grooved skin surface (a). The wider scalp follicle opening softly reaches the smooth scalp surface and gives way to thicker hair (b: right) and associated gland secretion, which, in the occasional absence of hair, can be seen as droplets in the follicular opening (b: left). Hair follicle openings are grouped by two or three (c; top shows a trio), but some openings may be filled by plugs (c, pointed in the middle), but a single opening may occur. When follicles are microdissected, internal structures can be observed with the scanning electron microscope (d, left), a magnifying glass (d, middle) or the light microscope (d, right). Each method brings about a new view. The earliest step for visible hair growth is when the fibre reaches the scalp surface (arrow on SEM, e).

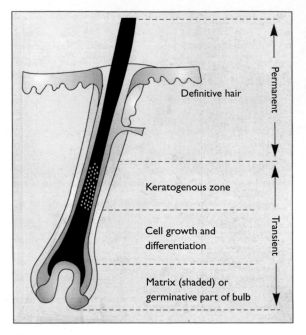

Definitive hair

Permanent

Keratogenous zone

Transient

Cell growth and differentiation

Matrix (shaded) or germinative part of bulb

Figure 1.3
Hair follicle. Schematic diagram to show the basic components.

sequence of activation and inhibition of adjacent cells that will or will not subsequently participate in the hair follicle formation. This process involves the total body surface except the palmar and plantar skin areas. As the body surface increases, there is a decrease in the actual density of follicles. It is generally accepted that under normal circumstances new follicles cannot develop in adult skin. The total number of follicles in an adult man has been estimated at approximately 5 million, of which about 1 million are on the head and perhaps 100 000 in the scalp. There appear to be no significant sexual or racial differences in follicle number.

In the face, follicle density displays a gradient from centre to periphery with more units in the midline. On the cheek and forehead, the average density of follicles of all

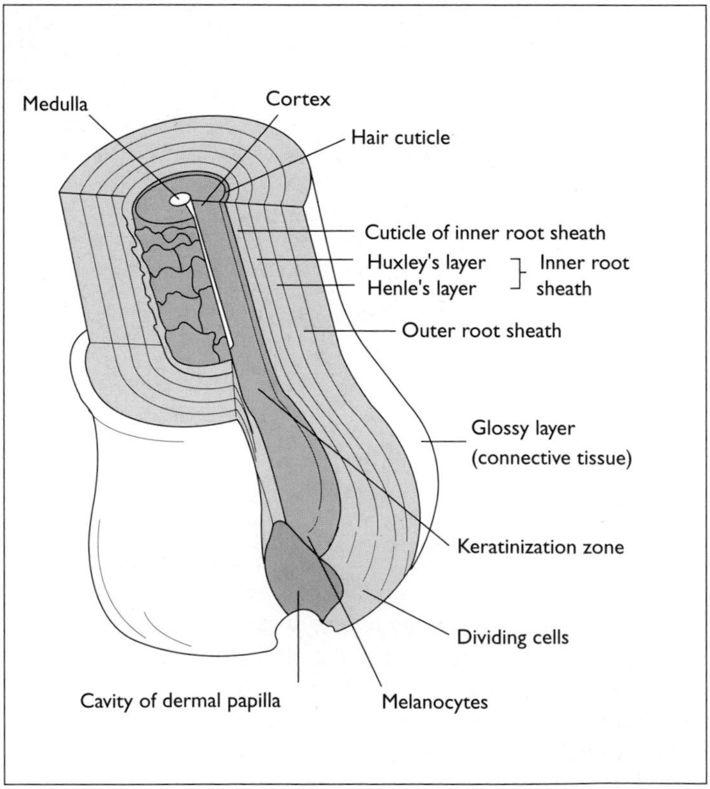

Figure 1.4
Hair follicle. Schematic diagram to show the basic structure.

Medulla

Cortex

Hair cuticle

Cuticle of inner root sheath

Huxley's layer   ⌐ Inner root
Henle's layer   ⌐ sheath

Outer root sheath

Glossy layer (connective tissue)

Keratinization zone

Dividing cells

Cavity of dermal papilla

Melanocytes

types is 800 per cm², of which about 50% have been found to produce vellus hairs actively in young adults, males and females alike. These values show a wide scatter between individuals (range from 300 to 1600 follicles per cm²) and there is also variation due to the observation methods. On the thigh and leg, the density of follicles of all types is much lower at 50 per cm², and on the chest, shoulder and back, the density of vellus hair ranges between 50 and 100 per cm². This again reflects the relative expansion of the skin surface after organogenesis of the follicular structure; scalp and head expand much less than chest and legs. The greatest density of vellus hairs occurs on the forehead where there are on average 400–450 per cm² in young adults, males and females alike. Females have a similar density on the cheek. Lower densities (50–100 per cm²) are found on the chest and back in both sexes.

On the scalp, a significant loss of hair follicles occurs with advancing age; in adults aged 20–30 years an average of 615 per cm² has been recorded, but between 30 and 50 years the mean density falls to 485, and by 80–90 years it is only 435 per cm². There are undoubtedly fewer follicles present in affected areas as androgenetic alopecia evolves from its young adult onset into middle and old age. Comparison of bald with hairy scalps for the whole range of 30–90 years gives mean values of 306 and 459 per cm², respectively. More recent methods of measurement have suggested lower densities: females 260 per cm²; males 250 per cm². The anagen percentage is usually >90% in males and >85% in females. The numbers vary according to the sampling and observation methods used: there is a biological variability but the extreme numbers are probably the result of inappropriate sampling and calculation methods (microscopy, biopsy or life, scalp photography, plucking and so on).

THE ACTIVE FOLLICLE

Dynamics

The bulk of any hair is formed by the cortical layer made up of elongated keratinized cells cemented together (Figure 1.5). In pigmented hairs these cells contain granules of melanin (Figure 1.6). These pigment-loaded lysosome-like structures are formed by a distinct type of cell, namely the melanocyte. The cortex is surrounded by a cuticle and may also have a continuous or discontinuous core or medulla. Although the hair cuticle is formed as a single cuboidal layer, the cells become flattened and progressively more overlapped (imbricated) as they move away from the hair bulb. The outer cells overlap with their free edges directed towards the tip, and they interlock with the cuticle of the surrounding inner root sheath (Figure 1.4). The inner root sheath consists, in addition to its cuticle, of Henle's and Huxley's layers; it is formed in pace with the hair and its keratinized cells are ultimately desquamated into the follicular infundibulum. Investing it is the outer root sheath, which is continuous with the superficial epithelium, and this is itself enclosed in a low-cellular, predominantly connective tissue layer formed of collagenous fibres, a few elastic fibres and fibroblasts. This cell layer in its deeper part may be responsible for dermal papilla replacement.

Cell formation in hair follicles has been studied by intracutaneous injection of tritiated thymidine into sites on the human scalp. In biopsy samples taken 40 minutes later, labelling of cells was observed in the lower half of the hair bulb, but not elsewhere. However, labelled cells were distributed diffusely throughout the area, and not in a well-defined basal layer along the papilla, and no labelled mitotic figures were observed. Six hours after injection, the number of labelled cells had increased,

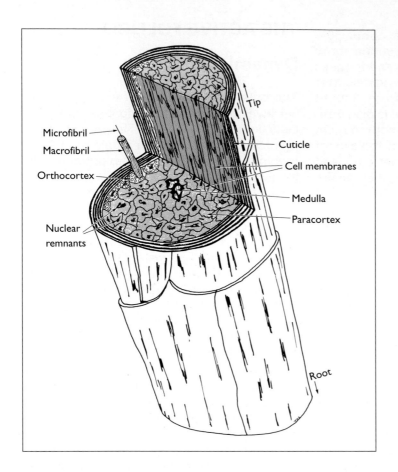

Figure 1.5
Hair structure.

labelled mitotic figures were seen and some movement was detected in cells of the outer bulb destined to become inner root sheath. Subsequently, a stream of cells moving into the cortex could also be detected, but it moved much more slowly. In general, these results confirm earlier suggestions that new cells are formed by division in the region of the bulb surrounding the dermal papilla, but they do not settle the question as to whether only cells adjacent to the dermal papilla are capable of division (Figures 1.3, 1.4, 1.7). The fact that the number of grains per cell is reduced as labelled cells move away from the basal matrix area suggests that further divisions take place. The assumption that at each division one daughter cell remains capable of further division

and attached to the dermal papilla is also questionable in the light of studies of the behaviour of cells in the basal layer of the superficial epidermis. As will be described later, the transient part of the hair follicle (Figure 1.3) is regularly regenerated by a hair cycling process. At each cycle, the hair follicle is reloaded with a new germinative population deriving from stem cells. Such cells are concentrated at the bottom of the permanent part of the follicle where they usually rest and divide from time to time after stimulation by the dermal papilla. Then, they generate a population of actively proliferating daughter cells (Figure 1.7). These transit amplifying cells divide and migrate during the initial steps of hair follicle regeneration. Whether such a build-up

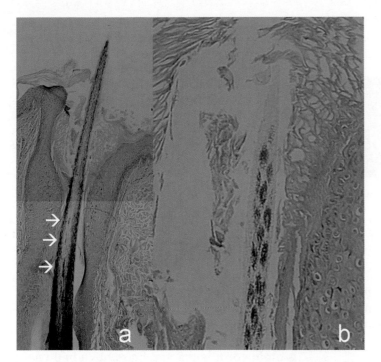

Figure 1.6
Scalp follicle of a black African subject. Pigment granules are abundant in the periphery of the hair cortex and less so in the centre. Dark spaces found in the middle of the hair reflect unpigmented medulla (arrows in a; light diffraction). The close-up of the hair cortex (b) shows the spindle-shaped cortical cells fully packed with pigment granules. The cuticle cells surrounding the hair cortex appear unpigmented.

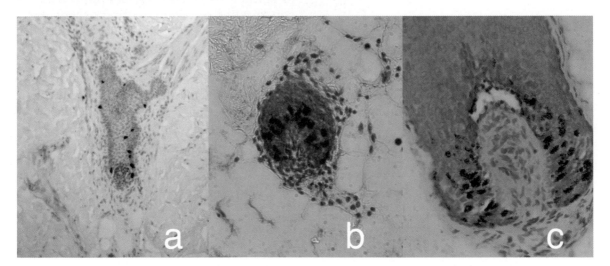

Figure 1.7
DNA synthesis in the human scalp follicles. Tritiated thymidine labelling of cells preparing for cell division (black dots) is initially observed in all the epithelial components of the regrowing hair follicle (a). Then the activity will concentrate in the newly formed hair bulb (b) and finally in the lower half of the mature hair bulb, i.e. the matrix of the continuously growing anagen hair. (c) Remarkably, there are no labelled cells in the dermal papilla and a few scattered cells in the dermis associated with microvascular structures.

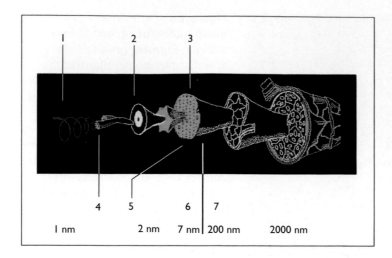

Figure 1.8
Hair subunit structures.
1, right-handed α-helix;
2, low-S; 3, high-S; 4, left-handed
coiled-coil rope; 5, matrix;
6, microfibril; 7, macrofibril.

of fresh cells can occur at any other times of the hair cycle – in all or some hair follicles – is not clearly documented, but, clearly, stem cell characteristics have been identified in some cells amidst the outer root sheaths (Figure 1.4) of mature hair follicles.

COMPOSITION OF HAIR KERATIN

Keratins are a group of insoluble cystine-containing helicoidal protein complexes produced in the epithelial tissues of verte-

brates. The main body of the hair is made up of an amorphous matrix (high-sulphur and ultra-high-sulphur proteins) in which the keratin fibres are embedded (Figures 1.8, 1.9). Because of the resistance of these protein complexes, the hairs have been said to contain hard keratins as opposed to the soft keratins of desquamating tissues. Even though the terms hard and soft keratins are still commonly used, one should clearly associate these peculiar physical properties of the hair fibre with the combination of proteins of different nature: a fibrillar rod made of the hair keratins embedded in an

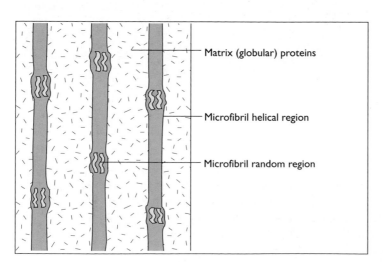

Figure 1.9
Fibrillar and matrix keratins of hair cortex.

amorphous matrix composed of high-sulphur proteins. In hair they make up the main body of the fibre. X-ray crystallography of hair gives a so-called α-diffraction pattern indicating an axial repeat of 0.51 nm units. If the hair is stretched or heated in water, it gives the β-pattern with an axial repeat of 0.33 nm. This bears some similarity to the 'feather pattern' characteristic of keratin in avian and reptilian tissues, which has a repeat of 0.31 nm. A fourth pattern, described as amorphous because it lacks discrete reflections, occurs in the keratin of the hair cuticle.

It was concluded from the X-ray diffraction pattern that the polypeptide chains of α-keratin have a geometrically regular secondary structure. The hypothesis was proposed that they are arranged in an α-helix with 3.6 amino acid residues in each turn of 0.54 nm. The 0.51 nm repeat could be explained if the helices are tilted, which led to the suggestion that they are intertwined to form a rope of two or three strands, and possibly even seven strands. The change to the β-pattern when hair is stretched can be explained by assuming that the helix is pulled into a straight-chain configuration.

Recent studies on keratin typing in various epithelia show clear differences between the hair follicle deep to the infundibulum and the epidermis. However, the significance of the variations has not yet been worked out.

Filaments known as microfibrils have long been recognized in keratinizing cells and are believed to bind up to form macrofibrils (Figures 1.8, 1.9). It is now realized that all cells contain filaments of several size ranges, including six major types of intermediate filaments, 7–10 nm in diameter. Keratins fall within this category. The current view is that there are several stages of organization as keratin filaments are progressively assembled from polypeptides, comprising a protofilament 2 nm in diameter consisting of two strands, a 3 nm protofilament of $2 \times 3 \times 2$ strands, a 4–5 nm protofibril of $2 \times 3 \times 4$ strands and a 10 nm filament of $4 \times 3 \times 8$ strands.

Chemical analysis of keratin is complicated because the preliminary procedures to render it soluble by breaking the disulphide links of the interchains could also cleave the peptides. Three soluble fractions can be obtained from wool: a low-sulphur fraction of molecular mass 45 000–50 000 Da, a high-sulphur fraction of molecular mass 10 000–28 000 Da and a high-glycine tyrosine fraction. Complete amino acid sequences have been determined for at least 21 wool proteins. Low-sulphur fractions contain the α-helices and account for the keratin filaments. The high-sulphur proteins are not keratins but are associated with the filaments to create a fibre–matrix complex.

Within the last decade considerable advances have been made in understanding the biochemistry of keratins and the mechanisms of their alignment into macrofibres. As typical examples we mention here fragile hair resulting from specific biochemical abnormalities: trichothiodystrophy is a defect of the amorphous sulphur-rich matrix proteins while monilethrix is always associated with abnormalities of hair keratins and subsequent conformational defects.

ULTRASTRUCTURE

The medulla

The cells of the medulla (Figures 1.4, 1.5) begin to show vesicles within their cytoplasm in the suprabulbar region. Such cells contain glycogen and may include melanosomes. Above the level of the epidermis, the cells appear to dehydrate and the vacuoles become air-filled. The protein composition of the medulla contains trichohyalin.

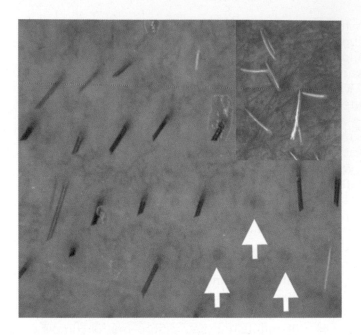

Figure 1.10
Clipped beard: pepper and salt hair with empty follicles (arrows).
The beard shows medullated hair fibres, both pigmented and unpigmented. The medulla appears as a central very bright stripe when examined under specific UV lighting (black and white insert).

The role of the medulla remains unknown. It is usually found in thicker hairs. It may be almost continuous in the thicker unpigmented beard hairs (Figure 1.10): a nice model of building a lighter fibre. Not all medullae degenerate and become air-filled. Therefore the medulla appears interrupted, especially due to reflection of light at the air-filled spaces; dark spaces do not always mean pigment deposition (Figure 1.6).

The cortex

In the zone just below the tip of the dermal papilla, the microfibrils can already be seen in the cells which give rise to the cortex. They rapidly aggregate to form clusters. In the upper bulb region, aggregates a few tenths of a micron (micrometre) wide can be seen as fibrils under the light microscope. At this level the fibrils are birefringent and give the oriented α-type X-ray diffusion pattern; thus, the synthesis of the basic structure is virtually complete. Subsequently, the denser sulphur-rich matrix develops, coincident with the intense sulphydryl reaction which indicates the presence of cysteine links. In contrast to the superficial epidermis and the inner root sheath, keratohyalin granules do not appear at any stage. On examination by electron microscopy, the mature cortex can be seen to consist of closely packed spindle-shaped cells (Figure 1.5) with their boundaries separated by a narrow gap (20–25 nm) containing a dense central plasma membrane or intercellular lamella (10–15 nm), believed to be proteinaceous and to cement the cells together. Within the cells most of the microfibrils are closely packed and orientated longitudinally in lamellae, though some remain in loose bundles. In transverse section these concentric lamellae have a characteristic 'thumbprint' appearance (Figures 1.11, 1.12).

The hair cuticle

The cuticle consists of five to ten overlapping cell layers, each 350–450 nm thick

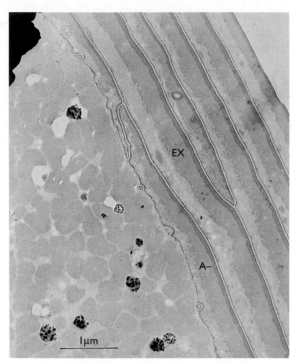

Figure 1.11
Hair fibre cross-section showing cortex with dark pigment granules to the left and layers of cuticle to the right. EX, exocuticle; A, A-layer of cuticle cell (electron micrograph, silver methenamine stain).

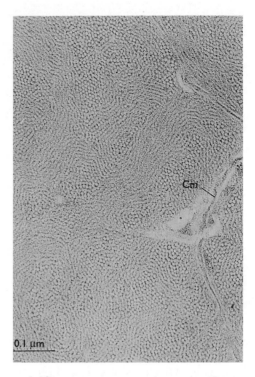

Figure 1.12
Hair cortex (electron micrograph, silver methenamine stain) showing intracellular bundles of microfibrils with dark background matrix protein. Cm, cell membrane.

(Figure 1.5). The mature cells are thin scales consisting of dense keratin which shows outer and inner zones of different densities. Between the cell boundaries is a narrow gap (30 nm) containing a dense central intercellular lamella. From the outside, the scales can be seen to be imbricated like the tiles on a roof. Over the newly formed part of the hair the scale margins are intact, but as the hair emerges from the skin they become jagged and progressively break off ('weathering').

The 'environmental' outer surface of each cuticular cell has a very clear A-layer, which is rich in high-sulphur protein; this protects the cuticular cells from premature break-down due to chemical and physical insults (Figures 1.11, 1.13).

Inner root sheath

Each of the three layers of the inner root sheath keratinizes (Figure 1.4), and though the rates of maturation are different, the patterns of change are identical. Filaments are about 7 nm thick and, in contrast to the hair cortex, amorphous trichohyalin granules appear in the cytoplasm. As the cells move up the follicle, the filaments become more abundant and the number and size of the granules increase. In the hardened cytoplasm, however, only filaments can be seen.

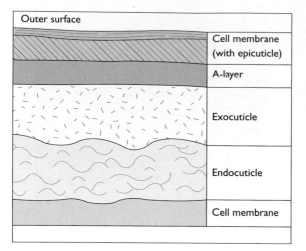

Figure 1.13
Diagrammatic representation of the hair cuticle cell structure.

The changes occur first in the outermost Henle's layer, then in the innermost cuticle and lastly in Huxley's layer, which is situated between them.

The inner root sheath hardens before the presumptive hair within it, and it is consequently thought to control the definitive shape of the hair shaft in health and in many genetic diseases with abnormal hair morphology.

Outer root sheath

In humans the outer root sheath is composed of two layers. In the outer, the cells gradually increase in number from root to tip. They produce membrane-limited granules, or cementosomes, which accumulate. Staining by anti-hair keratin monoclonal antibodies has suggested that the differentiating cells of the medulla, cortex, cuticle and inner root sheath display a similar keratin expression, but the innermost cell layer of the outer root sheath displays a unique expression. There is much specula-

tion on the potential direction of migration of cell streams in the outer root sheath during the various stages of the hair cycle.

CYCLIC ACTIVITY OF THE FOLLICLE

The duration of activity of follicles (Figures 1.14–1.17), or anagen, varies greatly with species, within the same species from region to region, with season and with age. For example, in the rat the dorsal hair is fully formed in 3 weeks and the shorter ventral hair in only 12 days, whereas in the guinea pig, anagen lasts for 20–40 days.

In human vellus follicles of both sexes, the periods of activity range from about 40 to 80 days. For terminal hairs in young Japanese males, the length of anagen has been estimated at 19–26 weeks on the leg, 6–12 weeks on the arm, 4–13 weeks on the finger, 4–14 weeks in the moustache, and 8–24 weeks in the region under the temple. Estimated averages of 54 and 28 days, respectively, have been made for the thighs and arms of Caucasoid males, and 22 days for each of these sites in females. It is known that in the human scalp, anagen may last for 3–7 years.

> **Each follicle goes repeatedly through the hair cycle during a lifetime. Reactivation of stem cells provides a new batch of fresh trichocytes, every cycle recapitulating much of its embryological development – 'youthful' new hair growth every few years, constantly!**

Activity (anagen) is followed by a relatively short transitional phase, catagen, occupying a few days in rodents and about

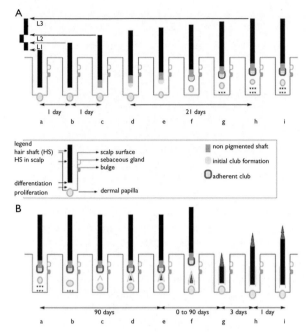

Figure 1.14
Diagrammatic representation of hair cycling of a human hair follicle: (A) from growth to rest and (B) from rest to growth.

The latest steps of the hair growth phase (anagen 6) during which hair is visible at the skin surface and growing are shown in A while the apparent rest phase of the hair cycle (telogen phase) is shown in B. During this phase a new hair cycle can be initiated. The legend (between A and B) helps the reader to orient himself within the various components of the human hair follicle which are essential to understanding growth and rest.

(A) From growth to rest.
The same hair follicle is represented at various times (days) at the very end of the growth phase. At the skin surface, there is normal pigmented hair production (days a–b and b–c) representing the constant daily hair production (L1 and L2).

Then, the pigmentation of the newly synthesized hair shaft (appearing at the bottom of the hair follicle) is decreased (c). This early event announces the regression of the impermanent portion of the hair follicle and is followed by terminal differentiation of cells in the proliferation compartment (d) and shrinkage of the dermal papilla (e). The latter starts an ascending movement together with the hair shaft as this characterizes the catagen phase (d–h; 21 days). The apparent elongation of the hair fibre (L3) reflects the outward migration of the hair shaft. What is left after disappearance of the epithelial cells from the impermanent portion of the hair follicle is first basement membranes followed by dermal connective tissue, usually referred to as streamers or stellae (***). The true resting stage begins when catagen is completed, i.e. when the dermal papilla abuts to the bottom of the permanent portion of the hair follicle. In the absence of physical interaction between dermal papilla and bulge, the next cycle (see B) is definitely compromised. As from now no hair growth is observed at the surface (h–i).

(B) From rest to growth.
During this stage, one notices absence of hair growth at the skin surface (a–g), but significant changes occur in the deeper parts of the hair follicle. The dermal papilla expands and attracts epithelial cells from the bulge (stem cell zone) in a downward movement (a–b). To create space, previously deposited materials have to be digested (a–b, ***) The epithelial cells then start differentiation in an orderly fashion, starting with the inner root sheath (c) and the tip of the cuticle and hair cortex of the newly formed unpigmented hair fibre (d).

The resting hair remains in the hair follicle for approximately 1 to 3 months (a–e); then the fixation is looser and finally the totally detached hair is shed (f). The shiny root end of the shed hair is the club. Before, during or after hair shedding there may be replacement by a new hair shaft (e–f–g). Indeed, under physiological conditions, the follicle proceeds immediately or only slowly with new hair production (from f to g; max. 90 days). In conditions like androgenetic alopecia a much longer interval before regrowth may be recorded. This results in empty follicular openings and plugging – see Figure 1.2(c). At the earliest stage of anagen (stage VI), a non-pigmented hair tip is seen first (h), followed by a thicker, more pigmented and faster growing hair fibre (i), depending on the many regulatory factors controlling the hair follicle.

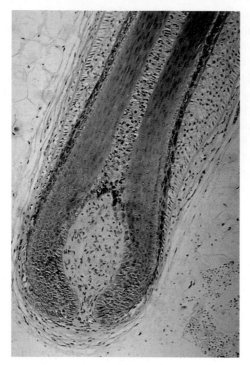

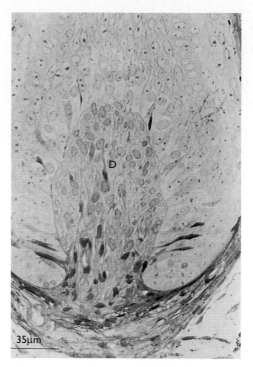

Figure 1.15
Hair follicle – anagen growth stage 6.

Figure 1.16
Hair follicle bulb – central dermal papilla (D) and surrounding matrix cell components.

2 weeks in the human scalp (Figures 1.18, 1.19), and a resting phase, or telogen. Towards the end of anagen, scalp follicles show a gradual thinning and lightening of pigment at the base of the hair shaft. The melanocytes in the region of the tip of the dermal papilla cease producing melanin, resorb their dendrites and become indistinguishable from the matrix cells. The middle region of the bulb now becomes constricted. Distal to the constriction the expanded base of the hair becomes keratinized as a 'club', and below this epithelial column can be seen the dermal papilla, which becomes released from its epidermal 'cover' (Figures 1.20–1.22). From the onset of catagen the connective tissue sheath of the follicle, in particular the vitreous membrane with its characteristic stain affinity

under the light microscope, thickens enormously and is associated with a characteristic corrugation in the epithelial strand. Subsequently, the club hair moves towards the skin surface, leaving a space that is filled up by undifferentiated epithelial cells forming an elongated column. After the ascent of the presumptive club, the epithelial strand shortens progressively from below and finally is reduced to a little nipple, and the secondary germ forms by the recombination of the old or new dermal papilla with newly formed epithelial cells. The latter probably derive from this resting stage, or telogen, and last only a few weeks in the human scalp. When the next hair cycle starts, the secondary germ forms probably from the stem cell bulge zone adjacent to the arrector pilorum muscle

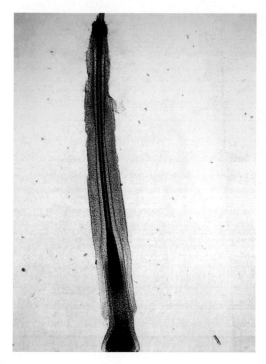

Figure 1.17
Plucked anagen hair with attached root sheaths.

attachment, elongates by cell division, grows downwards, becomes invaginated by the papilla and gives rise to the new bulb (Figure 1.23), from which arises the kera-

tinized dome of a new hair. After all cell attachments are lost, the 'old' club hair is ultimately shed, but, in the rat at least, it may be retained after emergence of the new hair, and on some body sites, particularly the leg, several successive telogen hairs may be retained before shedding. During this new stage, now called exogen, some enzymatic processes are probably involved, preparing for the final release of the old hair fibre and leading to hair shedding. Physiological or abnormal (premature, excessive or pathological) shedding can now be traced precisely on the scalp surface (Skinterface patent 2002; see measurement methods). When the hair shaft is very fine and the duration of growth is very short, passive accumulation of many exogen hairs may occur, leading to trichostasis. All hairs present in one follicle opening do not always reflect either the number of roots or the hair root activity!

Changes in antigen expression in the epithelial cells along with changes in the extracellular matrix of the dermal papilla may offer clues towards the elucidation of the dermal–epidermal interactions involved in the cyclic activity of the hair follicle.

In the adult human scalp the activity of each follicle is independent of its

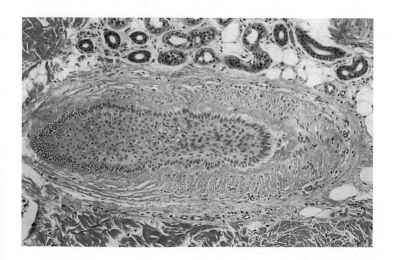

Figure 1.18
Hair follicle section in catagen phase.

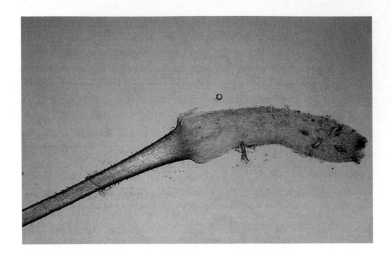

Figure 1.19
Plucked hair in catagen phase
(polarized light).

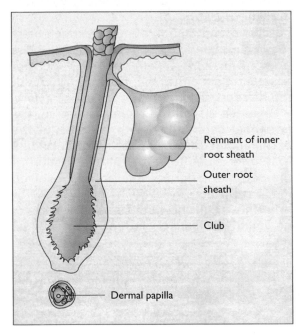

Figure 1.20
Telogen follicle showing the major components.

neighbours; such a pattern is known as mosaic. At any one time, on average about 13% of the follicles are in telogen, although the range is large: it has been recorded as 4–24%. Only 1% or less are in catagen. If there are about 100 000 follicles in the scalp and their period is about 1000 days, about 100 hairs ought to be released each day. In practice, the average recovery of shed hairs is usually rather less, and over 100 is regarded as high. Follicles throughout the body, as well as those on the scalp (Figure 1.24), are out of synchrony and, indeed, have different periodicities.

Each follicle is independent of its neighbours but has the same growth control characteristics

The guinea pig has been said to resemble humans in that moulting of the adult appears to take place in a mosaic pattern. However, in the newborn animal all follicles are simultaneously active, and it seems that for at least 50 days after birth, and probably for much longer, follicles producing a single fibre type show a measure of synchrony with each other, but are out of phase with those producing different fibre types. This finding is of interest, for in humans there is frequently a more or less synchronous moult of scalp hairs during the early months of life as well as the shed of lanugo hair during development. There is also evidence

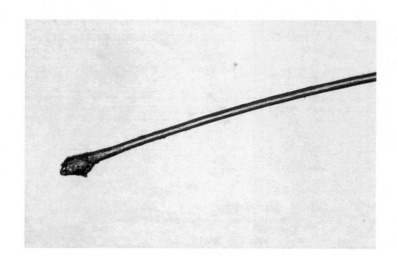

Figure 1.21
Plucked hair in telogen phase ('club' root).

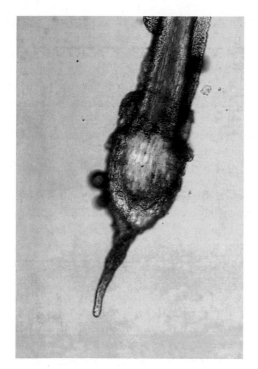

Figure 1.22
Plucked hair in telogen phase – 'club' root (polarized light).

of the passage of a growth wave from front to back in the scalp of newborn infants. Thus, it may be that in both the guinea pig and humans, asynchrony gradually develops from synchrony. The same is true after induction of hair growth either under the influence of a hair growth-promoting agent or after recovery from disease states (acute post-febrile telogen effluvium, alopecia areata; or after recovery from chemotherapy-induced hair loss). After some time without hair shedding due to synchronized hair regrowth, patients may be made afraid by the reappearance of the normal hair shedding.

Each hair follicle appears to have an intrinsic rhythm. In rats, this has been shown to continue when the site is changed or even, under some circumstances, when the follicle is transplanted to another animal in a different phase of the moult. Plucking of hairs from resting follicles brings forward the next period of activity, and such follicles continue out of phase with their neighbours, at least for a time. The nature of this intrinsic control and the mechanism by which epilation or wounding affects it are unknown. One hypothesis is that a mitotic inhibitor accumulates during anagen and is gradually used up or dispersed during telogen; another is that growth-promoting wound hormones are released by epilation. The finding that removal of residual club hairs after follicular activity has commenced

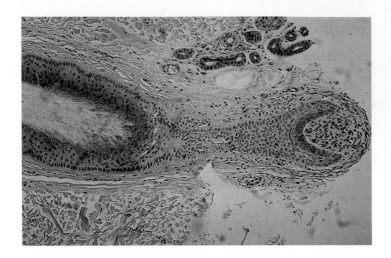

Figure 1.23
Hair follicle in early anagen phase (stage 2).

does not affect the anagen in progress but does advance the next eruption of hairs appears to be irreconcilable with the inhibitor hypothesis. Finally, under physiological conditions, there is clear evidence that telogen hair remains anchored to the follicle until it enters the exogen stage, i.e. after complete detachment (Figure 1.25).

Undoubtedly, changes in the hair cycle can be the basis of transient hair loss in humans. Some of the conditions formerly grouped under the description 'alopecia symptomatica', which can result from a variety of mental and physical stresses, involve the simultaneous precipitation of many follicles into catagen.

The term 'telogen effluvium' (or 'defluvium') was first used to describe cases of post-febrile alopecia in which shedding of club hairs began about 3–4 months after the fever and continued for 3–4 weeks. At the height of shedding, the telogen counts made from scalp biopsies ranged from 14% to 53%; regeneration was well under way 6 weeks later. As a specific example of this phenomenon, a prisoner who underwent a series of trials for murder began to lose hairs at the rate of over 1000 per day about 10 weeks after conviction. There were no histological abnormalities except an increased proportion of follicles in telogen. The nature of the neuroendocrine or other mechanisms by which the hair loss is brought about remains to be elucidated. The condition bears some similarity to post-partum alopecia. The benefits – whatever the basic mechanism, growth factor, immune regulation or hormonal influences – in terms of quality of growth gained during pregnancy have to be reimbursed but not in each and every case!

Telogen effluvium is now considered to be a non-specific response to a wide variety of acute physical or mental 'stresses'; it usually lasts for only a few months before returning to normal. After a first episode, hair growth patterns may be modified and some subjects complain they never recovered their initial hair status. It has been speculated that an acute induction of hair shedding may expose a large number of synchronized reinitiated follicles, i.e. more sensitive phases to the prevalent hormonal conditions. The committed follicles enter a new type of hair production and this may constitute a peculiar and acute mode of entry into an otherwise non-synchronized, chronic and progressive process of hair loss, e.g. androgenetic alopecia that affects both men and women.

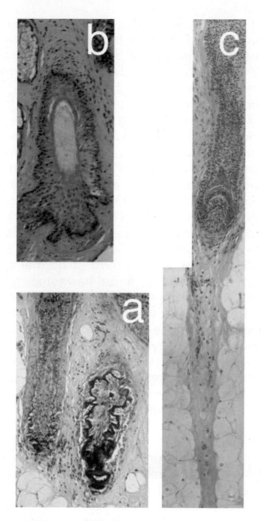

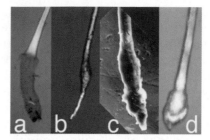

Figure 1.25
The incipient club hair is anchored to the surrounding trichocytes and hair sheaths during early catagen (a); the newly formed club hair shows a trail of still attached terminally differentiated cells (b, c) before final release as exogen hair (d).

Hormonal influences

It is important to make a clear distinction between the effects of a range of hormones on the follicular cycle, in evolutionary terms related to the adaptive function of moulting, and the particular role of androgens in the induction of sexual and other adult hair, an adaptation delaying until after puberty the associated sociosexual signals. Most dermatological problems centre around androgen-dependent hair. Knowledge of other hormonal mechanisms is, however, relevant to understanding not only the control of the moult cycle but also the problems of human hair loss in thyroid disorder and following pregnancy.

Irrespective of intrinsic control, the overall timing of the cyclic events also appears to be influenced by systemic factors, for follicles on homografts gradually come into phase with their hosts, and parabiotic rats gradually come to moult in phase with each other. This systemic control mechanism may embody components as yet unknown, but it could be accounted for by facts that can be demonstrated. In rats, oestradiol, testosterone and adrenal steroids delay the

Figure 1.24
Hair cycling is organ regeneration. In scalp sections, typical catagen (a) results in the old hair roots being squeezed out until they reach the level of adherent telogen or resting (b). Associated down growth and reconstruction of a new follicle (c) along the streamer, a path that is left over after the previous hair cycle, may be but is not always associated with full release of the previous hair shaft, leading to the exogen stage concurrent with early anagen. Most frequently in hair cycle disturbances, the two events are not associated: hair shedding occurs well before the new hair growth.

initiation of follicular activity, and oestradiol also delays the shedding of club hairs, so that the moult is accelerated by gonadectomy or adrenalectomy. Conversely, thyroid hormone advances the onset of follicular activity, and thyroidectomy or inhibition of the thyroid delays the passage of the moult.

Oestradiol has similarly been shown to delay the onset of follicular activity in the guinea pig. In the rat, hypophysectomy advances it, so the influence of the gonadal system appears to override that of the thyroid. The hypothalamus and the hypophysis may thus exert their influence by way of the thyroid, with the adrenal cortex and the gonads linking between environmental, reproductive and moulting cycles. To what extent these mechanisms operate in humans remains unknown.

Hormones also influence follicles in anagen. Studies in which rat hairs were pulse labelled with ^{35}S-cysteine showed that oestradiol and thyroxine each similarly reduced the duration of the active phase, their effects being additive when they were administered simultaneously. In contrast, whereas oestradiol decreased the rate of hair growth, thyroxine had the opposite effect. These findings suggest that the two hormones do not have the same point of action.

Human hair is profoundly affected by the level of unbound thyroid hormones. In some studies up to 10% of those who complained of hair loss were diagnosed as suffering from hypothyroidism on the basis of serum protein-bound iodine levels confirmed by radio-iodine tracer studies. Mean hair diameter in these subjects was reduced, whereas diameters in normal subjects had a symmetrical distribution, and there was a marked peak at 0.08 mm in all subjects with hair loss, especially in those with hypothyroidism, whose spread was much wider, with separate peaks at 0.04 and 0.06 mm. The proportion of roots in telogen has been shown to be abnormally high in hairs plucked from the occipital and parietal areas of hypothyroid subjects; treatment with thyroid hormone restored it to normal after 8 weeks.

The phenomenon of post-partum hair loss also appears to result from a change in growth supportive factors, e.g. hormonally mediated change in the cycles of scalp follicles. A loss of hairs at about two to three times the normal rate gives rise to a transient alopecia about 4–6 months after delivery. At this time the proportion of hairs in telogen can be as high as 50%, whereas in late pregnancy it may be less than 5%, which is only about a third of normal as a consequence of the altered hormonal conditions, particularly the rapid fall in oestrogen levels. The pattern of fluctuation in the anagen-to-telogen ratio was observed over three consecutive pregnancies in one subject over a period of 9 years; the change became less marked in each successive pregnancy. In most cases, however, the phenomenon is only poorly reproducible.

ANDROGEN-DEPENDENT HAIR

The growth of facial, trunk and extremity hair in the male, and of pubic and axillary hair in both sexes, is clearly dependent on androgens. The development of such hair at and after puberty is, in broad terms, and at least initially, in parallel with the rise in levels of androgen from testicular, adrenocortical and ovarian sources. The rise occurs in both sexes and is somewhat steeper in boys than in girls

That testosterone produced from the interstitial cells of the testis in male adolescence and that testicular activity is itself initiated by gonadotrophic hormones of the pituitary is unquestioned. However, the findings that growth hormone-deficient boys and girls are less than normally responsive to androgens, and that growth hormone is necessarily a synergistic factor to allow testosterone to be fully effective with respect to protein anabolism, growth promotion and androgenicity, imply that hypophysial hormones might also play a more direct role. In support of such a view is the evidence that the pubertal spurt in human body growth requires both growth hormone and androgen, and that the change from an 'infantile' to an adult hair pattern can be prevented by hypophysectomy and restored by prolactin in both the dog and the rat.

Direct evidence of the role of testicular androgen is provided by the fact that castration reduces growth of the human beard, whereas testosterone stimulates it in eunuchs and old men. Since very obvious facial and body hair is normally absent from women, it appears to require high levels of the hormone and, since it is usually deficient in cases of 5α-reductase deficiency, it seems that metabolism of the testosterone to 5α-dihydrotestosterone is mandatory. The role of androgen is further demonstrated in the treatment of hirsute women with the antiandrogen cyproterone acetate, which reduces the definitive length, rate of growth, diameter and extent of medullation of the thigh hairs. While the plasma androgen levels are lowered, the major part of the action appears to be by competition for the androgen receptors in the hair follicle.

Growth of pubic and axillary hair is also undoubtedly androgen dependent, as is that on the backs of hands, fingers, pinnae and the tip of the nose. This hair is deficient in testicular feminization, a condition in which genetic males develop as females because of a lack of intracellular androgen receptor, and in women suffering from adrenal insufficiency. However, it appears to be present in the condition type II incomplete hermaphroditism, in which genetic males lack 5α-reductase even though their plasma testosterone is normal. Therefore, it seems probable that growth of the lower pubic and axillary hair requires only low levels of androgen and is not dependent on 5α-reductase.

> **The hormonal principles that provoke sexual hair growth after puberty are similar to those that cause androgenetic alopecia on the scalp – the economy of nature!**
>
> **Much depends on how hormones are transformed in the target tissues and what is 'unlocked' at the level of regulatory genes**

Scalp hair differs in that its growth does not require any androgenic stimulus. However, in genetically ordained subjects, androgen is paradoxically responsible for post-pubertal hair miniaturization on the vertex of the scalp. Also, when skin androgen sensitivity is increased – as in Becker's naevus affecting the scalp (Figure 1.26) in a genetically susceptible individual – hair will be miniaturized at a much faster pace than in other scalp sites exposed to the same systemic hormonal factors. The existence of testosterone receptors in scalp hair follicles is implied by the fact that female diffuse alopecia can be alleviated by oral antiandrogens, especially when other signs of peripheral hyperandrogenism are present. Not only are androgen receptors present, as demonstrated by histochemistry of scalp biopsy specimens, but they also show active metabolism of androgens, as has been directly demonstrated in cultured dermal papilla cells. The additional necessity for 5α-reductase is suggested by the evidence that the male bald scalp has a greater capacity than the non-bald scalp to

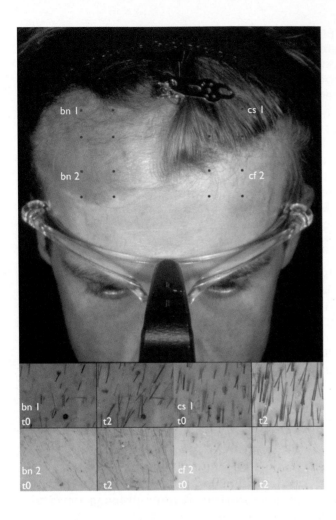

Figure 1.26

Becker's naevus affecting the frontal scalp. The affected side shows a more severe follicular miniaturization than the contralateral scalp. The hair follicles on the forehead are minimally affected by the increased androgen sensitivity. This illustrates that the biological response of hair follicles is determined by the skin field and that the presence of a Becker's naevus augments (positively in most body sites with hair growth potential or negatively in the scalp) this preconditioned androgen-dependent response. (princeps case reproduced from Van Neste D: Hair growth measurement in genetic hair disorders. Hair science and technology. Skinterface, Tournai, Belgium, pp 183–189.)

convert testosterone to 5α-dihydrotestosterone, that isolated hair roots have a similar capacity and that recession of the frontal hairline does not occur in cases of familial male pseudohermaphroditism involving 5α-reductase deficiency. However, the oxidative pathway may also be important, since the major metabolite produced by isolated hair roots in vitro is androstenedione.

If growth of hair on the face and body and deficiency of hair on the scalp are both androgen dependent, the question arises whether hirsutism and baldness are provoked by excess androgen or by an enhanced peripheral response. When hir-sutism is associated with other gross signs of virility or with menstrual disorder, it clearly has an endocrine pathology. Much more frequently, the hirsutism is described as idiopathic because there is no obvious 'central' hormonal disturbance. In idiopathic hirsutism the concentration of plasma testosterone is usually within or only slightly above the normal range; androstenedione is more often found to be elevated. The possibility that free androgen may be higher is suggested by the finding that sex hormone-binding globulin (SHBG) is, on average, lower. However, although such minor abnormalities are frequently associated with hirsutism, they cannot account for every case since about 40% of all patients appear to show all hormonal parameters within the normal range. The finding that hirsute women with no evidence of ovarian or adrenal dysfunction excrete about four times as much 5α-androstanediol as non-hirsute women suggests that increased 5α-reductase activity in the hair follicle might be involved; this is borne out by the demonstration that suprapubic skin from such patients, when incubated with tritiated testosterone, produces 5α-reduced metabolites at about four times the rate of skin from normal women.

The question as to whether male pattern baldness is associated with other signs of virility or abnormal androgen levels has been similarly debated. Evidence that it is correlated with hairiness of the chest appears to be contradicted by a failure to find any association with density of body hair, skin and muscle thickness, or rate of sebum excretion. However, the occasional finding that, despite normal plasma testosterone, bald men tend to have lower SHBG and higher salivary testosterone does suggest that they might enjoy more available androgen.

Most female diffuse alopecia is primarily androgenetic. While it may be associated with virilism and high androgen levels resulting from disorders of the adrenal cortex or ovaries, plasma androgens are more usually normal. However, as in males, there is a tendency for SHBG to be lower, although with a considerable overlap with the normal range.

The possibility that female pattern hair loss may also be expressed in the absence of androgens, or in the absence of androgen receptors, together with some genetic-epidemiological studies, challenges this view and may point to other biological factors implying androgens or not. Follicular commitment in certain scalp territories where a typical follicular miniaturization process will be phenotypically expressed under various suboptimal circumstances must be taken into account.

Since human hair itself so clearly differs between regions in its response to androgens, it is obvious that any possible animal models must be viewed with caution. The vibrissae of rats, the hairs of the gerbil ventral gland and, presumably, the mane of the lion or the mane and antler growth of the red deer are all androgen dependent. Even if male baldness is truly mimicked by the stump-tailed macaque, the model is not particularly accessible, and the wattled starling, which loses feathers from its head, can hardly be considered as a greatly superior alternative. Some progress might reasonably be expected from the transplantation experiments and the maintenance of human scalp grafts onto nude mice in order to monitor hair growth under experimentally controlled conditions, although this is a labour-intensive approach that is not rewarded with a 100% success rate. A much more clinically relevant modality is to run long-term properly designed and controlled studies in human subjects, using high-definition imaging techniques in order to monitor the in vivo hair growth replacement kinetics.

TYPES OF HAIR

Different types of hair may be produced by different kinds of follicle, and the type of hair produced in any particular follicle can change with age or under the influence of hormones. Animals characteristically have both an overcoat of stiff guard hairs and an undercoat of fine hairs, but many kinds of follicle and fibre have been described. Many species also have large vibrissae or sinus hairs, which are sensory and are produced from special follicles containing erectile tissue. There are no strictly comparable follicles in humans, but there are occasional, large, so-called tylotrich follicles with a structure suggesting a sensory function; they are most numerous in abdominal skin.

The infantile pelage of animals is usually fine, and such 'puppy' fur is retained in the adult if the young animal is hypophysectomized. In the absence of precise knowledge about species differences in pituitary hormones, the question as to whether growth hormones or prolactin induce the change to adult pelage may be unrealistic. Moreover, steroid hormones also influence the type of hair produced.

In humans, a prenatal coat of fine, soft, unmedullated and usually unpigmented hair, known as lanugo, is normally shed in utero by 36 weeks' gestation. However, lanugo may be retained throughout life in the rare hereditary syndrome hypertrichosis lanuginosa. Postnatal hair may be divided at the two extremes into two kinds: vellus hair, which is soft, unmedullated, occasionally pigmented and seldom more than 2 cm long, and terminal hair, which is longer, coarser, and often medullated and pigmented. However, there is a range of intermediate kinds. Before puberty, terminal hair is normally that limited to the scalp, eyebrows and eyelashes. After puberty, secondary sexual 'terminal' hair is developed from vellus hair in response to androgens. At the same time in some straight-haired individuals, the temporal hairs next to the beard area may become coarser and curly at puberty. Scalp hair is an effective sun-blocker and the first sign of hair regression, i.e. when thick pigmented terminal hair is replaced by thin unpigmented vellus hairs, in a young male is sunburn on the top of the head after usually well-tolerated outdoor activities!

Human vellus hairs act as very sensitive and subtle tactile nerve endings, and other hair fibres are important in specific conditioned reactions – nostril hairs in sneezing and eyelashes in blinking.

> **Human vellus hairs act as very sensitive and subtle tactile 'nerve endings'**

RACIAL AND INDIVIDUAL VARIATION

Wide, genetically determined variations in the pattern and amount of hair growth can be observed both between races and between individuals. The most striking differences are seen in scalp hair. It is a common observation that Mongoloids tend to have coarse, straight hair, Negroids curly hair (at the extreme the intertwined shafts rise to the 'peppercorn' pattern) and Caucasoids a range of textures and curl. According to several authors the macroscopic appearance of hair is related to its cross-section. Thus, Mongoloid hair is the most massive and is circular, Negroid hair is oval, and Caucasoid hair is moderately elliptical and finer than Mongoloid (Figure 1.27). Other evidence suggests that the shape of the follicle determines hair form: the Negroid follicle is helical, the Mongoloid is completely straight, and the Caucasoid varies between these extremes. However, even a straight Caucasoid follicle may produce a hair with an oval cross-section. Significant variations between populations can be shown for a number of other measurements such as medullation, cuticular scale count, kinking and average curvature. The shape of the hair may also be modified after diffuse hair loss such as occurs after acute telogen effluvium, as illustrated clinically in twins where straight hair was replaced by curly hair after post-febrile hair loss (Figure 1.28).

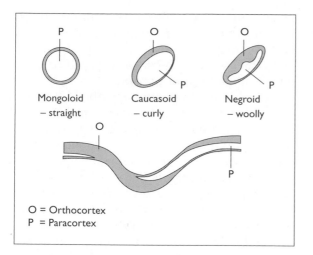

Figure 1.27
Racial hair types.

The hypothesis that hair form is controlled by only three or four genes (straight, wavy, spiral and peppercorn) is not currently accepted. On the one hand, while accepting that the genes have major as opposed to biometric or polygenic effects, it could be concluded that a number of genes are involved. On the other hand, it is more or less known that hair form is polygenic, but relatively few genes are involved.

Mongoloids, both male and female, have less pubic, axillary, beard and body hair than Caucasoids. The surface area covered by coarse beard hairs and the weight of hairs grown per day are less in Japanese than in Caucasoids, as are the mean number of axillary hairs and their daily growth. Not only the amounts of hair but also the patterns of distribution may vary between populations. Thus, the absence of hair on the foot combined with presence of hair on the thighs and lower leg is three times more frequent in blacks than in whites.

The growth of coarse hairs on the rim of the helix (hypertrichosis of the pinna) occurs between the ages of 17 and 45 years in many males, being particularly obvious

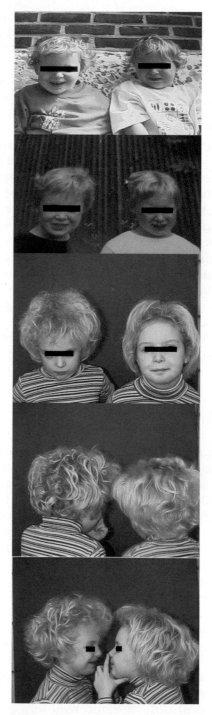

Figure 1.28
Identical twins with moderately curly or straight hair. After a severe acute episode of post-febrile telogen effluvium hair regrew very curly and was almost unmanageable.

among the Bengali and Singhalese. The character is well known to geneticists as a possible example of Y-linked inheritance. In other races, few or many coarse hairs may grow on the helix or on other regions of the pinna, usually after the third decade. The patterns have been classified but their modes of inheritance are unknown.

A syndrome of 'hairy elbows' (hypertrichosis cubiti) has been described. The mode of inheritance is uncertain. Hypertrichosis of the elbow region is noticed soon after birth. It reaches its greatest extent and severity at the age of 5 years and then may slowly regress.

Such individual variations in the patterns of hair growth can now be accurately recorded and correlated with other hereditary traits. They will be of undoubted genetic interest and may, like certain variations in the pattern of the eyebrows, prove to have clinical implications.

CHANGES WITH AGE

At puberty, terminal hair gradually replaces vellus, starting in the pubic regions. In both boys and girls the first pubic hair is sparse, long, downy, slightly pigmented and almost straight. It later becomes darker, coarser, and more curled and extends in area to form an inverse triangle. British observations have shown that boys have the first recognizable pubic hair at an average age of 13.4 years, and the full adult 'female' pattern at 15.2 years, about 3½ years after the start of the development of the genitalia. The corresponding mean ages for girls are considerably younger, namely 11.7 years and 13.5 years. In about 80% of men and 10% of women the pubic hair continues spreading until the mid-twenties or later. There is no absolute distinction between male and female patterns, only one of degree. Of 3858 normal young men, 4.7%

were found to have a horizontal upper border to the pubic hair, and a further 10.3% had a convex border. In a group of women aged 25–34 years, 3.7% were found to have an acuminate upper border.

Axillary hair first appears about 2 years after the start of pubic hair growth. The amount as measured by the weight of the fully grown mass continues to increase until the late twenties in males as well as in females, but in females it is less at any age. The mean amounts grown per day increase from late puberty until the mid-twenties and thereafter decrease steadily.

Facial hair in boys first appears at about the same time as the axillary hair, starting at the corners of the upper lip, spreading medially to complete the moustache and then spreading to the cheeks and beard. Some areas on the midline never grow hair like the upper lip, glabella and chin areas.

Terminal hair development is continued in regular sequence on the legs, thighs, forearms, abdomen, buttocks, back, arms and shoulders. The patterns of distribution of terminal hair on the neck, chest, back and limbs have been clearly differentiated and classified. In some cases the lack of hair growth and the absence of acne at puberty have suggested the existence of acne-free naevus or hair-free zones. The extent of terminal hair tends to increase throughout the years of sexual maturity, but most patterns occur over a wide age range. The adult pattern is not achieved until the fourth decade, when the androgen levels are already somewhat lower than in early adult life. Moreover, aural hairs do not appear until late middle age, and detailed observations of coarse sternal hair in men showed that the hairs continue to increase in length and number from puberty to the fifth or sixth decade.

Certain follicles of the scalp may regress with age to produce only fine short vellus hair (Figure 1.29). This condition of patterned baldness is inherited and requires

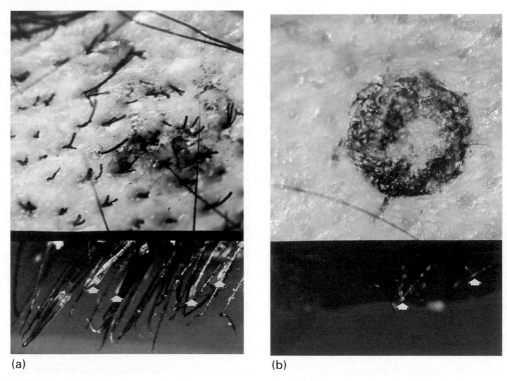

(a)   (b)

Figure 1.29
Hair growth evaluation. In most males there are a number of scalp follicles growing terminal hairs.
(a) Top – on the face; bottom – profile with arrows pointing to telogen clubs. Under the influence of
androgens, these follicles will grow a regressive-type follicle producing barely visible vellus hairs.
(b) Top – on the face; bottom – profile with arrows pointing to atrophic vellus anagen roots and
telogen clubs.

male hormone. It is prevented by castration before puberty, though not substantially reversed by castration in maturity. Approximately one-third of men of Caucasoid stock develop, during the third and fourth decades, sharply defined patches of alopecia in the peroneal area of the lower leg and often smaller patches on the calves. Some never grow hair on those areas.

SEASONAL CHANGES

As mentioned above, evidence that human hair growth varies with season has been noted by many observers. Clear and statistically significant data on seasonal varia-tion have been provided by a study of young Caucasian men in the UK. These changes probably reflect the importance of the change from the summer to the winter coat in homeotherms, mainly in relation to body temperature control. Clear and statistically significant data on seasonal variation have been provided by several studies in Europe.

> **Human hair growth may show seasonal changes at different sites – late spring/early summer growth being maximal in temperate climates**

There was an increase of telogen in scalp hairs culminating in September and reaching the lowest levels in December. This appeared to follow with a slight lag-phase the peak temperatures noted in July and the peak irradiation noted in June. These data were generated using the phototrichogram technique. The proportion of scalp follicles in anagen, as determined by plucking hairs, reached a single peak of over 90% around March and fell steadily to a trough in September. This pattern appeared to be shared by all areas of the scalp.

The numbers of shed hairs collected by the subjects closely followed the pattern of activity of the follicles. Hair loss reached a peak around August/September, when the fewest follicles were in anagen. At this time, the average loss of hairs was about 60 per day, more than double that during the previous March and compatible with the observed increase from 10% to 20% in the proportion of follicles in telogen.

The diameter of growing scalp hairs exhibited no significant seasonal fluctuations, though the trends were similar to those of thigh hair diameter.

The rate of beard growth showed very significant seasonal variation. It was lowest in January and February, and from March it increased steadily to reach a peak about 60% higher in July.

The rate of growth of thigh hair showed a similar seasonal pattern to that of the beard. The mean rate from February to March was 0.27 mm/day. It then rose to reach a plateau of about 0.3 mm/day from June to September and then declined steadily for 6 months. The percentage of follicles in anagen showed a remarkable and quite different pattern. It appeared to be lowest in March and August, and highest in May/June and November/December. The pattern is exactly what would be expected if the follicles were undergoing a spring moult and an autumn moult, in common with many other mammals of the temperate zone. The diameter of thigh hair showed a similar pattern to that of the follicular changes, though the differences were less pronounced.

The seasonal variation in the rate of growth of beard and thigh hair probably reflects circannual changes in circulating androgens or other hormonal fluctuations under the influence of photoperiod. It is possible that the peak in hair fall associated with the increase in the percentage of follicles in telogen in the scalp is similarly related to testosterone levels, but such an explanation is insufficient to account for the apparent changes in the hair follicles in the thigh. Other hormonal factors regulated by the photoperiod probably play a major role in determining the seasonal renewal of the human hair follicles.

As can be understood from this overview of basic science, many gaps remain as to our understanding of hair growth and its regulation. The many current hair biological studies and the development and standardization of hair evaluation methods will provide more appropriate information to assist those involved in developing and assessing new treatments.

FURTHER READING

Blume U, Ferracin I, Verschoore M, Czernielewski JM, Schaefer H (1991) Physiology of the vellus hair follicle: hair growth and sebum excretion, *Br J Dermatol* **124:** 21–28.

Chuong CM, Hou L, Chen PJ, et al (2001) Dinosaur's feather and chicken's tooth? Tissue engineering of the integument, *Eur J Dermatol* **11:** 286–292.

Pagnoni A, Kligman AM, El Gammal S, Stoudemayer T (1994) Determination of density of follicles on various regions of the face by cyanoacrylate biopsy: correlation with sebum output, *Br J Dermatol* **131:** 862–865.

Robinson M, Reynolds AJ, Gharzi A, Jahoda CA (2001) In vivo induction of hair growth by dermal cells isolated from hair follicles after extended organ culture, *J Invest Dermatol* **117:** 596–604.

Stenn KS, Paus R (2001) Controls of hair follicle cycling, *Physiol Rev* **81:** 449–494.

Sundberg JP, King LE, Bascom C (2001) Animal models for male pattern (androgenetic) alopecia, *Eur J Dermatol* **11:** 321–335.

Van Neste D, Randall VA (eds) (1996) *Hair research for the next millennium* (Amsterdam, Elsevier).

Van Neste D, Blume-Peytavi U, Grimalt R, Messenger A (2003) *Hair science and technology* (Tournai, Skinterface).

2 Hair examination and investigation

On being presented with a patient complaining, for example, of pruritus or a blistering eruption, most clinicians are fully competent to carry out a careful clinical examination and to use appropriate histological, biochemical and other laboratory investigations if required. The details of specific techniques for studying the pathogenesis of hair diseases seem for many clinicians and pathologists to be shrouded in mystery, mainly because the methods concerned are not within the province of any one speciality. This section considers the clinical methods required for studying hair growth and the microscopic methods for detailed examination of hair shafts and hair follicles.

History taking is of paramount importance in assessing hair loss. A patient complaining of balding or hair loss may in fact have an increased shedding rate, a decrease in hairs per unit area, a decrease in hair diameter or a combination of these. Sometimes this may be worsened by a substantial shortening of the hair cycle, a delay in hair regrowth, or a decrease in hair pigmentation or intrinsically pale hair at the outset. By careful questioning, it is possible to assess the factors which guide one into particular lines of investigation and differential diagnosis. It is important that these factors should be quantified in order to assess accurately the progress of hair disease and also to assess the changes induced by treatment. As the total hair mass is directly related to cumulative growth, one practical modality that can be easily applied in the hair clinic is to capture the global coverage of scalp skin (Figure 2.1). Thorough standardization of scalp hair preparation will transform a clinical image into a proper documentation for the analysis of scalp skin coverage, as illustrated here in male pattern baldness during the detailed analytical correlation studies within a target site (white spot on the top of the head, top panel; Figure 2.1). In a series of recent validation and investigative studies the scalp coverage scoring (SCS; Skinterface patent PCT/EP01/06970) method could be applied for various clinical purposes in male pattern baldness studies. Indeed, as SCS is able to detect natural worsening of androgenetic alopecia (AGA) in less than 1 year, the method has been used to check the severity of AGA subjects both in real time in vivo

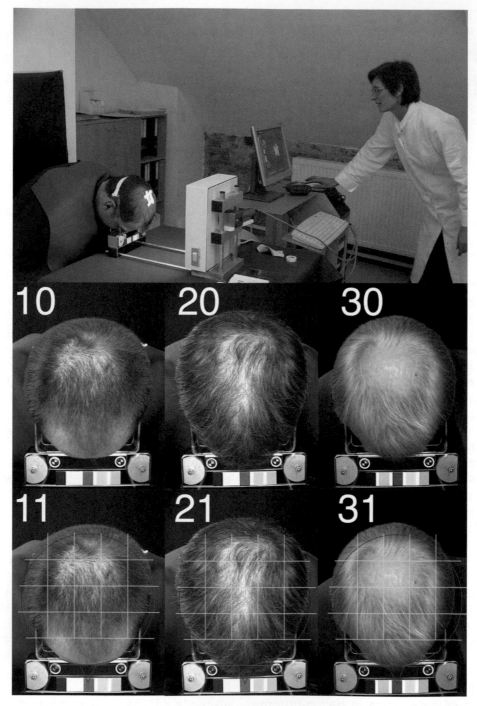

Figure 2.1
A standardized way to capture a global view of the top of the head and to evaluate scalp coverage in male pattern baldness. Each area as seen through the reference grid (yellow squares) is rated against a density ruler and generates a scalp coverage scoring (SCS method; Skinterface patent PCT/EP01/06970).

and on global pictures (see Figure 2.1). Accordingly, SCS has become a practical tool to measure drug effects during international multicentre phase II–III clinical trials for measuring changes rather than relying on impressions by the clinical investigator. Global methods require some time to detect changes, as the measurement is based on cumulative growth. Other methods also rely on the same phenomenon but measure in greater detail some aspects of growth.

For example, in AGA and hirsutism, changes in the anagen or telogen count, linear growth rate, thickness of hair, and its medullation and pigmentation are detectable before the affected individual is able subjectively to observe the changes. Hair growth may be assessed by several easy clinical investigations. Daily hair growth may be measured with a graduated rule after shaving the skin. With some limitations due to hairstyle, the durations of anagen of the growth cycle can be calculated by dividing the overall length of an uncut hair by the daily growth rate. To be absolutely correct, this would mean in some cases not cutting the hair for at least 5–7 years! In some circumstances it is only necessary to know the relative proportion of telogen and anagen hairs. This remains a less-refined evaluation and may be assessed by plucking hairs – using an exhaustive sampling technique such as the unit area trichogram – to examine the roots, or by scalp biopsy and performing serial sectioning or a folliculogram. It should be noted that only telogen hairs with clubs already processed for being released, i.e. exogen hair, are removed by combing or washing – anagen, and catagen-telogen scalp hairs are bound too firmly to be removed by these procedures (Skinterface patent PCT/EP02/06434). More refined, totally painless quantitative techniques have now been developed for counting shedding thick and thinning hair per unit

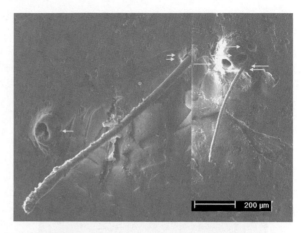

Figure 2.2
A non-invasive method to capture specifically shedding hair. Thin (right panel) and thick (left panel) shedding hair was collected in a subject with male pattern baldness. Single arrows identify follicular openings containing hair – anagen or telogen – while double arrows point to exogen follicles releasing the fully differentiated club hair (Skinterface patent PCT/EP02/06434).

area (Figure 2.2); the process could be applied even without clipping the scalp hair!

> **Trust the patient complaining of chronic hair shedding even in the absence of clear-cut balding. Such patients or those presenting with diffuse hair loss must undergo a total body examination, and hair growth should be assessed properly**

LENGTH OF THE HAIR CYCLE – EXAMINATION OF HAIR ROOTS

The length of the hair cycle can be studied by observation over long periods of time

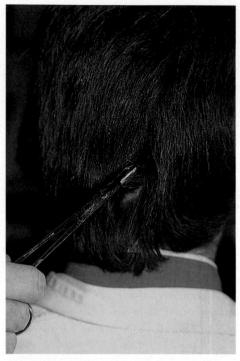

Figure 2.3
Method of scalp hair sampling for
anagen/telogen counting and root microscropy.

of hair root status. This gives information on the length of the growth cycle (anagen = total length/daily growth) and the percentage of growing roots. Hair roots are examined by plucking hairs (Figures 2.3–2.8). The shafts should be grasped firmly and extracted briskly in the direction of their insertion. This ensures that the roots are not deformed. Surgical needle holders are used, the blades being covered with fine rubber tubing or cellophane tape to ensure a firm grasp (Figures 2.3, 2.4). Approximately 50 hairs are extracted in order to reduce sampling errors. The roots are examined under a low-power microscope (Figure 2.5). The root morphology is stable and hairs can be kept for many weeks in dry packaging before analysis. Normal telogen counts are 13–15% on the vertex, but this figure varies from site to site, with age, with physiological androgen influences and with many other factors. The appearance of the root is also important: shrivelled and atrophic roots are a feature of protein-calorie malnutrition (PCM).

and accurate identification of individual hairs. It is more convenient to assess overall growth, using hair length and daily linear growth in conjunction with an assessment

Histological techniques

It is not always possible to obtain representative samples of hair by plucking,

Figure 2.4
The forceps used for hair sampling
as in Figure 2.3.

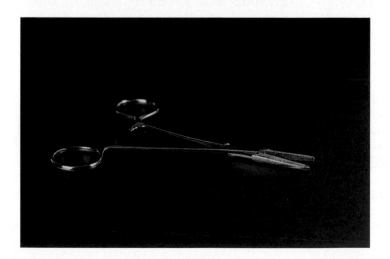

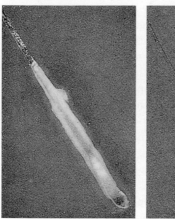
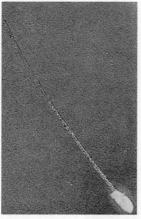

Figure 2.5
Hair root microscopy – anagen stage 6 (left) and telogen (right) roots.

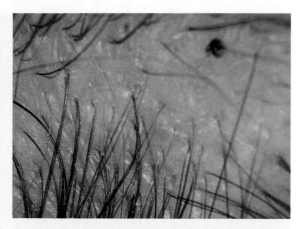

Figure 2.7
Scalp showing slight follicular haemorrhage at the site of hair plucking.

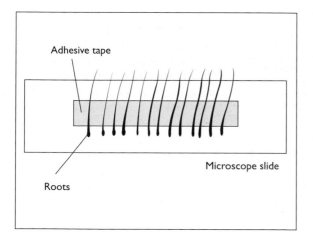

Figure 2.6
Plucked hairs prepared for microscopy.

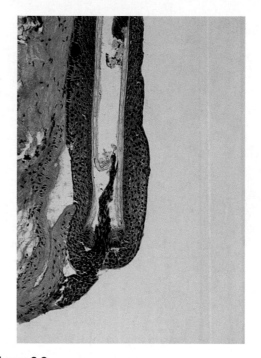

Figure 2.8
Follicular components removed from the haemorrhagic follicle in Figure 2.7.

particularly when examining the balding scalp or when assessing regrowth while the shafts are too short to grasp. In order to overcome this problem, several investigators have devised histological and morphometric techniques (Figure 2.9). Standardization has been carried out in the stump-tailed macaque and other primates which develop AGA like that in *Homo sapiens*. Serial horizontal sections of skin are measured along the length of the folli-

cles, and a folliculogram is constructed to compare different areas of the scalp, using follicle length and developmental stage as

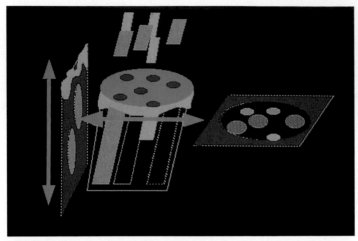

(a)

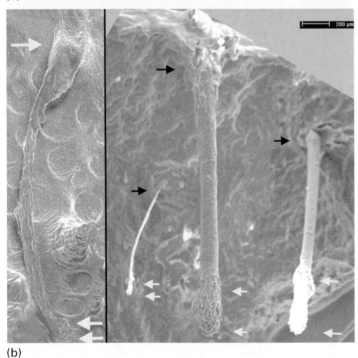

(b)

Figure 2.9

(a) Histological techniques for viewing scalp biopsies – longitudinal or transverse sections. Centre, schematic scalp punch biopsy bearing 6 hairs (3 thin, 3 thick) from 6 individual follicles opening at the scalp surface. The section can be made either horizontally (at right angles to the axis of the hair follicle) or vertically (following the axis of the hair follicle). On longitudinal sections (left) only a few follicles can be seen at a time and usually only part of the follicle is visible. It is therefore necessary to examine a large number of serial sections in order to obtain an overall view of follicular activity. On transverse sections (made 1–1.5 mm below the dermal–epidermal junction) all follicular units can be observed at once (right). The diameter of the hair follicle correlates with that of the fibres (centre) and the stage in the hair cycle can be easily identified. The most miniaturized follicles would require serial sections in the upper segment, as they do not always reach a 1–1.5 mm depth.

(b) Scanning electron microscopy view of anagen (left panel) and telogen (right panel) roots in a three-dimensional display after an original scalp preparation method for the folliculogram analysis. Depth, i.e. from the basis of epidermis (single arrow; white for anagen and black for telogen roots) to the deepest part of the root (double arrows) in the microdissected scalp, together with shape and hair thickness, reflects the growth status of the individual hair roots. These relate directly to the hair productivity: a thick, deeply set anagen root will produce a thick, long and clinically significant hair, as opposed to the miniaturized root, more frequently in telogen as it relates to a shorter duration of anagen. Besides depth, the size of the club also reflects miniaturization (distance between white arrows in right panel).

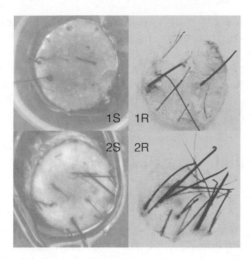

Figure 2.10
Surface view and root view of scalp hair and follicle roots after 1 year of oral treatment with finasteride or placebo.

In two subjects with equal hair density at baseline (as determined by a photographic technique) biopsies were taken from a predefined scalp target after 1 year of oral treatment with finasteride (1 mg/day) or placebo. Samples were processed to show surface views (1S = placebo; 2S = finasteride) and hair follicle roots (1R = placebo; 2R = finasteride). Finasteride results in a majority of thicker, deeply set, mostly anagen roots while placebo shows more atrophic, miniaturized anagen roots and with even a higher proportion in telogen.

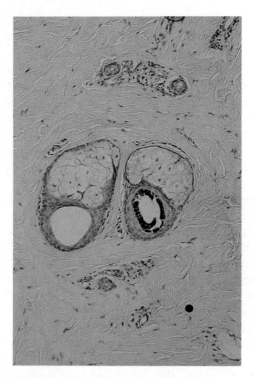

Figure 2.11
Transverse section of hair follicle structures at the level of the sebaceous duct.

indices. As the roots convert from terminal to vellus, their length decreases. This has been used to display the different patterns and change of growth with therapy. A similar approach has been proposed for men with male pattern baldness, comparing the scalp follicles after 1 year of oral treatment with finasteride or placebo (Figure 2.10).

Telogen effluvium was originally studied by scalp histology, demonstrating increased telogen roots, in combination with a standardized combing technique and counting the shed hairs. These control data revealed that 90% of the normal population shed fewer than 75 hairs per day.

The Headington technique has made detailed studies of hair roots possible by means of horizontal sections of scalp taken with 4–6 mm punch biopsies (Figure 2.11). This method defines the transverse appearance of the root in its different growth phases. Vellus hairs, which are arbitrarily defined as having a diameter less than 0.03 mm, are not seen below the entry of the sebaceous duct. Anagen hairs are recognized by the inner root sheath and absence of keratinocyte necrosis in the tricholemma. Catagen hairs have a distinctive thickening of the basement membrane in the lower external root sheath. Telogen follicles have a bulbous configuration and have lost their inner root sheath. With this technique, a 6-mm punch biopsy will yield 22–30 follicular units or 60–80 terminal hairs. Once the orientation using this technique has been mastered, considerable data can be gleaned on the total number and density of follicular units, follicular structures and their developmental stage, and hair shaft diameters. In controls over 90% of the follicles were in anagen and there were less than 10% vellus hairs. Similar results have now been obtained with the contrast-enhanced phototrichogram (CE-PTG) technique so that the growth process can be monitored in vivo without destroying scalp tissue.

Root volumes were first calculated using horizontal sections of skin. This method assumed that the volumes between sections approximated to truncated cones and that the total volume comprised the sum of the slices. The volume of the matrix was calculated by subtracting the volume of the papilla from the total root. By these means it was estimated that in normal hair the papilla was $338 \times 10^3 \, \mu m^3$ and contained 1220 cells, and that the matrix was $3370 \times 10^3 \, \mu m^3$ with 139 cells in mitosis. It was found that the volume of the matrix was proportional to the height of the papilla. A constant relationship was found between the volume of the dermal papilla and the volume of the fully grown hair in rats and mice. In humans, the ratio between the volume of the hair matrix and the dermal papilla was found to be 15 in controls and 18 in male pattern baldness, indicating homogeneous hypotrophy in the latter. In some disease states, a thin hair grows from an abnormally severe atrophy of the dermal papilla. In such a case, for example, trichorhinophalangeal (TRP) syndrome, the ratio VM/VP is 32. This points to the predominant importance of the size of the dermal papilla to condition the pattern of hair growth. Indeed, in the TRP syndrome there is production of extremely thin hairs even though a significant amount of epithelial tissue is available. An earlier method estimated root volume by linear displacement of water in a calibrated capillary micropipette under a low-power microscope. The estimation of root volume and protein content are directly proportional, correlating well with reduction in body weight.

Follicle kinetics

Hair growth is the end result of the combination of cell proliferation and the maturation process. As the entire cell is eliminated and structurally conserved, it can be assimilated to a holocrine secretion by the hair follicle, this occurring in bursts of activity lasting for several months or years. Therefore, at the tissue level, the ultimate measure of growth is by examination of the matrix cell kinetics. There are two methods of estimating kinetic activity: proliferative indices and metaphase arrest. The former are counts of the number of cells actively dividing at a given time and the latter is a count of the number of cells entering mitosis during a given period. The proliferative indices provide the simpler methods measuring the proportion of cells at a particular phase within the cell cycle. The synthetic (S phase) and mitotic (M phase) are the most easily detected and can be measured by the labelling index (S phase) and the mitotic index (M phase).

Mitotic index

Mitotic figures can be counted on wax-embedded sections. The mitotic index is the number of mitotic figures observed, divided by the total number of cells counted. There are four phases of mitosis: prophase, metaphase, anaphase and telophase. The early and late stages are difficult to identify and criteria for distinction must be defined clearly. It has been estimated that the replacement time of the entire germinative matrix is as short as 23 hours.

Labelling index

Cells synthesizing DNA (S phase) will incorporate ³H-thymidine, which can then be visualized by autoradiography (Figure 2.12). After autoradiographic development the label appears as silver grains over the nucleus due to the emission of β particles. Unfortunately, even after the subtraction of background radiographic interference, there are still many pitfalls in this technique. The method can be performed in vitro by incubating skin slices in medium containing ³H-thymidine (92 MBq/ml for 2.5 hours) and has also been performed in vivo, using intradermal injections of 184 MBq/ml of ³H-thymidine and carrying out biopsies after fixed intervals. Unincorporated thymidine is rapidly cleared and only cells in the S phase will incorporate the injected thymidine. For dynamic studies, results must be extrapolated from several individuals as multiple injections of ³H-thymidine are very toxic. The labelling index is the proportion of labelled cells in a sample of 1000 cells counted and provides a static appreciation of a dynamic event.

> **When hair matrix kinetics are inhibited without total arrest, hair diameter narrowing may be evident and is the easiest way to quantitate growth inhibition**

Metaphase arrest

Cells can be arrested in metaphase by the administration of a stathmokinetic agent. Early studies on sheep were performed using systemic colcimid to study growth in different seasons. Cells with metaphase nuclei are counted and expressed as a proportion of the whole (metaphase index). Vincristine, which inhibits the production of the mitotic spindle, is probably the best agent; it has been used to examine hair growth in pig skin, but not in human hair. A dose–response curve needs to be calculated prior to its use, and this has only been done for squamous epithelia. The rate of increase of the metaphase index is proportional to the number of cells entering mitosis and

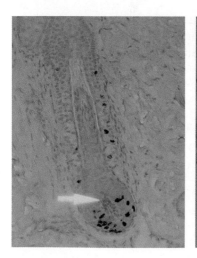
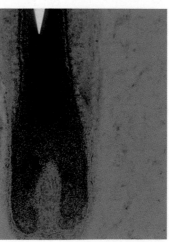

Figure 2.12
Anagen hair roots stained to show sites of DNA synthesis with radiolabelled thymidine (left, arrow) and protein synthesis with radiolabelled cystine (right, arrow) incorporation.

therefore to the birth rate of cells in the time between injection and sampling the tissue. The metaphase index, therefore, differs from the labelling index, which only gives a static measurement with no information concerning cell production. The metaphase arrest technique provides a measure of the rate of cell production. It is a more accurate and enlightening method and should be used to study hair follicles.

HAIR SHAFT LENGTH AND DIAMETER MEASUREMENTS

The hair shaft is measured using the parameters of length and diameter, and with these measurements the volume can be calculated from the formula $\pi r^2 l$, where r is the radius and l the length. The weight of hair is a comparable measure to volume but must be carefully standardized for shaving technique, washing and removal of epithelial debris. The easiest method to measure length is to bleach or shave the hair and measure the subsequent growth of undyed hair or stubble. Shaving does have the advantage of removing telogen hairs but may result in some discomfort when in-

growing hairs result from an inappropriate technique. Therefore, some laboratories prefer clipping close to the scalp surface with sharp scissors. Plucking hairs is not a useful manoeuvre as it introduces a variable lag in growth until the shaft has grown through the skin, and animal experiments suggest that plucking may alter linear hair growth and synchronize the random anagen growth phase for a while.

There are two widely used methods for measurement of linear growth: calibrated capillary tubes (Figure 2.13) and macrophotography. Both of these methods are used after shaving, are repeatable and offer good correlation between observers. The capillary tube technique is easy and cheap, requiring only an accurately graduated tube. Macrophotography requires apparatus to ensure that magnification and orientation are kept constant and that processing does not introduce any alterations in magnification. It does offer the advantage of clinical speed. The hairs are pressed flat against the skin with a transparent window in front of the camera optics to ensure that the entire length is visualized. The addition of oil further sharpens the contrast between pigmented hairs and scalp background. When the contrast between hair and scalp

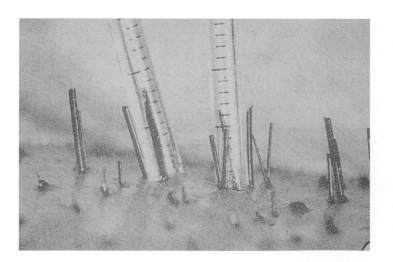

Figure 2.13
Hair growth measurement using graduated scale capillary tubes.

is decreasing (for example, white hairs or vellus hairs in Caucasians and black hair on dark-skinned individuals), most photographic methods (and derivative methods such as video recording or CCD capturing) were found less appropriate than those using a contrast enhanced method. The correlations between hair counts, staging and hair thickness measurements with the photographic procedure were shown to be identical with those generated by histology using serial sectioning of scalp samples from top to bottom. The discrepancies between methods were considered neither biologically nor clinically relevant. After a long period of technological development we have now devised a high-quality procedure, the clinical application of which for hair growth measurements has become an important tool for communication between physician and patient: numbers are invaluable for discussing the diagnosis, prognosis and therapeutic options with the patient.

Reference points on the hair shaft can also be made by autoradiography after incorporation of radioisotopes such as ^{14}C-glucose and ^{35}S-cystine. ^{35}S-Cystine is not taken up by the bulb but seems to enter the keratogenous zone directly. In the mouse, using ^{35}S-cystine, appreciable radioactivity can be seen after 2 minutes, but detectable activity is measurable within 30 seconds, which suggests immediate uptake. After 2 days the majority of the radioactivity is in the hair shaft above the keratogenous zone and, after 6 days, it is above the surface of the skin. No radioactivity within the follicle is measurable after 16 days. Using ^{35}S-methionine intravenously, orally and by inunction to a defined area on the dorsum of the guinea pig, some authors have found identical patterns of shaft labelling with each form of administration. The ^{35}S-cystine method may be used in humans, the radiolabel being injected intradermally into the site to be

studied; other routes of administration are not appropriate.

Hair clippings can be used to determine length or diameter and may be measured using a graduated eyepiece graticule mounted in a low-power microscope. Micrometers cannot be used as hair is too soft and will yield to low compression forces. The hairs should be mounted on a glass microscope slide using Canada balsam or Depex – a high-viscosity plastic which sets as hard as glass on exposure to air. Alternatively, the hair can be floated on water in a Petri dish and the individual hairs drawn up into a syringe needle to measure the diameter in two dimensions. This may be important in elliptical sections since a diameter variation between 77 and 39 μm (mean maximum and minimum dimensions) can be found in normal hairs. Various investigators have measured hair diameters at several sites from the bulb to the shaft and found that, if measurements are made above the outer root sheath, the hair diameter is constant throughout the shaft, though greater in anagen than in telogen. Measurements of scalp hair show a constancy in diameter over the proximal 40 mm. It should be noted that telogen hairs taper towards the bulb.

Measurement of the diameter of hair may be complicated by swelling due to humidity and by the oval cross-section of hair shafts. Although we have not found these to introduce errors when a mean diameter of several hairs is required, several devices have been constructed to overcome these problems. Individual cells have been used which hold individual hairs with glue and hooks and allow rotation under a microscope. It has long been known that the shaft diameter is not uniform along its length. This was determined from a representative number of major and minor diameters measured along a 20 mm fibre. During a comparative study using scalp CE-PTG and microscopic measurements of hair diameters, we realized that microscopy performed less well. Surprisingly, we observed that very thin hair may resist and eventually escape at various stages the clipping–sampling–display process! Also, when the clipping technique is used, for whatever purpose, make sure that all elements are taken into account, from the sampling until the display. Other techniques involve the use of vibration resonance and laser beam diffraction.

Hair weight may be used as an index of hair growth in both humans and animals. The weight will be affected by oils and scales, and standardized methods must be established. This method appears to be suitable for measuring the small reductions in hair growth obtained with low-dose antiandrogen therapy in hirsuties.

HAIR SHAFT MORPHOLOGY – VELLUS HAIR INDEX

Androgenic stimulation of hair roots mediates the conversion of vellus into terminal hair and vice versa. Because of this, one can use the ratio of vellus to terminal hairs as an index of hair growth in hirsuties. An area of skin is shaved (approximately 5 cm × 5.5 cm, but there is no need to accurately define the field), the hair shafts are examined microscopically and the proportion of vellus hairs is noted. The index is derived by comparing the results from hirsute and non-hirsute women, but it is unknown at present whether it is adequately sensitive to detect subtle alterations as a result of antiandrogen therapy. A huge measurement programme (over 64 000 hair diameter measurements) was recently completed by one of us (D. Van Neste) in balding male subjects. Although 8% more thick hair was present after finasteride as compared with

placebo, the study was unable to show statistically significant differences in clipped hair diameter distribution between finasteride and placebo treatment (12 months' study). This suggested that follicles that were dormant at baseline could become productive of thin hair, a modified bioresponse that will never be detected by relative testing, as contrasted with the clinical improvement documented by global and analytical methods on predefined areas!

> **Repeat measurements using an accurate method in a clearly defined target population of follicles are critically important and directly relevant to the dynamics of the clinical condition**

Compound measurements

The phototrichogram is a composite measurement of several of the growth parameters described above (Figures 2.6 and 2.9a). It was developed in order to formulate a more dynamic expression of growth. The term has been used by several authors to describe their different concepts, some of the techniques measuring transverse diameters and hair cycle status on biopsied tissue.

A less-invasive means involves collating multiple measurements of the number of hairs per unit area, shaft diameter and growth, and root-cycle stage. A specifically designed microscope is used with ×60 magnification. This is placed on the skin surface, which acts as the stage. Two eyepieces are used: one with a micrometer scale calibrated down to 0.25 mm and the other containing a reticulum defining an area of 4 mm^2. This area is then shaved and re-examined for length of growth after

5–10 days. Root status is measured, as before, by plucking. Using this technique, data have been collected regarding the normal pattern of growth in the newborn child, prepubertal children, adults, pregnant women, pubic hair and axillary hair. Stencils have been used to delineate the area for repeatability. Some investigators have modified the trichogram by including an intense washing and combing programme for 3 days, including the sample day, prior to plucking the hairs individually from a larger area of 35–45 mm², and also by measuring the shaft diameter in two planes.

> **Trichogram measurements were useful research tools – they are fraught with variable variables. Unless exhaustive samples are taken from a specific target with a non-invasive technique, trichograms would better be abandoned for clinical research purposes!**

A more recent development is the use of enhanced contrast between hair and scalp so as to allow hair counts with photographic methods (differential interaction of light with hair and skin). If properly calibrated, the measures are as precise as with a light microscope. The advantage of photographic approaches is that they are totally non-invasive and that a representative target sample (around 100 hair follicles) can be analysed readily and monitored repeatedly over time (Figures 2.14, 2.15).

Hair pluckability

From studies of children suffering from PCM it has long been known that the hair in this condition is not fully pigmented, and is thin, sparse, straight and easily plucked. Therefore, hair has been suggested as an easily obtainable tissue source for assessment of PCM using anagen/telogen ratios, shaft diameter and bulb morphology. The so-called trichotillometer is a plucking device which comprises a spring dynamometer with a clamp to hold individual hairs and a scale graduated at 1.4 g intervals from 0 to 62 g. This device measures epilation forces. The mean epilation force required to pluck 10 hairs has been assessed in normal and malnourished children and has been found to correlate well with the serum albumin level. The normal epilation force is >36 g, whereas in kwashiorkor it is <19 g. This measure correlates well with shaft diameter, which is also a good index of 'hair growth'. The use of this technique, which requires little training and no laboratory facilities, is encouraged. Regional epilation forces have been measured for hair from the scalp, eyebrows, cilia, axillae and pubic area. However, this technique still needs to be rigorously evaluated on normal hair to determine variations with growth status (anagen or telogen) and with diameter, since the relatively 'crude' technology has a wide margin of experimental error. Recent studies also indicate that a telogen hair can require more extraction force than an anagen hair. Therefore, easy-to-use methods must be critically considered before extensive use in the clinic.

> **The relative data generated by hair root status methods are poor indicators of alopecia or scalp dysfunction**

A novel approach has been shown to extract, specifically, loosely attached hair from a precise field. The technique is even

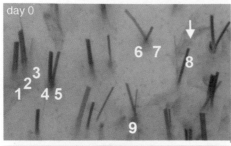

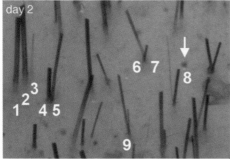

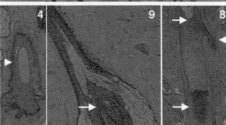

Figure 2.14
The contrast-enhanced phototrichogram (CE-PTG) technique (upper panels) matches perfectly histology (lower panels) for hair growth measurement.

Evaluation of hair growth with the phototrichogram. At time 0 (day 0), the hairs are clipped close to the scalp surface and photographed. After a given time (48 hours in the authors' experience, day 2) the same scalp site is photographed again.

Substantial elongation at day 2 reflects hair growth and indicates anagen in thick (1, 2, 5) and thin (7) hair. Moderate elongation reflects catagen in a thinning hair (3). No elongation reflects resting in thick (4) and thinning hair (6). After shedding the thick (4) or the typical tiny (9) resting hair, an empty follicle in the exogen stage will remain visible (8 arrows at day 0 and day 2 and upper arrow in histology 8, lower panel). The formation of new follicles can be seen only with histology (8). The newly formed follicles show initial stages of anagen. The lower arrow points to a thick, miniaturised hair follicle, while the upper right arrowhead shows a thin, miniaturised hair follicle. Tracking of such empty follicles with CE-PTGs will show newly growing hair in some days or weeks (see later).

easier to apply than the trichotillometer (one hair at a time) and reflects, under physiological conditions, exogen hair only per unit area (see Figure 2.2). Current evaluations with this method in various pathological conditions show that loosely attached or dystrophic anagen hair can also be extracted from inflammatory scalp disorders without or with scarring. This opens up a new field of clinical investigation: not only the method but also the interpretation of the numbers and their translation in a message that speaks to the patient must be fully documented and sensitive enough to clinically relevant changes over rather short periods of time (6 months to 1 year; see below).

Growth pattern analysis

Most mammals have synchronized hair growth which permits seasonal moulting. Hair growth in rats which spreads in a cephalocaudal direction may be observed by administering a dye that colours the hair shaft. This is clearly not an acceptable treatment for use in humans, who do not obviously moult. In a human clinical setting it is more useful to measure the changing pattern of hair growth. The patterns of androgen-dependent hair growth on the body (hirsutism) and on the scalp (AGA) have been formally defined, and grading systems formulated according to the

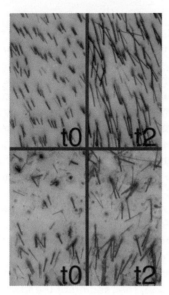

Figure 2.15
The contrast-enhanced phototrichogram
(CE-PTG; t0 = day 0 and t2 = day 2) technique
shows great differences in hair growth potential
in these two female patients complaining about
chronic diffuse hair loss.

Besides growth and thinning, they differ in
natural contrast, orientation, numbers of empty
follicles and decreased numbers of follicular
openings in the two lower panels as compared
to the two upper panels. The detailed analysis of
a scalp surface tells a lot about the past history
and future potential of the hair follicles.

varying degrees of severity. These scores
are easy to determine but are subject to
considerable observer bias. Breaking down
the complexity of 1 image = 1 number,
we devised a scoring method on smaller
fields (up to 18 fields; see Figures 2.1, 2.16)
with built-in controls for 3-D orientation
between subject and observer, matching all
degrees of density and all hair colour variations. The cumulative growth of hair will be
estimated indirectly by making the scalp
skin detection more difficult. A properly
trained clinician has first-hand information
to check whether the prescribed regimen

helps the patient or not. The more expert
methods may further refine the hair
dynamic status.

HAIR AND HAIR FOLLICLE MICROSCOPY

Hair shaft microscopy is essential for the
diagnosis of many abnormalities, particularly fungal disease and congenital and
hereditary hair shaft disorders, and to
assess hair weathering.

In the diagnosis of fungal diseases of hair,
plucked hairs are mounted in 20% aqueous
potassium hydroxide solution. If the
microscopy is to be carried out within
30 minutes, then the addition of 40%
dimethylsulphoxide (DMSO) may speed the
clearing time. DMSO may cause false-nega-
tive results beyond this time since hyphal
destruction occurs. The kerion type of infection may show only arthrospores on the
proximal part of the plucked hair shaft
despite massive inflammatory changes in
the skin.

Optical microscopy

Routine light microscopy of hair shafts is
essential for the diagnosis of diseases such
as hereditary and congenital shaft abnormalities. To assess intrinsic shaft changes,
only the proximal 1–2 cm of plucked hairs
should be examined since more distal
changes may be extrinsic and due to non-
specific weathering. Hairs may be mounted
dry if they are required for further studies,
but in routine transmitted light microscopic
examination, the surface of dry-mounted
hairs will scatter light. More detail is seen
and higher magnification is possible if a
standard mounting medium is used;
potassium hydroxide and water are not

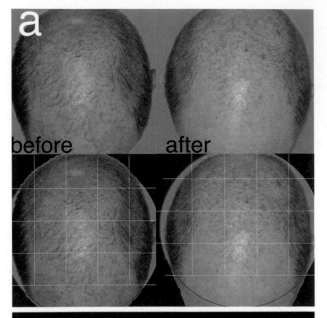

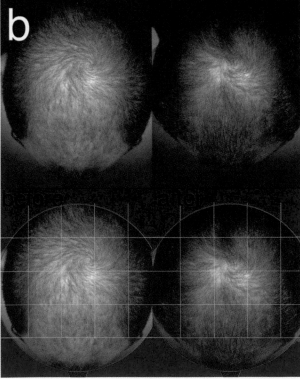

Figure 2.16

Scalp coverage scoring (SCS): a clinically useful tool for scalp hair monitoring.

(a) Upper four panels: the comparative examination of two global photographs showing the top of the head documents a dramatic worsening after 6 months of placebo lotion (upper panel). The placement of an external reference (lower panel) rapidly detects that the angle of view was not exactly the same at the two time points. When identical target sites are re-evaluated there is still a worsening of the SCS, reflecting the clinical condition, but the figures are more accurate.

(b) Lower four panels: when the photographs are taken exactly in the same position, the reading of the lower panel ascribes a more dramatic improvement to the central areas, i.e. the more significantly androgen-sensitive sites showing a significant improvement of the scalp coverage. A regrowth as impressive as this one may occur within 6 months after withdrawal of oral corticosteroid therapy.

satisfactory. 'Colour' changes seen by routine light microscopy may be due to pigment alterations, or structural changes not transmitting light and thus giving dark areas. If reflected light is used, then the dark areas in structural diseases such as pili annulati become light. Pigmentation changes are not altered by this technique. Careful examination using routine light microscopy provides most of the information required in clinical practice.

Polarization microscopy may provide extra information regarding the biochemical make-up of the hair and fine structural changes may become more obvious. Using this method it is possible to determine the refractive index and the birefringence of fibres (the numerical difference between the the refractive indexes parallel and perpendicular to the hair axis), a physical phenomenon caused by the orientation of internal structures in the hair. In the examination of hair from patients with a neuroectodermal symptom complex (trichothiodystrophy), polarizing microscopy has revealed striking bright and dark regions on viewing the hair between crossed polarizers. Turning the microscopic stage approximately 10° (5° on each side of the position of maximum extinction) reverses the bright and dark areas. Between crossed polarizers with the hair axis parallel to the vibration direction of the polarizer (maximum extinction, or 0°), the hair shows lines – 'tiger' or 'zigzag' hairs. This abnormality is associated with profound sulphur and high-sulphur (matrix) protein deficiency. Polarization microscopy has been used in many structural abnormalities of hair. The colour changes of polarization show up the abnormalities seen under transmitted light with greater clarity.

The subtlety of optical microscopic methods can be enhanced by various specialized techniques. The scale pattern can be examined in detail by examining a hair cast or impression of the hair in a suitable plastic material. An impression made by rolling the hair in the medium enables the whole circumference to be viewed. Interference microscopy, using monochromatic sodium light, greatly facilitates the examination of minute surface changes.

Electron microscopy

Optical microscopy is limited in resolution to approximately 0.2 μm and has a narrow depth of focus. Transmission electron microscopy is capable of very high resolution (down to 2 nm for biological materials) and has a depth-of-image focus that is greater than the normal specimen thickness (approximately 100 nm). Routine electron microscopic preparation may be suitable for examination of hair follicles, but the presence of keratinized hair within the follicle and the nature of hair structure make it necessary to modify routine procedures to obtain the best resolution and meaningful results. Glass knives give poor sectioning; a diamond knife is necessary for cutting ultrathin sections of hair without distortion. This is a very skilful procedure that is not always available in electron microscope laboratories. Hair displays a homogeneous electron density and must be stained with a heavy metal to show anatomical detail. Uranyl acetate and lead citrate enable the overall structure to be seen, and dodecatungstophosphoric acid gives added detail of cortex matrix proteins and cortical cell membranes. For transverse sections of hair fibres, ammoniacal silver or the silver methenamine stain, which specifically stains cystine, gives more contrast by highlighting the cystine-rich exocuticle and cortical matrix protein (Figure 2.17). Other electron histochemical techniques already usefully applied to tissue from many other organs have not yet been fully exploited in hair follicle disease; these include the identification

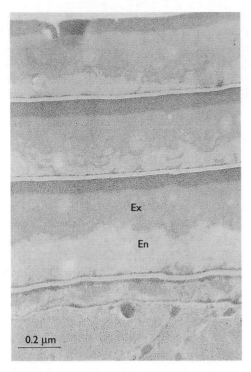

0.2 μm

Figure 2.17
Hair fibre cross-section (electron micrograph, silver methenamine stain) showing three cuticular cells (upper two-thirds) and cortex with pale pigment granules (lower part). Ex, exocuticle; En, endocuticle.

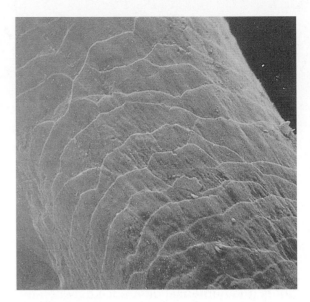

Figure 2.18
Normal hair near root end showing overlapping surface cuticular cells (scanning electron micrograph).

and localization of enzyme systems and antigen–antibody reactions.

Scanning electron microscopy is very diverse in its modes of operation and gives a wealth of information about surface architecture (Figure 2.18), elemental composition (if an X-ray microanalytical attachment is available), crystalline make-up, and electrical and magnetic properties of specimens. However, scanning electron microscopy or the more refined colour scanning is a research tool, and it cannot be stressed too greatly that all the detail needed by the clinician regarding hair microstructure can be obtained by optical microscopic methods. Also, elemental analysis remains interesting in selected cases (e.g. green hair) as a research tool and cannot be considered as a

diagnostic technique to support prescription of specific nutrient supplements or intake of oligo-elements. This use is commercial and relates to pseudo- or non-scientific purposes.

Follicular microscopy

The biopsy technique must be considered carefully if useful histological results are to be obtained. The biopsy must extend deep into the subcutaneous fat to avoid cutting off the hair bulbs (Figure 2.19). The epidermal surface of the excised tissue should be apposed to a rigid piece of paper to avoid curling of the tissue and immediately placed in fixative. If necessary, it can be glued or pinned to the paper if longitudinal follicular cutting is desired, since follicles have a great propensity for bending prior to hardening, leading to cross-cutting in the dermis. Punch biopsies (6 mm) and horizontal sectioning at various levels give more dynamic information about the hair cycle status at the site from which the tissue was taken.

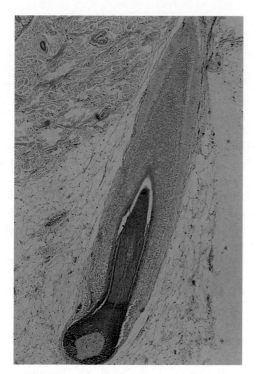

Figure 2.19
Hair follicle in anagen stage 6 – the deeper
components are seen to be in the subcutaneous
fat.

After processing, the embedded tissue
requires careful orientation prior to cutting
to maximize the chance of obtaining longitudinal follicular sections. Routine paraffin-
wax-embedded tissue has never been
entirely satisfactory for visualizing cytological detail within the follicle. Where possible,
tissue should be fixed and embedded as for
routine electron microscopy and 1 μm sections cut to give greater cytological clarity.

**Scanning electron microscopy of
hair is interesting and educational,
but note that microstructural
changes of importance in clinical
practice can be seen quickly, easily
and cheaply with routine optical
microscopy!**

Haematoxylin and eosin staining reveals
the general detail of the various cell layers
in the follicle. Other histochemical stains
may specifically enhance the appearance of
various cell layers. The lower border of the
internal root sheath takes up the Giemsa
stain, which stains the keratinized internal
root sheath specifically dark blue. The
intrafollicular hair cuticle stains with tolui-
dine blue and rhodamine B, first becoming
visible as a thin, blue layer surrounding the
presumptive hair. The van Gieson stain
gives a yellow colour to the hair and the
club in telogen roots. The tissue surrounding the club is brownish red with PAS stain
while rhodamine B stains the cuticle a faint
blue colour and the surrounding tricholem-
mal layer brilliant red.

Useful screening techniques for abnormal
hair keratins are the fluorescence methods
using either acridine orange or thioflavine T.
Normal hair keratin fluoresces blue with
dilute acridine orange, whereas altered keratins, such as the tip of hairs in trichorrhexis
nodosa, dystrophic hairs in kwashiorkor, or
weathered fibres, fluoresce red or orange.
The peracetic oxidation and thioflavine L
fluorescent method stains the disulphide
bonds in cystine, enabling sites of mature
keratin to be detected in the exocuticle or
cortex. S–H bonds can be specifically detected by a fluorogenic maleimide N-(7-
dimethyl-amino-methyl-coumarinyl)-
maleimide (DACM), which fluoresces only on
combining with an S–H bond. This method
requires frozen tissue. It has the advantage
that the emission maximum of DACM does
not overlap with any of the aromatic residues
of proteins such as tryptophan.

The first steps have now been taken in the
dermatological application of confocal
microscopy. This method allows examination of thick specimens because focusing to
a very narrow level of tissue can be
achieved. With a specific adaptation confocal
microscopy can be utilized in vivo and can
visualize hair follicles to a depth of 100 μm.
Further progress is expected in this area.

Also, sophisticated in vivo approaches using UV or laser light, ultrasound and other techniques will generate useful information. The clinical perspective will require a longer time to sort out what can be useful in terms of diagnostic or prognostic information.

FURTHER READING

Barth JH (1991) Investigations of hair, hair growth and the hair follicle. In: *Diseases of the hair and scalp*, 2nd edn (Oxford, Blackwell Scientific Publications), pp 588–606.

Birch MP, Messenger JF, Messenger AG (2001) Hair density, hair diameter and the prevalence of female pattern hair loss, *Br J Dermatol* **144**: 297–304.

Leonard C, Sperling MD (2001) Hair density in African Americans, *Arch Dermatol* **135**: 656–658.

Leroy T, Van Neste D (2002) Contrast enhanced phototrichogram pinpoints scalp hair changes in androgen sensitive areas of male androgenetic alopecia, *Skin Research and Technology* **8**: 106–111.

Rushton DH, de Brouwer B, De Coster W, Van Neste DJJ (1993) Comparative evaluation of scalp hair by phototrichogram and unit area trichogram analysis within the same subjects, *Acta Derm Venereol (Stockh)* **73**: 150–153.

Van Neste D (1993) Hair growth evaluation in clinical dermatology, *Dermatology* **187**: 233–234.

Van Neste D, de Brouwer B, De Coster W (1994) The phototrichogram: analysis of some factors of variation, *Skin Pharmacol* **7**: 67–72.

Van Neste D, Fuh V, Sanchez-Pedreno P et al (2000) Finasteride increases anagen hair in men with androgenetic alopecia, *Br J Dermatol* **143**: 804–810.

Whiting DA (1993) Diagnostic and predictive value of horizontal sections of scalp biopsy specimens in male pattern androgenetic alopecia, *J Am Acad Dermatol* **28**: 755–763.

3 Hair loss/hair dysplasias

In this chapter are included a variety of abnormalities in which hair is obviously less than normal or is shed in greater than normal quantities with or without overt thinning. Many structural entities described here may have normal amounts of hair or not, depending on a variety of secondary factors, e.g. excessive weathering.

CONGENITAL AND HEREDITARY ALOPECIA

Total or partial absence of hair of developmental origin occurs in a great variety of clinical forms, either as an apparently isolated defect or in association with a wide range of other anomalies.[1-3] A logical classification ought to be based on detailed histological and genetic investigations, but these, unfortunately, have seldom been carried out. Provisionally, a purely clinical

> **One in four babies is born 'bald' – more than 1 year may be required for congenital hair faults to become clinically obvious as hair grows**

classification is useful to enable the clinician at least to understand the clearly defined types.

CIRCUMSCRIBED ALOPECIA

Circumscribed alopecia of congenital origin is usually the result of a local aplasia of all layers of the skin or an epidermal naevus (Figure 3.1). However, aplasia of the hair follicles in an otherwise grossly normal skin eventually with normal development of other appendages can also occur.

TOTAL ALOPECIA

As an isolated abnormality

Total alopecia as an isolated defect is usually determined by an autosomal recessive gene (Figure 3.2). Dominant or irregular dominant inheritance may occur in some families. The two genotypes seem to be phenotypically indistinguishable, but detailed investigation may reveal differences. The term 'total' is relative, but if any hairs are present they are extremely few. Many isolated cases and families reported under the

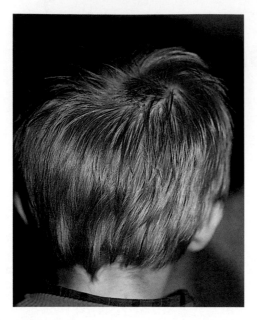

Figure 3.1
Scalp epidermal naevus.

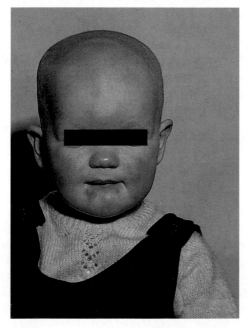

Figure 3.2
Congenital scalp hypotrichosis (total).

diagnosis of congenital alopecia are found on review of the original reports to be examples of other syndromes; many are hidrotic ectodermal dysplasia.

The hair follicles are absent in adult life, even when the fetal hair-coat was normal. Sebaceous glands are smaller than normal. When a few stray hairs have survived, the structure of the shaft appears to be normal.

Clinical features

The scalp hair is often normal at birth but is shed between the first and sixth months, after which no further, or very irregular, growth occurs. In some cases the scalp was totally hairless at birth and has remained so. Eyebrows, eyelashes and body hair may also be absent, but often there are a few pubic and axillary hairs and scanty eyebrows and eyelashes. Teeth and nails are normal and general health, intelligence and life expectancy are unimpaired.

With associated defects

Total or almost total alopecia is unusual in hereditary syndromes.

Progeria

Scalp and body hair is totally deficient.

Hidrotic ectodermal dysplasia

Total or almost total alopecia is associated with palmar plantar keratoderma and thickened, discoloured nails. Any hairs that are present are structurally normal but are often of finer diameter than the average.

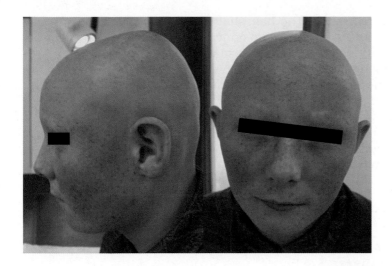

Figure 3.3
Atrichia with keratin cysts. Normal scalp and body hair in the newborn is lost permanently as a result of defective hair replacement. Microscopic follicular cysts, as present here but clinically unnoticeable (histology not shown) may take some years to become clinically visible. Reproduced with permission from: Van Neste D, Leroy T, de Ramecourt A, Hair removal and hair follicle targeting. In: *Hair Science and Technology*, pp 401–412.

Moynahan's syndrome

This autosomal recessive syndrome, described in male siblings, is associated with mental retardation, epilepsy and total badness of the scalp. The hair may regrow in childhood between 2 and 4 years of age.

Atrichia with keratin cysts[4–7]

This rare syndrome, comparable with the condition found in certain hairless mice, has been reported mainly in girls, but the mode of inheritance is unknown (Figure 3.3). One can speculate that it is an X-linked mutation. Total and permanent alopecia develops after the first hair-coat is shed. At any age between 5 and 18 years numerous small, horny papules appear, first on the face, neck and scalp, and then gradually over the greater part of the limbs and trunk. Histologically the papules are thick-walled keratin cysts. Atrichia with cysts has been described with mutations in the vitamin D receptor, suggesting that both these entities may be in the same genetic pathway that controls postnatal cycling of the hair follicle.

Baraitser's syndrome

This autosomal recessive syndrome presents as almost total alopecia following the loss of some downy scalp hair present at birth. Mental and physical retardation may be associated.

HYPOTRICHOSIS

Congenital hypotrichosis of sufficient degree to cause social embarrassment but not to reach clinical referral is not uncommon and is probably determined by an autosomal dominant gene. Severe degrees of congenital hypotrichosis without associated defects are rare. Dominant inheritance has been recorded, but many cases have occurred sporadically. There are a number of distinct syndromes.

Hypotrichosis is a common feature of many hereditary syndromes, usually in association with other ectodermal defects.[1] In the majority the hair is not only sparse but is structurally abnormal. Where hypotrichosis is the most prominent manifestation and the structural defect is distinctive and well characterized, it has given its name to the syndrome, as in monilethrix and pili torti. In other syndromes the scanty scalp hair is a minor and sometimes inconstant manifestation, and the shaft defect is usually less specific, although clinically often gross. The follicles are sparse and reduced in size, and the hair shafts are brittle and hypopigmented. The nature of the disturbance in keratinization is not known.

> **Congenital hypotrichosis is a diagnostic mixture of cases with decreased follicular numbers: smaller follicles or 'fragile' abnormal hairs, or all of these, which must be assessed in every case**

Clinical features

When hypotrichosis occurs as an isolated abnormality, the scalp hair at birth is normal in quantity and quality, but is shed during the first 6 months and is never adequately replaced. It is sparse, fine, dry and brittle and seldom exceeds 10 cm in length. The eyebrows, eyelashes and vellus hair may be absent, sparse or normal. In rare cases, improvement or recovery has taken place at puberty, though the condition is usually permanent.

In some families the hair is normal until the age of 5 years or later, when growth becomes retarded and the scalp is progressively denuded to the extent that baldness is almost total by the age of 25 years.

Many of the hereditary syndromes of which hypotrichosis is a constant or frequent feature are listed in Table 3.1. In the majority the hair is not only sparse but fine and brittle, and is often hypopigmented.

The hair shafts are often defective but may show no consistent well-characterized structural abnormality. There are also many syndromes, as yet incompletely defined, in which hypotrichosis is associated with other defects.

> **There are many unique hypotrichotic syndromes – this field is a bit like philately and cries out for modern genetic studies**

Hypotrichosis with keratosis pilaris

The hair is apparently normal at birth, but after the 'birth-coat' has been shed, between the second and sixth months, it fails to grow satisfactorily and remains sparse, short, brittle and poorly pigmented. Eyebrows and eyelashes may be normal or sparse. Keratosis pilaris is present on the occipital region and neck, and sometimes on the trunk and limbs. Nails, teeth and general physical development are normal. The hairs show no beading or other distinctive abnormality. Keratosis pilaris may occur with increasing hair loss and atrophy (Figures 3.4–3.6).

Hypotrichosis with keratosis pilaris and lentiginosis

This develops with hypotrichosis at or just after puberty and progresses until the menopause. Axillary and pubic hair is completely lost. There is keratosis pilaris of the scalp and axillae, brittleness and longitudinal striation of the nails, and centrofacial lentiginosis.

Table 3.1 Alopecia or hypotrichosis in hereditary syndromes

	Main clinical features	Hair characteristics
Hidrotic ectodermal dysplasia	Nail thickened, striated, discoloured; palmoplantar keratoderma	Scalp hair sparse and fine; may be totally absent
Progeria	Normal first year, then severe retardation of physical growth; senile appearance; thin, dry wrinkled skin, bird-like features	Total alopecia
Monilethrix	Keratosis pilaris, mainly on occiput and nape of neck	Normal at birth; later brittle, beaded hair 1–2 cm length; microscopy diagnostic; may improve spontaneously with age due to hair thickening
Pili torti	Hair defect main or only manifestation; onset first noted in 2nd or 3rd year	Hair sparse and brittle; 'spangled' in reflected light; microscopy diagnostic
Anhidrotic (hypohidrotic) ectodermal dysplasia	Usually male; reduced sweating; sunken nose; conical teeth; smooth, finely wrinkled skin	Sparse, dry, fine, short scalp hair and eyelashes; hair may sometimes be normal but with decreased density
Rothmund–Thomson syndrome	Erythema cheeks, hands, feet from 3 to 6 months, followed by poikiloderma; light sensitivity	Scalp hair sparse; eyebrows, eyelashes, and body hair very sparse
Werner's syndrome	Scleroderma-like changes on face and extremities; cataracts	Premature greying before age 20; progressive alopecia from adolescence
Hallermann–Streiff syndrome	Dyscephaly, aplasia of mandible; dwarfism	Normal at birth; later sparse with patchy alopecia; often sutural
Marinesco–Sjögren syndrome	Cerebellar ataxia; mental retardation; cataract; short stature	Scalp hair fine, sparse, short; hypopigmentation

Table 3.1 Continued

	Main clinical features	*Hair characteristics*
Netherton's syndrome	Both sexes; atopic eczema may flare with peanuts	Sparse, brittle; often 'bamboo-hairs', trichorrhexis invaginata or nodosa
Cartilage-hair hypoplasia	Dwarfism, skeletal abnormalities	Sparse, brittle, fine and light in colour, but hair may be normal or totally absent
Trichorhinophalangeal syndrome (type 1–11)	Pear-shaped nose	Hair sparse, fine, brittle (may be normal)
AEC syndrome	Ankyloblepharon, ectodermal dysplasia, cleft lip and palate	Hair sparse, coarse, wiry
EEC syndrome	Ectodactyly, ectodermal dysplasia, cleft lip and/or palate	Hair sparse, twisted and irregular surface (multiple canal)
Follicular atrophoderma	Depressions at follicular orifices; basal cell naevi	Sparse and fine
Menkes' syndrome	Retarded growth; symptoms of cerebellar degeneration	Sparse, brittle, poorly pigmented; twisting microscopically

Data modified from Rook AJ and Dawber RPR (eds), *Diseases of the Hair and Scalp* (Oxford, Blackwell Scientific Publications, 1998).

For detailed descriptions of the above and rarer syndromes see Sinclair et al[1] and Sinclair and De Berker.[3]

Eyelid cysts, hypodontia and hypotrichosis

This congenital triad is extremely rare and usually sporadic.

Trichorhinophalangeal (TRP) syndrome

Two types of TRP syndrome have been reported: one is familial and shows autosomal dominant inheritance, and the other is sporadic in nature (Figures 3.7–3.12).

Prominent findings are pear-shaped nose and the gradual deviation of the distal phalanges. Other changes have been recorded by morphometric studies of the maxilla, and the hips have been reported to be modified. Phalangeal bone changes are diagnostic with the pictures described as 'chapeau de gendarme'.

Hypomelia, hypotrichosis, facial haemangioma syndrome

This 'pseudothalidomide' syndrome, which is probably determined by an autosomal

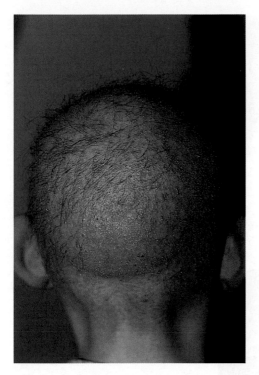

Figure 3.4
Keratosis pilaris decalvans with severe hair loss.

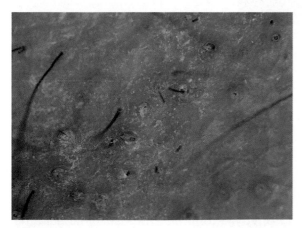

Figure 3.5
Keratosis pilaris decalvans – marked follicular keratosis evident.

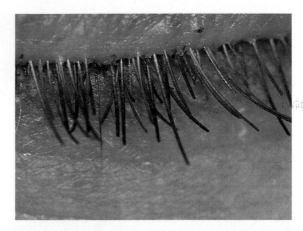

Figure 3.6
Keratosis pilaris decalvans – as in Figure 3.5, at eyelid margin.

recessive gene, is the association of gross reduction defects of the limbs, a mid-facial capillary naevus and sparse silver-blond hair.

Marie–Unna type hypotrichosis

This rare but very distinctive syndrome (Figures 3.13–3.18) is determined by an autosomal dominant gene. Affected individuals may be normal at birth or be completely or almost completely hairless. Hair becomes or remains sparse or absent until about the third year when coarse, flattened, irregularly twisted hair appears on the scalp. This coarse hair is gradually lost with the approach of puberty as follicles are progressively destroyed by an atrophic process. The hair loss is greatest around the scalp margins and on the vertex (Figures 3.13, 3.14), but may be patchy. Lashes, eyebrows and body hair are sparse, and often virtually absent from birth. Occasionally, sporadic cases similar to Marie–Unna syndrome occur with severe hair loss (Figure 3.15). General physical and mental

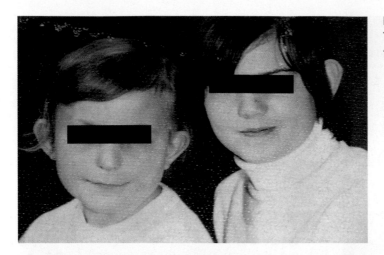

Figure 3.7
Trichorhinophalangeal syndrome
facies in affected siblings.

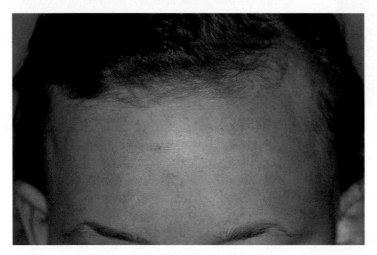

Figure 3.8
Trichorhinophalangeal syndrome –
some degree of hypotrichosis.

development are normal. Scanning electron microscopy shows that the hair shafts are coarse, irregularly twisted and fluted; this is usually diagnostic in its uniqueness (Figure 3.18). In some cases the coarse, wiry black hair, before hair is lost, looks rather like a wig.

Hypotrichosis in disorders of amino acid metabolism

In many disorders with amino aciduria, the hair is hypopigmented and often also fine, friable and sparse. Fine sparse hair may occur in phenylketonuria, arginosuccinic aciduria, hyperlysinaemia and homocystinuria.

A number of case reports associate hypotrichosis with a variety of ectodermal

> **Severe 'widespread, familial' hypotrichosis in childhood and early adult life with a small number of long, coarse, 'wiry' scalp hairs usually means Marie–Unna syndrome**

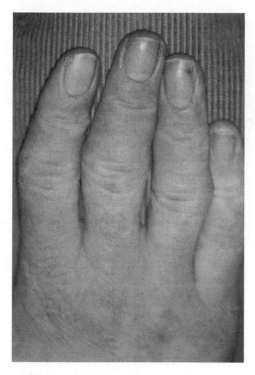

Figure 3.9
Trichorhinophalangeal syndrome –
characteristic hand deformity.

defects. Some cases may represent partial forms of recognized syndromes but it is probable that many additional distinct syndromes remain to be identified and characterized.

Differential diagnosis of hypotrichosis

Microscopy of plucked hairs will exclude the more distinctive structural defects such as pili torti, monilethrix and pili annulati. Other ectodermal defects should be carefully sought and relatives examined.

CIRCUMSCRIBED ALOPECIA OF CONGENITAL ORIGIN

The differential diagnosis of circumscribed alopecia of developmental origin presents little difficulty if a reliable history is available. Without it, alopecia areata and the acquired cicatricial alopecias must be considered:

1. The commonest forms are naevoid. Epidermal naevi (Figure 3.19) are usually devoid of hair and present as warty or smooth but slightly indurated plaques. A zone of non-cicatricial alopecia sometimes develops around melanocytic naevi.
2. Aplasia of all layers of the skin gives rise to a congenital defect (Figure 3.20),

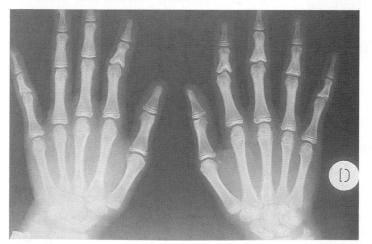

Figure 3.10
Trichorhinophalangeal syndrome –
radiograph of hands in Figure 3.9.

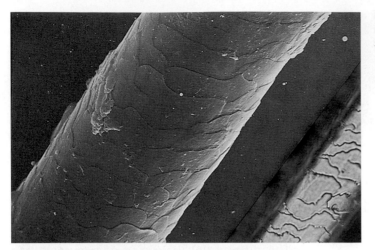

Figure 3.11
Hair cuticle changes in trichorhinophalangeal syndrome (scanning electron micrograph above; light micrograph below).

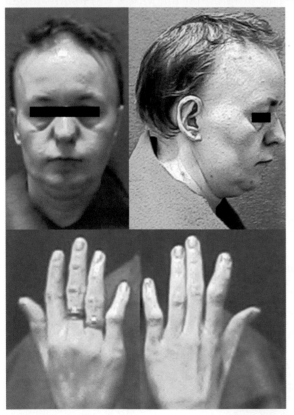

Figure 3.12
Trichorhinophalangeal syndrome. Same patient as in previous pictures seen at the age of 34 years; further worsening of hair loss and hand deformation. In male subjects this pattern can be mistaken as common baldness.

usually a circular or rectilinear area of scarring somewhat depressed below the scalp surface and commonly on the vertex.

3. Irregular areas of cicatricial alopecia not preceded by obvious inflammatory changes produce the syndrome known as pseudopelade. Pseudopelade may develop during early infancy in association with certain hereditary syndromes, e.g. incontinentia pigmenti and Conradi's syndrome.

4. Circumscribed non-cicatricial alopecia is uncommon. It is the result of hypoplasia or aplasia of a group of follicles. The scalp is clinically normal and histologically shows no change other than a reduced number of follicles. The follicles present are usually small and of vellus rather than terminal type. The first hair-coat is normal and the patches develop between the third and sixth months, but if they are small and not completely bald, they may not be noticed until considerably later.

Several clinical forms occur. In *vertical alopecia*, a small and often irregular patch of alopecia is present on the vertex at birth. It can be confused with aplasia cutis, but the skin is normal apart from the absence of

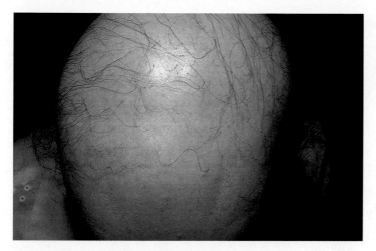

Figure 3.13
Marie–Unna syndrome – remaining hair is wiry.

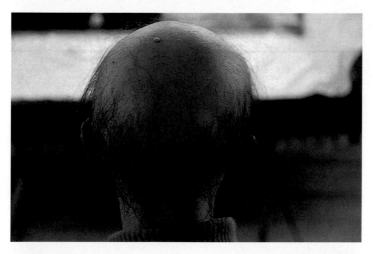

Figure 3.14
Marie–Unna syndrome.

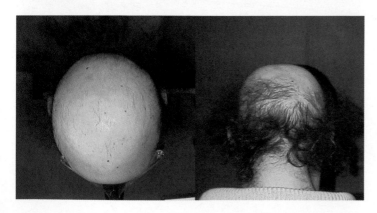

Figure 3.15
Marie–Unna syndrome. Occasionally, a pattern very similar to the familial Marie–Unna hypotrichosis with severe hair loss may occur in a sporadic case; the presence of nail defects may point to a genetic heterogeneity
Reproduced with permission from: Van Neste D, Hair growth measurement in genetic hair disorders. In: *Hair Science and Technology*, pp 183–189.

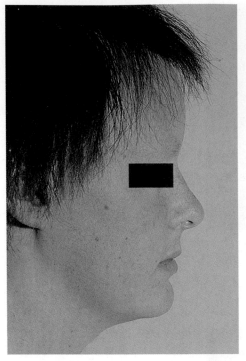

Figure 3.16
Marie–Unna syndrome.

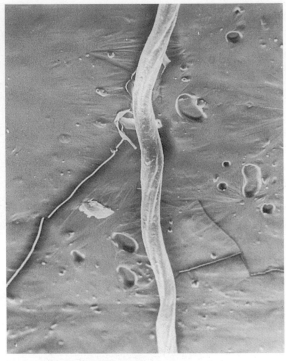

Figure 3.18
Marie–Unna syndrome – scanning electron
micrograph of affected hair.

Figure 3.17
Marie–Unna syndrome – light
micrograph of affected scalp hair.

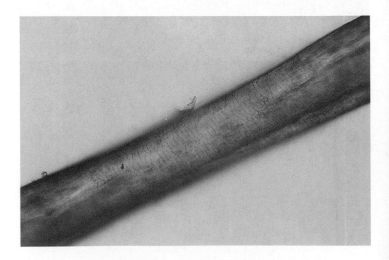

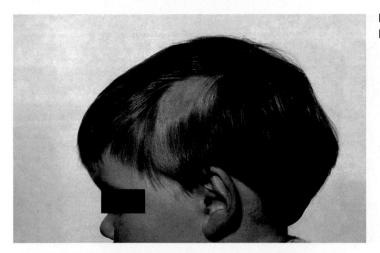

Figure 3.19
Epidermal naevus.

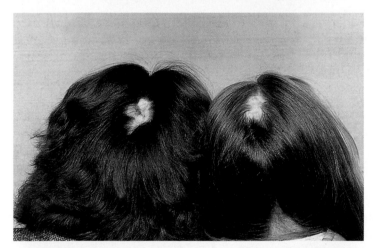

Figure 3.20
Aplasia cutis in sisters.

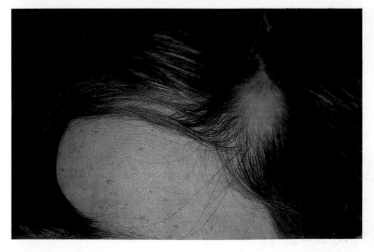

Figure 3.21
Triangular alopecia.

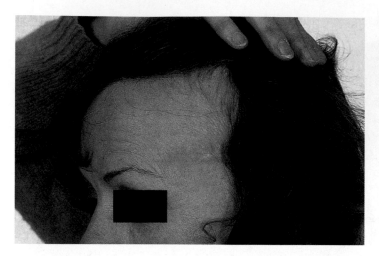

Figure 3.22
Another example of triangular alopecia.

appendages. In *sutural alopecia*, which is one component of the Hallermann–Streiff syndrome, multiple patches overlie the cranial sutures. In the usual form of *triangular alopecia* a triangular area overlying the frontotemporal suture just inside the anterior hairline (Figures 3.21, 3.22), and with its base directed forwards, is completely bald or covered by sparse vellus hairs. Rarely, similar triangular patches have occurred on the nape of the neck.

Single or multiple small patches of total alopecia or hypotrichosis may occasionally occur in other sites but are often inconspic-

uous. The rare congenital dermoid cyst may regress to a flat, non-scarred, circular, bald patch (Figure 3.23).

ABNORMALITIES OF HAIR SHAFT

Structural defects of the hair shaft may be sufficiently obvious to cause significant cosmetic disability, or they may render the hair abnormally susceptible to injury by minor trauma (excessive weathering). They may also be the result of hereditary or acquired

Figure 3.23
Dermoid cyst of scalp.

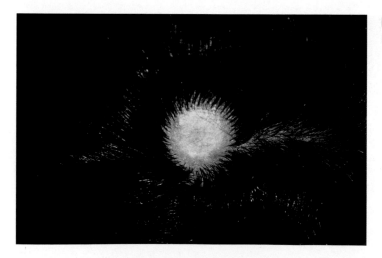

metabolic disorders, thus giving valuable clues in the diagnosis of these disorders.

The most convenient classification of anomalies of the shaft divides them into those which are associated with increased fragility, and those which typically are not. This distinction is useful, because only the former present clinically as patchy or diffuse alopecia.

> **Routine light microscopy is mandatory in cases with abnormal hair no matter how little is left! – polarization highlights the defects**

Structural defects with increased fragility

Monilethrix (beading of hair)

The term 'monilethrix' (Figures 3.24–3.31) was first used early in the 20th century. Nevertheless, in some early reports, and even in some more recent ones, microscopic similarities have led to the confusion of monilethrix with other shaft defects, e.g. trichorrhexis nodosa (when weathering is severe) or pili torti.

The hereditary nature of monilethrix was recognized soon after the condition was first identified. Autosomal dominant

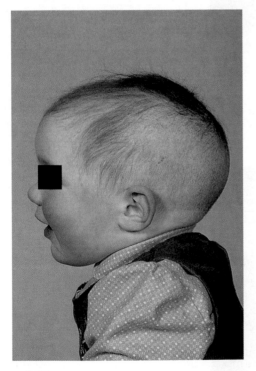

Figure 3.24
Monilethrix.

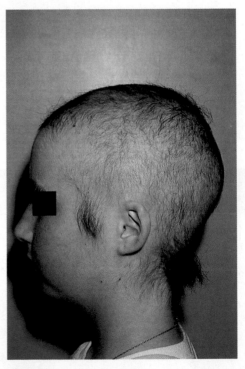

Figure 3.25
Another example of monilethrix.

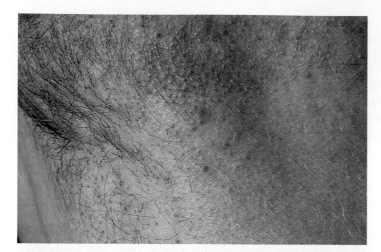

Figure 3.26
Monilethrix – showing hair loss and follicular keratotic 'plugs'.

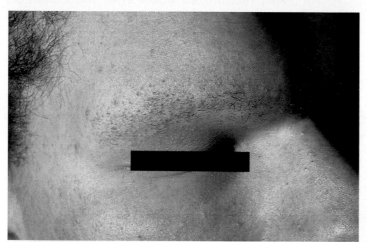

Figure 3.27
Monilethrix – eyebrows affected.

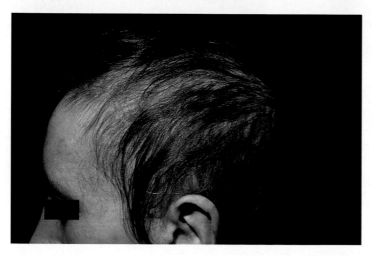

Figure 3.28
Monilethrix – some hair regrowth during pregnancy.

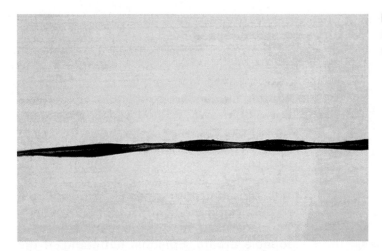

Figure 3.29
Monilethrix – beaded hair (light
micrograph).

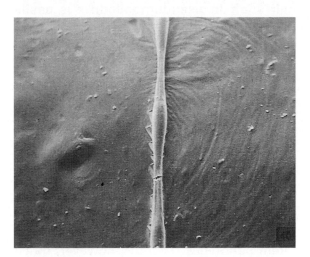

Figure 3.30
Monilethrix – beaded hair (scanning electron
micrograph).

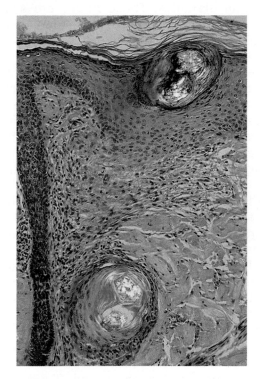

Figure 3.31
Monilethrix – section showing follicular beading
(left) and hyperkeratosis (right). (HE staining.)

transmission has been demonstrated in
numerous large pedigrees. The alleged
occurrence of normal carriers of the dominant gene has not been proven, for a parent
with only 5% of abnormal follicles is easily
passed as normal. The gene appears to
have high penetrance but variable expressivity. Several pedigrees have suggested an
autosomal recessive trait. The abnormal
gene is found on the long arm of chromo-

some 12 and is responsible for the production of type II keratin (12q11-q13). Various
mutations within a keratin gene (hHb6, hHb1)
have been described; in one described

family in which both parents had monilethrix, three of the children were very
severely affected because they were
homozygous for a particular hHb6 mutation.

> **Short or broken scalp hair with
> prominent keratosis pilaris is
> almost always monilethrix**

Pathology
The hair shaft is beaded and breaks easily.
Elliptical nodes 0.7–1.0 mm apart have the
normal thickness or slightly less than
normal diameter. These nodes are separated by narrower internodes (Figures 3.29,
3.30). Hair breaks at internode spaces. The
width of the nodes and the distance
between them show some variation within a
single family. By scanning electron microscopy the nodes and some of the internodes
show a normal imbricated scale pattern, but
most internodes show longitudinal ridging.
The internodes break not only because they
are narrower but also because the cortical
keratinous protein within the longitudinal
cells is irregular in its distribution. If this
does not withstand physical factors, such as
bending and twisting, well, it cracks and
weathers very prematurely.

Histologically the follicle shows wide and
narrow zones (Figure 3.31), corresponding
to the nodes and internodes, and keratosis
pilaris, but the general structure of the follicle is otherwise normal. On electron microscopic examination, changes are visible in
the zone of keratinization. The cell membranes of the deeper hair shaft cuticular
cells are thrown into folds, particularly at
the narrower internodes where breakage
occurs. The thinnest hairs can even break
inside the scalp. The broken hair shafts do
not find an easy way out of the infundibulum. They disrupt the outer root sheath.
This gives rise to a kind of foreign body

granuloma, a characteristic feature of the
red occipital papules.

Attempts have been made to investigate
the mechanism of node formation and to
relate it to the diurnal rate of hair growth.
Different studies are conflicting. Some have
shown no growth-related nodal pattern, and
others have shown a 24–48 hour growth per
nodal complex.

Intermittent administration of an antimitotic agent can give rise to zones of constriction alternating with zones of normal diameter, mimicking monilethrix. Moniliform hairs
can also occur at the incipient stages of
alopecia areata. Episodic flattening of the
hair shaft in pseudomonilethrix is easily
distinguished.

Electron microscopic studies have shown
that an increased susceptibility of the hair
shaft to the effects of the trauma – premature weathering – is an important factor in
the failure of the hair to grow to normal
length.

Clinical features
Monilethrix shows considerable variation
in age of onset, severity and course (Figures
3.24–3.28). There is not yet sufficient information to establish whether these variations
are in part consistently correlated with different genotypes. There is, however, much
variation even within the more commonly
reported autosomal dominant form.

The hair may be obviously abnormal at
birth but is most commonly normal, and is
progressively replaced by abnormal hair
during the first months of life. In other cases
the normal hair is succeeded by horny follicular papules from the summit of which
emerge fragile beaded hairs. The follicular
keratosis and the abnormal hairs are most
frequent on the nape and occiput but may
involve the entire scalp (Figure 3.26). In
typical cases the short stubble of brittle
hairs and rough horny plugs give a distinctive, almost diagnostic appearance. The

eyebrows (Figure 3.27) and eyelashes, pubic and axillary hair, and general body hair may be affected in some cases.

Some investigators have suggested that the association with oligophrenia and with nail and tooth defects is significant. It is possible that such associations may be a feature of the recessive phenotype, since oligophrenia and poor physical development have been noted also in siblings with monilethrix. Juvenile cataract may also occur.

Reports of abnormalities of amino acid metabolism are conflicting. Argininosuccinicaciduria has been described, but a technical error in the study was subsequently detected. The urinary amino acid pattern is usually normal in the autosomal dominant type or in isolated cases. An apparent excess of aspartic acid and of arginine in the urine has been reported.

Treatment
None is available but oral retinoids can induce some hair regrowth,[8] but this may be the result of effects on follicles obstructed by keratosis pilaris. Reduction of hairdressing trauma may be followed by some improvement, because of a lessening in the 'weathering' from chemical and physical insults. In many patients the condition persists with little change throughout life, though spontaneous improvement or complete recovery has occurred, and improvement during pregnancy has been reported (Figure 3.28). Griseofulvin or oral and topical retinoids have also temporarily restored some normal hair growth.

Pseudomonilethrix

It is not uncommon to see patients who complain that their hair is of poor quality or brittle, and if the patient in question is a young child, microscopy of the hair to exclude the classical shaft defects is a routine procedure. It should be a routine procedure also in the older child or adult. The syndrome termed 'pseudomonilethrix' was first reported from South Africa in individuals of European or Indian descent. The status of the syndrome is uncertain; some of the shaft deformities are almost certainly artefactual (Figures 3.32–3.34).

Alopecia develops from the age of 8 years onwards and the lack of hair in affected individuals can be shown to be the result of a defect, the inheritance of which is determined by an autosomal dominant gene,

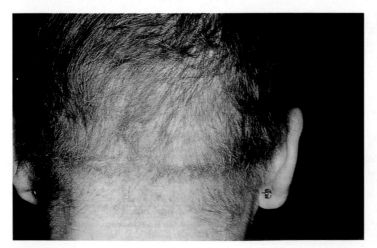

Figure 3.32
Pseudomonilethrix.

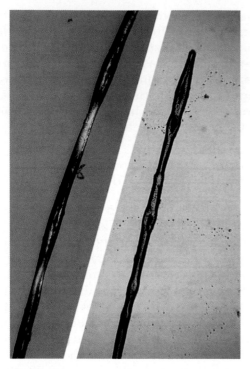

Figure 3.33
Pseudomonilethrix hairs – polarized light (left)
and transmitted light (right).

which renders the hair so fragile that it readily breaks with the trauma of brushing, combing or other hairdressing procedures. On microscopy one, or occasionally two, of three abnormalities can be seen: (1) pseudomonilethrix in the form of irregular nodes, which on electron microscopy prove to be the protruding edges of depressions in the shaft; (2) irregular twists of 25–200° without flattening of the shaft; and (3) breaks with brush-like ends in otherwise normal shafts. There is no keratosis pilaris. Most authorities now believe that the microscopic changes in pseudomonilethrix are artefactual; they can be produced in normal hairs by trauma from tweezers or forceps or by compressing overlying hairs between two glass slides. The indentation in one shaft caused by an overlying hair exactly mimics the appearance of pseudomonilethrix. In congenitally soft or fragile hair, pseudomonilethrix may occur very prominently as a significant disease-related artefact.

> **Pseudomonilethrix is a microscopic artefact that may be very prominent in a variety of 'fragile' hair dystrophies**

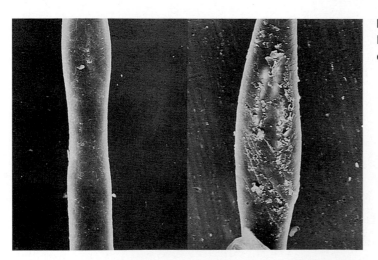

Figure 3.34
Pseudomonilethrix hairs (scanning
electron micrographs).

Pili torti (twisting of hair)

The hairs are flattened and at irregular intervals completely rotated through 180° around their long axes (Figures 3.35–3.38). Scanning electron microscopy has made it clear that twisted hairs occur in many distinct forms, and that the twisting may be associated with a number of other shaft defects. Occasional twists of varying angle should not be taken to be the distinctive genetically 'fixed' abnormality of pili torti. Many dystrophies and distortions of the follicular zone of keratinization will vary the hair shaft 'bore', sometimes showing <180° irregular twists.

> **The term 'pili torti' should be limited to congenital or hereditary syndromes in which multiple hair twists (180°) are the predominant sign. Irregular twists are common in many syndromes with other hair faults**

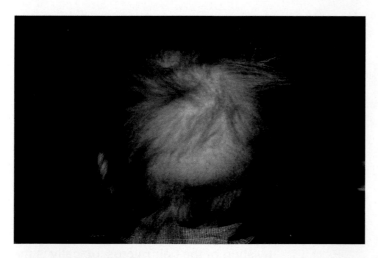

Figure 3.35
Pili torti.

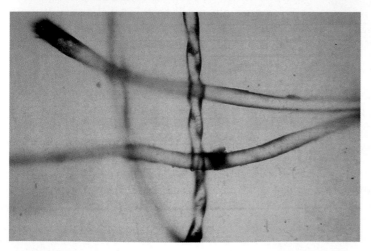

Figure 3.36
Pili torti – dry-mounted hairs showing twisting and some weathering.

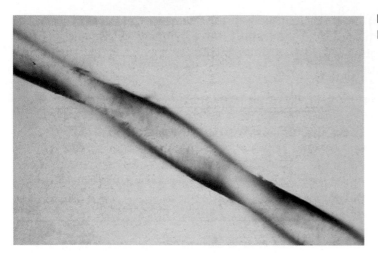

Figure 3.37
Pili torti – hair-twisting.

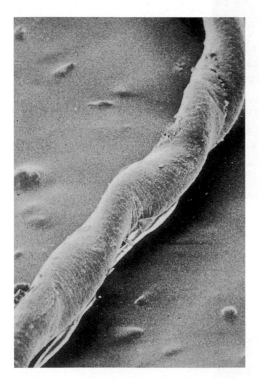

Figure 3.38
Pili torti – hair-twisting (scanning electron micrograph).

There are several syndromes of which twisted hair is a feature:

- *Menkes' syndrome:* light coloured, twisted hair as a manifestation of a hereditary defect of intestinal copper transport. The inheritance is of an X-linked recessive type. Female carriers may be mildly affected. The disease has been mapped in genetic terms to Xq13. It is caused by a defect of an ATPase that is responsible for Cu^{2+} transport. The twisting of the hair microscopically is the same as in pili torti, and the amino acid analysis of the defective hairs shows a severe disturbance of the high-sulphur protein synthesis.
- *Björnstad's syndrome:* twisted hair with sensorineural deafness. Probable autosomal dominant inheritance.
- *Bazex syndrome:* twisted hair, hypotrichosis, basal cell carcinomas of the face and follicular atrophoderma.
- *Crandall's syndrome:* twisted hair and deafness associated with hypogonadism. Probable sex-linked recessive inheritance.

- *Hypohidrotic ectodermal dysplasia:* twisted hairs with characteristic facies and dental defects.
- *Pseudomonilethrix:* twisted hair associated in the individual or the family with apparently beaded hairs of autosomal dominant inheritance.

When patients with these syndromes are excluded, only those with 'pure' pili torti remain, but there is evidence that these cases do not constitute a homogeneous entity. The hairs show considerable variation from patient to patient in their ability to withstand breaking and pulling; i.e. the hairs in some patients weather badly, but in others they do not.

Mental retardation, pili torti and trichorrhexis nodosa with hair keratin deficient in crystine may rarely be linked together. However, dystrophic pili torti may occur with a normal cystine content.

Improvement in hair length may develop after puberty when 'classical' pili torti of early onset occurs as an isolated defect, and in these cases inheritance is usually by an autosomal dominant gene. There are many reports of apparently sporadic cases. However, there are also cases in which the siblings of consanguineous parents have been affected, and in which recessive inheritance can be suspected.

Local inflammatory processes which distort the follicles can result in distorted and twisted hairs. Such hairs can be found around the edges of patches of cicatricial alopecia or along the wound edges after brain or cosmetic surgery on the scalp. Acquired pili torti type changes may be produced by oral retinoids, but this hair is more 'kinked' than twisted.

The earlier reports emphasized that the affected hairs were flattened and twisted through 180° around their long axes at irregular intervals along the shaft. The load–extension curve (breaking stress analysis) resembles that of the wool of merino sheep, the hairs breaking more easily than normal. Histologically the only abnormality is curvature of the hair follicles. With the scanning electron microscope the cuticle of the hair shaft appears normal, though severe weathering changes are not uncommon, and the 'bore' of the hair is typically oval and elliptical in cross-section.

Clinical features

The hair is usually normal at birth, gradually being replaced by abnormal hair by the third month, or not until the second or third year. There is a wide variation from case to case in the fragility of the hair, and hence in the clinical picture. Affected hairs are brittle and may break off at a length of 5 cm or less, or grow longer in areas of the scalp least subject to trauma. There may therefore be only a short, coarse stubble over the whole scalp or circumscribed baldness, irregularly patchy particularly on occipital areas. Affected hairs have a 'spangled' appearance in reflected light since the irregularly flattened hairs together reflect light at different angles.

Other ectodermal defects may be associated with pili torti. Keratosis pilaris is the most common, but nail dystrophies, dental abnormalities, corneal opacities and mental retardation have all been linked. Corkscrew hair is microscopically clinically separate.

The diagnosis should be suspected if the hair is brittle and dry. The typical spangled appearance in reflected light is present only if the hair is at least moderately severely affected, yet is not so brittle that it breaks to leave only a sparse stubble. Microscopic examination of several hairs must be made to confirm the diagnosis.

Björnstad's syndrome/ Crandall's syndrome

In these syndromes pili torti is associated with sensorineural hearing loss. The loss of hair usually begins in infancy, but may not be noticed until the age of 8 years. There is a correlation between the severity of the hair defect and the degree of hearing loss. On microscopy the hair shafts show longitudinal ridging and irregular twisting. The mode of inheritance is probably autosomal recessive.

Examples have been recorded of the associated findings of secondary hypogonadism with deficiency of luteinizing and of growth hormones. The pedigree suggests that inheritance of this syndrome is autosomal recessive.

Netherton's syndrome

The original observations recorded bamboo-like nodes in the fragile hairs of a girl with 'erythematous scaly dermatitis'. It has gradually become apparent that ichthyosis linearis circumflexa and 'bamboo hairs' (trichorrhexis invaginata) are two features of a single syndrome (Figures 3.39–3.41). Most

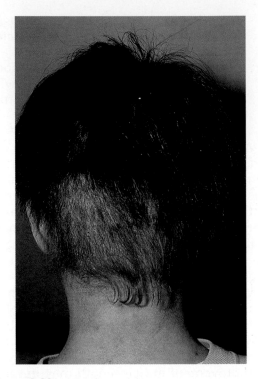

Figure 3.39
Netherton's syndrome.

cases of Netherton's syndrome have had ichthyosis linearis circumflexa (ILC), but some have ichthyosis vulgaris or both conditions or ichthyosiform erythroderma.

Figure 3.40
Netherton's syndrome – hair showing a bamboo node.

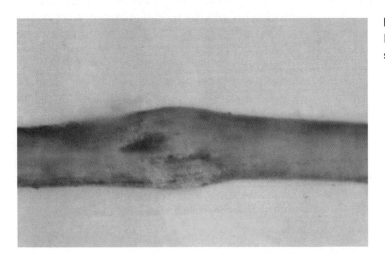

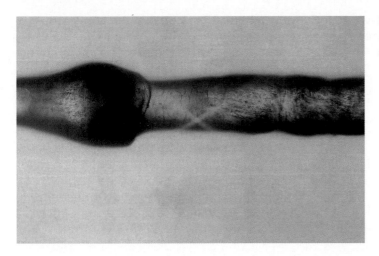

Figure 3.41
Netherton's syndrome – hair
showing an invaginate node.

All cases of ILC in which hair changes
have been carefully sought have been
found to show them. ILC is thus the most
constant feature of the syndrome, with hair
shaft defects of various types and degrees
of severity. Until the nature of the underlying abnormality is fully understood,
the eponym 'Netherton's syndrome' is
acceptable.

The inheritance of Netherton's syndrome
appears to be determined by an autosomal
recessive gene of variable expressivity.
Girls are affected more than boys.

> **The two diagnostic signs of
> Netherton's syndrome are ichth-
> yosis linearis circumflexa and hair
> nodes of invaginate and 'bamboo'
> type**

Pathology
The histological changes have until recently
been considered not to be diagnostic, but it
has now been shown that in the figurate
lesions there is eosinophilic degeneration of
cells in the upper malpighian layers. The
eosinophilic material, probably a glycopro-
tein, is also seen in the overlying parakera-

totic horny layer. In the electron microscope
the severity of the localized disturbance of
keratinization is consistent and distinctive:
the desmosome tonofilament complex is
reduced, membrane coating granules are
lacking and dense round bodies are present.
The horny layer loses its lamellar structure.

Scanning electron microscopy of the hair
shafts shows focal defects which produce
the development of torsion nodules, invaginated nodules (trichorrhexis invaginata) and
trichorrhexis nodosa. If the invaginate node
'breaks' within it, the appearance of the hair
may resemble a golf tee at its tip (de Berker
sign).

Clinical features
The patient may present primarily either
with cutaneous changes or complaining of
sparse and fragile hairs. Generalized scaling
and erythema are present from birth or
early infancy, but the degree, extent and
persistence of the erythema are very variable. In some cases the erythema may be
slight and transient. On the trunk and limbs
the fine, dry scales are associated with poly-
cyclic and serpiginous eruption, the horny
margin of which slowly changes its pattern.
Atopic manifestations are superimposed in
a significant minority of cases, in some

cases associated with increased level of IgE and intolerance to 'type 1' allergens as in nuts.

Trichorrhexis nodosa (weathering of hair)

Introduction

Trichorrhexis is best regarded as a distinctive response of the hair shaft to injury, the so-called 'weathering' of hair (Figures 3.42–3.48). If the degree or frequency of the injury is sufficient, it can be induced in normal hair. The cuticular cells become disrupted, allowing the cortical cells to splay out to form nodes (Figures 3.42–3.48). If the hair is constitutionally abnormally fragile, however, trichorrhexis may follow relatively trivial injury and, in this case, the breakage is seen closer to the scalp surface of the emerging hair. The trauma of hairdressing procedures has often been incriminated. Scratching may produce identical changes in the hairs in the genitocrural region, and the severity of experimentally induced trichorrhexis nodosa is related to the degree of trauma in patients with or without pre-

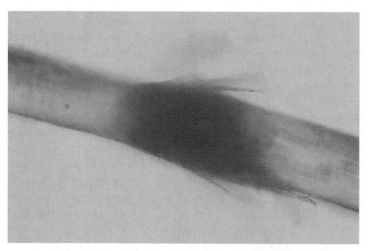

Figure 3.42
Trichorrhexis nodosa – dry-mounted hair (light micrograph).

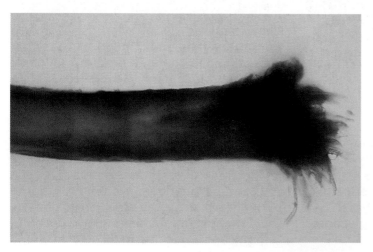

Figure 3.43
Trichorrhexis nodosa – hair showing 'paintbrush' tip.

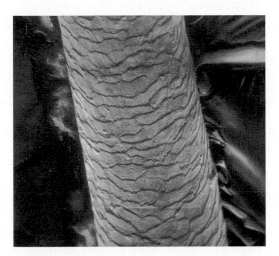

Figure 3.44
Trichorrhexis nodosa – hair at root end, largely unweathered (scanning electron micrograph).

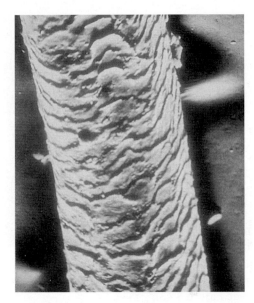

Figure 3.45
Trichorrhexis nodosa – hair shaft showing early surface cuticular weathering.

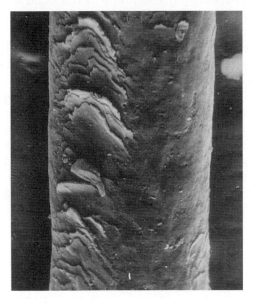

Figure 3.46
Trichorrhexis nodosa – hair shaft distal to Figure 3.45 showing loss of many surface cuticular cells.

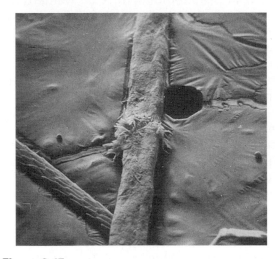

Figure 3.47
Trichorrhexis nodosa – hair shaft showing a node.

existing trichorrhexis. The cumulative effect of brushing, sea bathing, 'sandpapering' and sunlight has been shown to lead to seasonal recurrences each summer. The use of

alkaline soaps in the beard area may also be responsible.

Congenital and hereditary defects of the hair shaft can be predisposing factors in the

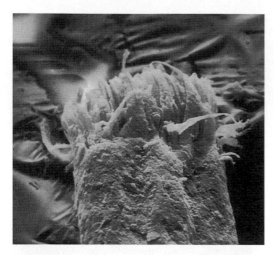

Figure 3.48
Trichorrhexis nodosa – hair showing paintbrush tip (see Figure 3.43).

formation of trichorrhexis nodosa. It may occur in pseudomonilethrix, in Netherton's syndrome or with pili annulati. Trichorrhexis nodosa is a feature of the rare metabolic defect argininosuccinic aciduria, in which it is associated with mental retardation. In this condition there is a deficiency of the enzyme argininosuccinase.

Trichorrhexis nodosa may occur in certain families as an apparently isolated defect of the hair. Node formation and fracture are induced by minimal trauma and develop during the early months of life. Very rarely, electron histochemical studies show evidence of a disorder in the formation of the hair. Electron histochemical study has shown evidence of a disorder in the formation of α-keratin chains within the globular matrix of the hair cortex with respect to cystine.

In simple trichorrhexis nodosa the shaft may appear normal by light or electron microscopy except at the nodes, or the shaft, apart from the proximal 1 cm, may show signs of abnormal 'wear and tear'. At the nodes the cuticle bulges and is split by longitudinal fissures. If fracture occurs transversely through a node, i.e. trichocla-

> **Trichorrhexis nodosa is always acquired, but many intrinsic hair faults may be predisposing factors to its formation**

sis, the end of the hair resembles a small paintbrush.

Clinical features
In trichorrhexis nodosa complicating a congenital defect of the hair shafts, the hair breaks so easily that large or small portions of the scalp show only broken stumps, and alopecia may be quite gross. In the much commoner conditions in which trauma plays a proportionately larger role and the predisposing inadequacy of the shaft a proportionately smaller one, there are three principal clinical presentations. First, the patient may present with proximal trichorrhexis nodosa, which is often discovered incidentally and only a few whitish nodules are seen near the ends of scattered hairs. Secondly, if many hairs are affected, the patient may complain that the hair is rough, dull or brittle. The third clinical form is well described but very rare; in a localized area of scalp, moustache or beard, some hairs are broken, and others show from one to five or six nodules.

Diagnosis
The congenital forms must be differentiated from other shaft defects. The distal acquired form may simulate dandruff or even pediculosis. In all cases diagnosis depends on careful microscopy. Excessive physical and chemical (cosmetic) trauma must be avoided, apart from shampooing.

Trichothiodystrophy

The term trichothiodystrophy (TTD) was coined to describe brittle hair with an

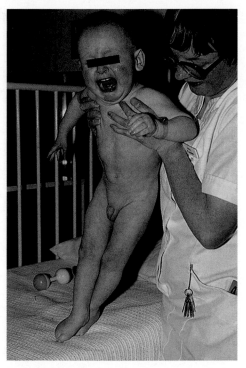

Figure 3.49
Trichothiodystrophy child – hair signs and spasticity are evident.

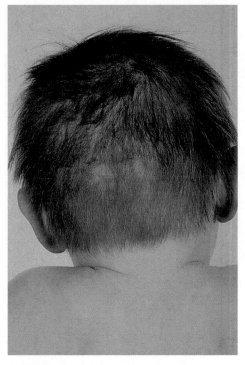

Figure 3.50
Trichothiodystrophy – short, brittle hair.

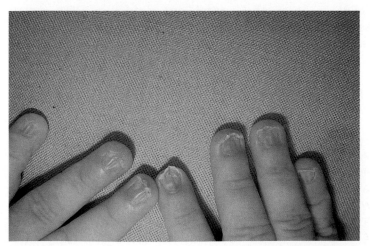

Figure 3.51
Trichothiodystrophy – thin nails with koilonychia.

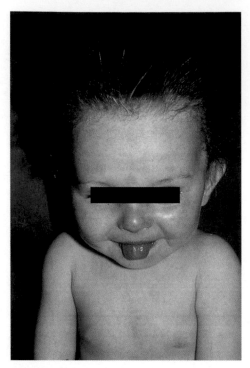

Figure 3.52
Trichothiodystrophy with photosensitivity.

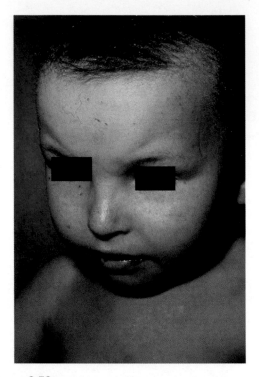

Figure 3.53
Trichothiodystrophy with photosensitivity (same patient as in Figure 3.52 seen 8 years later).

abnormally low sulphur content. It is not yet certain whether the different syndromes of which it is a feature represent a single rather variable entity, or distinct entities sharing this feature (Figures 3.49–3.58).

Various syndrome complexes associated with brittle hair have been associated with trichothiodystrophy:

1. Brittle hair, intellectual impairment, decreased fertility and short stature (BIDS).
2. Ichthyosis and BIDS (IBIDS).
3. Photosensitivity and IBIDS (PIBIDS). This light sensitivity may be the association of TTD with a cellular defect of DNA repair equivalent to xeroderma pigmentosum (XP). In such cases, however, the ichthyosis appears to be different from that of IBIDS. Therefore, in the absence

of more in-depth information as to the basic mechanisms, a more pragmatic classification has been proposed with categories A to F (Table 3.2). However, the search for defective DNA repair should still be performed in all cases

TTD thus belongs to a group of disorders that includes Cockayne's syndrome as well as XP. There is a defect in the nucleotide excision repair system, especially in the transcription factor TFIH.[9] TFIH has two functions: DNA repair and DNA transcription. When neoplasms develop as in XP, DNA repair is faulty. In TTD, only transcription is abnormal.

Where it has been possible to establish the mode of inheritance this has been of autosomal recessive type.

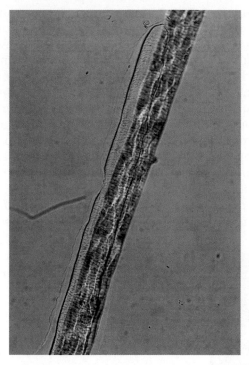

Figure 3.54
Trichothiodystrophy – characteristic striped
appearance of hair under polarized light.

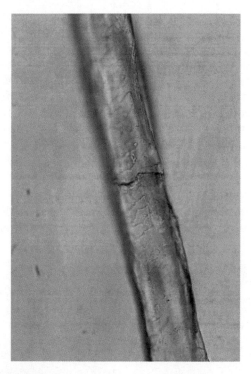

Figure 3.55
Trichothiodystrophy – hair showing transverse
fissure (trichoschisis).

Table 3.2 Guidelines for classification of trichothiodystrophy

A	Isolated congenital hair defect
B As type A +	Nail dystrophy (unreported by 1994)
C As type B +	Mental retardation
D As type C +	Growth retardation
D′ As type D +	Decreased fertility in family studies
E As type D′ +	Ichthyosis
E1	Lamellar ichthyosis (congenital type)
E2	Ichthyosis vulgaris (acquired type, as usual in F)
F As type E2 +	Light sensitivity
	Evaluation of DNA repair
	Complementation studies with xeroderma pigmentosum cells
	Defect similar to that in xeroderma pigmentosum complementation group–D

> **In any neuroectodermal syndrome always do scalp hair light microscopy no matter how vestigial the hairs appear – if TTD, BIDS, IBIDS or PIBIDS is the diagnosis, the hair will show it; a few minutes' simple observation to categorize complex cases!**

Pathology

The hair is brittle and weathers badly. With trauma it may break cleanly (trichoschisis; Figures 3.55, 3.56) or may form nodes somewhat resembling trichorrhexis nodosa, but without conspicuous exposure of individual spindle cells. The hairs are flattened and can be twisted into various appearances – rather like a ribbon or shoelace (Figure 3.57). By scanning electron microscopy the hairs are seen to be flattened, and sometimes folded over themselves (ribbon-like). The shaft is irregular with ridging and fluting and the cuticular scales are patchily absent. Under the polarizing microscope the hairs show alternating bright and dark zones (Figure 3.54). Using transmission

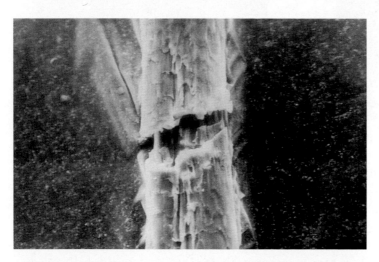

Figure 3.56
Trichothiodystrophy – hair showing transverse fissure (scanning electron micrograph).

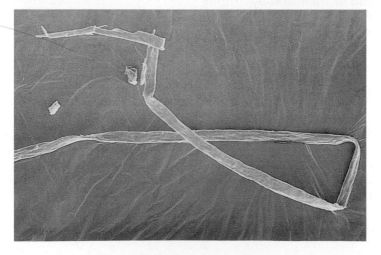

Figure 3.57
Trichothiodystrophy – weathered ribbon-like hair.

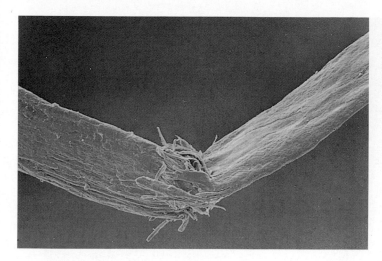

Figure 3.58
Trichothiodystrophy – trichorrhexis nodosa appearance.

electron microscopic methods, a quantitative decrease in high-sulphur protein in the hair shaft and a failure of this protein to migrate to the exocuticular part of the cuticle cells have been shown. Biochemistry has clearly shown the deficient synthesis of the usual high-sulphur and ultra-high-sulphur proteins and the appearance of new low molecular mass proteins. The supposed mechanism of this disease is a defect in a regulatory gene controlling different functions in different tissues. This may also explain the involvement of the central nervous system and the decreased fertility.

Clinical features
The hair is sparse, short and brittle, but the degree of alopecia varies considerably (Figures 3.49, 3.50, 3.52, 3.53). There may be lamellar ichthyosis. The nails are often dystrophic, soft and curved into flat spoon shapes (koilonychia; Figure 3.51). Mental and physical development may be normal, but one or both may be slightly, moderately or severely retarded. Until further cases have been studied the relationship between the syndromes showing trichothiodystrophy is a matter for speculation.

Marinesco–Sjögren syndrome

This rare syndrome of autosomal recessive inheritance also includes cerebellar ataxia, dysarthria, retarded physical and mental development and congenital cataracts. The teeth are abnormally formed and the lateral incisors may be absent. The nails are flat, thin and fragile. The hair is sparse, hypopigmented, short and brittle. On microscopy transverse fractures – trichoschisis – can be seen at the sites of impending fracture. In polarized light the hair is irregularly birefringent. Scalp biopsy shows normal anagen follicles, but with incomplete keratinization of the internal root sheath.

Structural defects usually without increased fragility

Pili annulati (ringed hair)

This abnormality of hair is characterized by hairs showing alternate light and dark bands along their length ('sandy' appearance), but which are otherwise normal (Figures 3.59–3.61). The inheritance of ringed hair has been shown in many

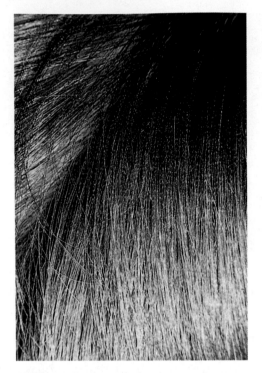

been shown to be associated in some members of a family, but the two conditions segregated.

With the light microscope abnormal dark bands alternate with normal light bands (Figure 3.60). The bright appearance of the abnormal bands in reflected light is due to air spaces in the cortex (Figure 3.61). The rate of growth has been measured and

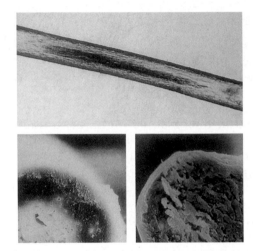

Figure 3.59
Pili annulati – 'sandy' hair appearance.

Figure 3.61
Pili annulati – abnormal band (above); scanning electron microscopy of hair cross-sections below – left, normal dense cortex; right, cortex filled with spaces.

extensive pedigrees to be determined by an autosomal dominant gene, though autosomal recessive inheritance has been detected rarely. Blue naevus and ringed hair have

Figure 3.60
Pili annulati – hair banding; dark sections abnormal (transmitted light microscopy).

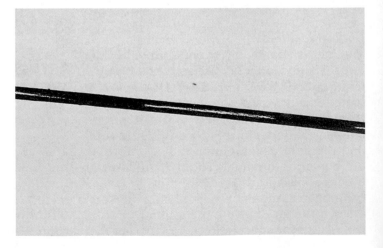

found to be 0.16 mm/day, which is less than half the average normal rate. Breaking stress analysis has shown no significant abnormality in ringed hair, but fractures are always in the normal bands.

Electron microscopic studies have shown that the clusters of air-filled cavities randomly distributed throughout the cortex in the abnormal bands (Figure 3.61) lie between macrofibrils within cortical cells and in the case of larger cavities may appear to replace the cortical cells. Hairs from one family showed an abnormal surface cuticle that showed a 'cobblestone' appearance on scanning electron microscopy. Electron histochemical methods have confirmed this finding: cuticle cells are thrown into folds. The abnormal alternating bands appear to be produced at random and not cyclically in relation to specific periods of growth.

It has traditionally been thought that pili annulati is due to an alternating primary keratin defect, though recently it has been suggested that there are earlier follicular faults in the basement membrane zone.

> **In pili annulati the hair is usually clinically normal, apart from an overall 'sandy' appearance**

Clinical features
Ringed hair may be associated with a very variable degree of fragility. When the fragility is slight and relatively few hairs are affected, the condition may be discovered only when deliberately sought. If many hairs are affected and fragility is great, then short hair may attract attention in early life and the 'banded' and sandy appearance of the shafts in reflected light can be readily detected. Axillary hair is occasionally affected.

The diagnosis is readily established on microscopy of affected hair. It is important to differentiate between intermittent medulation and pili annulati – in the latter the dark sections are cortical as opposed to the central location of the medulla.

Prognosis
The prognosis is good in the sense that the severity of the defect does not increase with age.

Woolly hair

Woolly hair is more or less tightly coiled hair occurring over the entire scalp (Figure 3.62) or part of it (Figures 3.63, 3.64), in an individual not of black African origin.

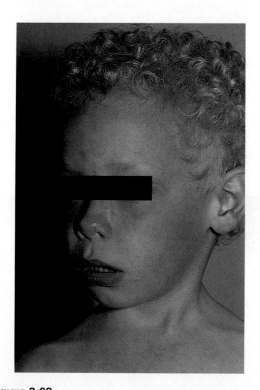

Figure 3.62
Woolly hair – 'Negroid' appearance in a Caucasoid individual.

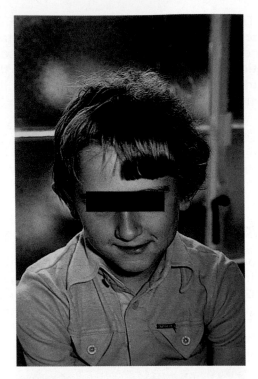

Figure 3.63
Woolly hair naevus.

Woolly hair is a feature that has been much confused by many authors. The classification most commonly adhered to has four types:

1. Hereditary woolly hair. The inheritance of this disorder is determined by an autosomal dominant gene.
2. Familial woolly hair. The genetic evidence is inconclusive but the condition has occurred in siblings whose parents were normal. Autosomal recessive inheritance is probable.
3. Symmetrical circumscribed allotrichia appears to be a distinct syndrome.
4. Woolly hair naevus. This is a circumscribed developmental defect, present at birth, and apparently not genetically determined (Figures 3.63, 3.64).

Hereditary woolly hair
In some pedigrees the shaft diameter in affected individuals is reduced, and the hair is fragile and may show trichorrhexis nodosa. Excessively curly hair is evident at birth or in early infancy. It has sometimes been described as black African in appearance, though the actual coiling may be less than this (Figure 3.62). The degree of variation in severity within a family is inconstant. The hair shaft may be twisted. In some cases the hair is brittle and breaks readily.

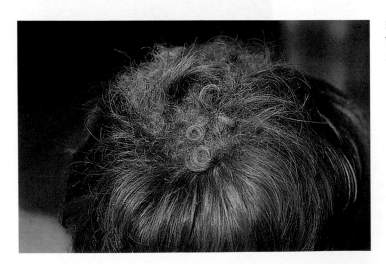

Figure 3.64
Woolly hair naevus – same subject as in Figure 3.63.

Familial woolly hair

There is a marked reduction in the diameter of hair shafts, which may be poorly pigmented. The hair is brittle and by scanning electron microscopy shows signs of cuticular weathering. So few cases have been reported that generalizations are unwarranted. In some cases fine, tightly curled, poorly pigmented hair is present from birth, the hair never achieving a length of more than 2 or 3 cm.

Symmetrical circumscribed allotrichia

Among cases reported as woolly hair naevus are some which have been termed 'whisker hair' but which are identical with the cases previously reported as symmetrical circumscribed allotrichia. From adolescence onwards, the hair in an irregular band extending around the edge of the scalp from above the ears towards the occipital region becomes coarse and whisker-like. Many people believe that whisker hair is synonymous with acquired progressive kinking. As symptoms develop at puberty and occasionally coincide with the development of male pattern baldness, an androgen-dependent mechanism is possibly indicated. Whether this is due to direct action on the follicles or on the interadnexal dermis remains to be determined.

Woolly hair naevus

The hair in the affected region of the scalp is finer than elsewhere. Electron microscopy of the abnormal hair shows the absence of cuticle; trichorrhexis nodosa may be present. The hair in a circumscribed area of the scalp is tightly curled from birth or early infancy (Figures 3.63, 3.64). The size of the affected areas usually increases only proportionately with general growth. The abnormal hair may be slightly paler in colour than that of the rest of the scalp. In over half of the reported cases an epidermal naevus has been present, but not on the same site. Woolly hair naevus has also been associated with ocular defects.

Acquired progressive kinking of the hair

Acquired progressive kinking (APK) of the scalp hair appears to be extremely rare, but in many cases may not be recorded. It is probably synonymous with whisker hair. Some have confused it with the woolly hair

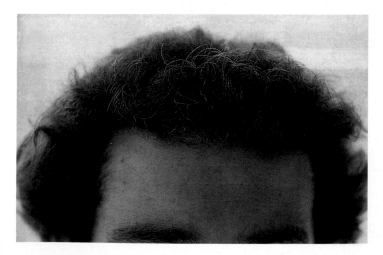

Figure 3.65
Acquired progressive kinking of hair.

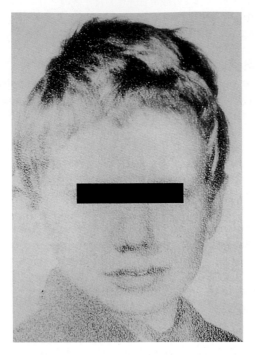

Figure 3.66
Same subject as in Figure 3.65 – straighter hair
3 years earlier.

naevus, but APK is differentiated clinically
by its onset in adolescence or adult life and
its progressive extension over a period of
years (Figures 3.65, 3.66).

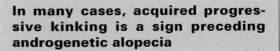

In many cases, acquired progressive kinking is a sign preceding androgenetic alopecia

Aetiology and pathology
The aetiology of APK is unknown. There is
as yet no evidence that it is genetically
determined. The hairs in the affected region
of the scalp may be finer or coarser than in
the normal scalp, and they show irregularly
distributed kinks and half-twists. The duration of anagen is reduced in some cases.

Clinical features
The patient gradually becomes aware that
the hair in one region of the scalp is becoming kinked and that a progressive change in
texture is occurring. On examination the
hair on one or more regions of the scalp is
wiry, kinked and unruly, rough, and lustreless. There are no sharply defined boundaries between normal and abnormal hair. In
some of the cases described, the acquired
kinking precedes the development of
common male baldness. In women, the
same entity may simply be a small minority
of APK hair in the midst of normal hair.

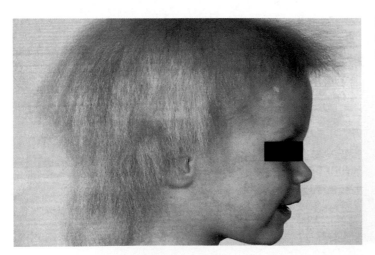

Figure 3.67
Cheveux incoiffables – uncombable
(unruly) hair syndrome.

Uncombable hair syndrome

This syndrome is also known as spun glass hair, cheveux incoiffables or pili trianguli et

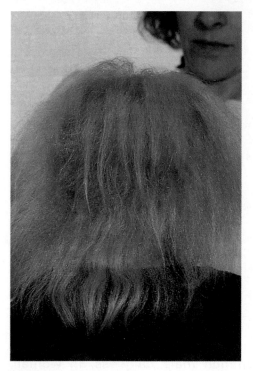

Figure 3.68
Another example of cheveux incoiffables.

canaliculi. It is a very distinctive hair shaft defect, which appears to have been first described by Dupré and co-workers (Figures 3.67–3.72), but many more cases have since been reported. The mode of inheritance is probably autosomal dominant.

Pathology
Microscopically the hairs may appear more or less normal. Histological examination of horizontal sections of the scalp in the scanning electron microscope clearly shows the triangular or kidney-shaped (Figure 3.71) configuration of the shaft, and also a well-defined longitudinal depression or canal (Figure 3.70). The term 'pili trianguli et canaliculi' has been proposed for these defects. The pili canaliculi are present in all cases, pili trianguli in the majority and some torsions in a few. It has been suggested that the misshapen dermal papilli alters the shape of the internal root sheath, which hardens (before the central forming hair) in a triangular cross-sectional shape. The hair shape then hardens into a shape complementing the root sheath.

Clinical features
The abnormality may first become obvious from 3 months to 12 years of age. The hair

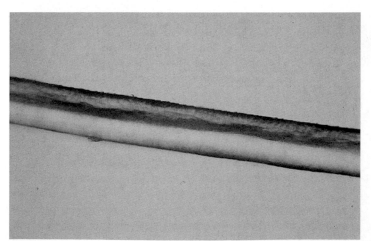

Figure 3.69
Hair shaft in cheveux incoiffables – canalicular 'gutter' along one side (light micrograph).

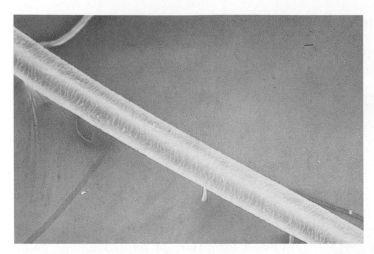

Figure 3.70
Hair shaft in cheveux incoiffables –
canalicular 'gutter' along one side
(scanning electron micrograph).

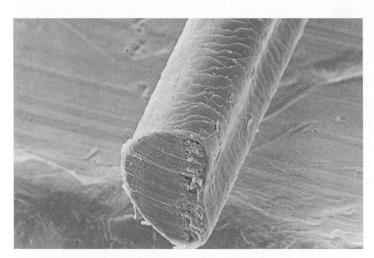

Figure 3.71
Hair shaft in cheveux incoiffables
showing longitudinal 'canal' and
kidney-shaped, almost triangular
cross-section (scanning electron
micrograph).

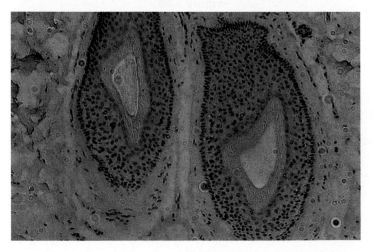

Figure 3.72
Hair follicle histology in cheveux
incoiffables – triangular cross-
sections of follicles are evident.

is normal in quantity and sometimes also in length, but its wild, disorderly, unruly appearance totally resists all efforts to control it with brush or comb (Figures 3.67, 3.68). In some cases these efforts lead to the hair breaking, but increased fragility is not a constant feature. The hair is often a rather distinctive, silvery blond colour. The eyebrows and eyelashes are normal.

The clinical appearance is usually distinctive. By light microscopy the diagnosis cannot be reliably established unless triangular hairs are seen. The appearances in the electron microscope are distinctive. No treatment is known although oral biotin therapy has been suggested.

Straight hair naevus

In straight hair naevus the hairs in a circumscribed area of Negroid scalp hair are straight, and are round in cross-section (Figure 3.73). The abnormal hair may be associated with an epidermal naevus. In the scanning electron microscope the cuticular scales may appear small and their pattern disorganized. This has been suggested as a localized form of cheveux incoiffables, but the hair microscopic changes are not triangular or canalicular.

Loose anagen hair syndrome

This distinctive condition features anagen hairs that are loosely anchored and easily pulled from the scalp.[10] The majority of patients are children aged 2–9 years, mostly girls (Figure 3.74); familial groups suggesting autosomal dominant inheritance have been described. The hairs pulled out are misshapen without an external root sheath. Histology reveals premature keratinization

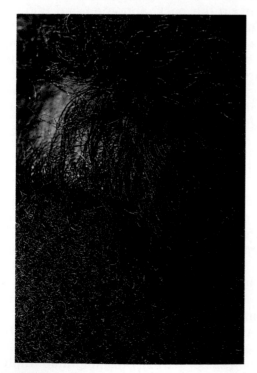

Figure 3.73
Straight hair naevus.

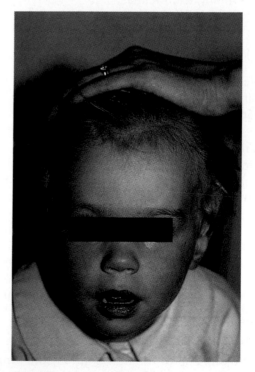

Figure 3.74
Loose anagen hair syndrome.

of the inner root sheath layers of Huxley and Henle. Trichograms show 98–100% anagen hairs with no telogen hairs.

Other abnormalities of the shaft

Trichoclasis

Trichoclasis is the common 'greenstick' fracture of the hair shaft. Transverse fractures of the shaft occur, partly splinted by intact cuticle. Cuticle, cortex and sulphur content are abnormal. This sign may be seen in a variety of congenital and acquired 'fragile' hair states.

The condition termed 'trichorrhexis blastysis' – unusual facies, failure to thrive, unexplained diarrhoea and abnormal hairs – shows scanning electron micrographs resembling trichoclasis.

Trichoptilosis

Trichoptilosis is longitudinal splitting of the hair shaft tip. Patients often refer to the condition as 'split ends'.

Aetiology
Trichoptilosis is the commonest macroscopic response of the hair shaft to the cumulative effects of chemical and physical trauma. It can readily be produced experimentally by vigorous brushing of normal hair, and it occurs in the nodes of the pili torti. It is one component of the 'weathering' process and is seen in long hair in normal individuals and any congenital 'brittle hair' syndrome.

Pathology
The distal end of the hair shaft is split longitudinally into two or several divisions. Other microscopic evidence of hair damage may be present.

Clinical features
Trichoptilosis is often an incidental finding in a woman who complains that her hair is dry and brittle. Trichorrhexis nodosa and trichoclasis are often present in the same patient. Central trichoptilosis, a longitudinal split in the hair shaft without involvement of the tip, sometimes occurs, particularly in knotted hair (trichonodosis).

Treatment
Careful explanation is necessary to encourage the patient to avoid further cosmetic trauma, which inevitably leads to recurrence.

Circle hairs

Circle and spiral hairs occur in middle-aged men on the back, abdomen and thighs as small dark circles next to hair follicles. They are an unusual form of ingrown hair lying in a coiled track just below the stratum corneum and can be easily extracted. Keratin follicular plugging is not associated (compare the keratosis pilaris and rolled and 'corkscrew' hairs of scurvy).

Trichomalacia

Trichomalacia is a patchy alopecia in which some follicles are plugged and contain soft, deformed, swollen hairs. The changes result from the repeated trauma of a hair-pulling tic; many histological studies in trichotillomania confirm this opinion.

Pathology
Above the bulb the cells of the hair shaft appear to be disconnected and the hair is shapeless or partially disintegrated. High in the follicle the shaft is thin and may be

coiled. Biopsy specimens show partially avulsed hair roots which are deformed and twisted, and clefting between matrix cells and between hair bulb and outer connective tissue sheath. There is no inflammatory reaction. The changes are said to be pathognomonic of trichotillomania. The clinical features are consistent with those of trichotillomania.

Trichoschisis

Trichoschisis is a clean, transverse fracture across the hair shaft through cuticle and cortex; the fracture is associated with localized absence (loss) of cuticular cells (Figures 3.55, 3.56). It is said to be a characteristic microscopic finding of the many syndromes associated with trichothiodystrophy. It probably represents a clean fracture through hair with decreased high-sulphur matrix protein content and particularly a similar decrease in the exocuticle and A-layer of cuticular cells. It may be prominent in the sulphur-deficiency syndromes, but it should not be seen as specific or pathognomonic.

Pohl–Pinkus constriction

In some individuals a zone of decreased shaft diameter coincides in time with a surgical operation or an illness, or the administration of folic acid antagonists or other drugs that inhibit mitosis. It was first described in the 19th century. The proportion of hairs so affected is variable and it seems probable that hairs in early anagen are most susceptible to a period of hypoproteinaemia or disturbed protein synthesis.

These constrictions in the hair shaft have been considered to be analogous to the transverse lines of the nails (Beau's lines), which also coincide with periods of ill health. Longer narrowings, resembling

monilethrix, may occur with 'bolus' doses of cytotoxic drugs that do not lead to anagen effluvium.

> **Pohl–Pinkus hair nodes are equivalent to Beau's nail lines**

Tapered hairs

Tapered hairs may occur in association with many other structural abnormalities of the hair shaft. They can arise in association with any process inhibiting cell division in the hair matrix. Severe inhibition leads to fracture if the narrowing of the fibre is marked. If the matrix inhibitory influence is temporary, the hair may widen again, giving a local 'dumb-bell-like' appearance in the emerging shaft, for example, due to cytotoxic drugs, and not leading to complete anagen effluvium. This may be due to re-entry of a group of blocked cells into the cycling transient amplifying cell population. An alternative type of tapered hair is the so-called 'embryonic' or 'young' anagen hair – short hairs with tapered pointed tips seen particularly in trichotillomania but also in acquired progressive kinking. If many such 'young' anagen hairs are seen, this usually represents a phase post-dating a period of acute hair shedding.

Bayonet hairs

Bayonet hairs are characterized by a 2–3 mm spindle-shaped, hyperpigmented expansion of the hair cortex just proximal to a tapered tip and may be associated with hyperkeratinization of the upper third of the follicle. This change is probably related to the first type of tapered hair described above.

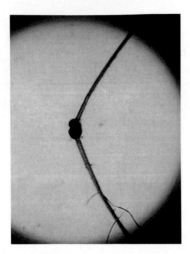

Figure 3.75
Trichonodosis – hair knotting.

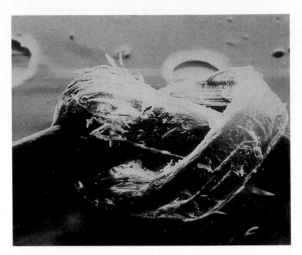

Figure 3.76
Trichonodosis (scanning electron micrograph).

Trichonodosis (knotted hairs)

This knotting of the hair shafts is induced by trauma (Figures 3.75, 3.76). Short curly hairs of relatively flat diameter are most readily affected. Knots are found most frequently in Negroid hair and in short, curly Caucasoid hair, but only rarely in long, straight hair.

Pathology
The only abnormalities are secondary to the knotting and are localized to that part of the shaft which forms the knot. By scanning electron microscopy the cuticle shows longitudinal fissuring and fractures, and cuticle scales are lost (Figure 3.76).

Clinical features
Trichonodosis is usually an incidental finding, for it is inconspicuous and must be deliberately sought. One or few hairs are affected. The trauma of brushing or combing may cause the shaft to break at the site of the knot.

Trichostasis spinulosa

This is probably a normal, age-related phenomenon in which successive telogen hairs are retained in predominantly sebaceous follicles.

Aetiology
Due to the pigmentation of the horny plug it is thought that trichostasis is no more than a variant of the open comedo, but this does not appear in skin sites from which acne is usually absent. It has been noted that most comedones contain from 1 to 10 or more vellus hairs. Trichostasis is found most commonly in the middle-aged or elderly. It is said by most authors to occur particularly on the nose and face, but others have found it to be not uncommon on the trunk and limbs.

Pathology
The affected follicles contain up to 50 vellus hairs embedded in a keratinous plug. A mild perifolliculitis is often present. The condi-

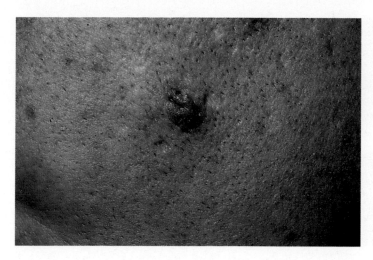

Figure 3.77
Trichostasis spinulosa – inflamed facial lesion.

tion must be differentiated from the 'multiple hairs' of Flemming–Giovannini, in which up to seven hairs grow from a composite papilla with a common outer root sheath.

Clinical features
Those reported to be affected have ranged in age from 17 to over 60. The lesions, which closely resemble comedones, may occur predominantly on the nose, forehead and cheeks (Figure 3.77), or the face may be spared and the nape, back, shoulders, upper arms and chest may be affected. The lesions vary greatly in number. On inspection with a hand lens the 'comedones' seem to be unusually prominent and in some cases a tuft of hairs may be seen projecting through the horny plug.

Treatment
Keratolytic preparations have often been recommended, but the present authors have found them to be of little value. The most effective treatment is topical retinoic acid, which should be used as in the treatment of acne. Depilatory wax has also been successfully employed.

Multiple hair

The term *pili multigemini* describes an uncommon developmental defect of hair follicles as a result of which multiple matrices and papillae form hairs which emerge through a single pilosebaceous canal (Figure 3.78). The incidence of multigeminate hairs in the general population is unknown. Numerous follicles showing this defect have been seen in a patient with cleidocranial dysotosis.

Pathology
From two to eight matrices and papillae, each with its internal root sheath, form hairs which are often flattened, ovoid or triangular in configuration and may be grooved. In the follicular canal contiguous hairs may adhere, bifurcate and then re-adhere, depending on the variable proximity of the matrix cells and their differentiation programme.

Clinical features
Multigeminate follicles occur mainly on the face, especially along the lines of the jaw. Tufts of hair may be seen emerging from a

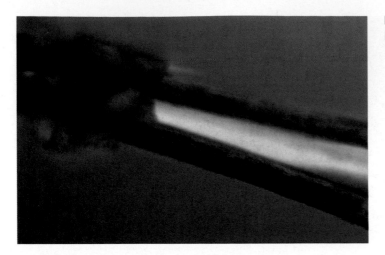

Figure 3.78
Pili multigemini (polarized light).

few or many follicles. Their discovery is often a matter of chance, but the patient may complain of recurrent inflammatory nodules that leave scars. Treatment is unsatisfactory. If the hairs are plucked, they regrow.

Peripilar keratin casts (pseudonits)

Peripilar casts (see Chapter 5) are tubular masses of amorphous (keratinous) material of varied size that surround the hair shaft. They are cast from within the hair follicle infundibulum and before they separate may bulge out from the follicular openings, the so-called parakeratotic comedones. Some casts are of internal root sheath origin. They are easily differentiated from nits because, in contrast to the latter, peripilar keratin casts are mobile along the hair shaft. Treatment with atopical lotion of retinotic acid has been reported to improve the condition. Regular brushing and combing help to shed the casts along the length of the hairs.

Weathering of the hair shaft

All hair fibres undergo some degree of cuticular and secondary cortical breakdown from root to tip before being shed during the telogen or early anagen phase of the hair cycle. The slower the rate of hair growth, the more proximally will the weathering be seen. The term 'weathering of hair' has been limited by some authorities to structural changes in the hair shaft due to cosmetic procedures. Indeed, both in vivo and in vitro studies carried out by cosmetic scientists have shown the type of damage that procedures such as combing, brushing, bleaching and permanent waving can cause. However, in considering the degeneration of hair fibres, cosmetic and other influences such as natural friction, wetting and ultraviolet radiation are so interwoven that it is more useful in practice to define weathering as the degeneration of hair from root to tip due to a variety of environmental, including cosmetic, factors. Scalp hair, having a long anagen phase and being subject to more frictional damage and cosmetic treatment, shows more deep cuticular and cortical degeneration than fibres from other sites.

Weathering of the scalp hair has been studied in greater detail than hair from other sites (Figures 3.42–3.48). At the root end, surface cuticle cells are closely apposed to deeper layers. Within a few centimetres of the scalp, the free margin of these cells lifts up and breaks irregularly. Increasing scale loss leads to surface areas denuded of cuticle. Many fibres show complete loss of overlapping scales well proximal to the tip. This is particularly common on long hair shafts, which frequently have a frayed tip. Proximal to terminal fraying, longitudinal fissures may be present between exposed cortical cells. Hairs subjected to considerable friction damage may show transverse fissures and some nodes of the type seen in trichorrhexis nodosa. Hair that has been bleached or permanently waved may show shaft distortion. The severest changes are mostly seen near the distal part of the hair shaft in normal scalp hair.

Trichorrhexis nodosa is the severest form of weathering. Many of the changes seen in normal hair towards the tip are visible more proximally in congenitally weakened hair and in trichorrhexis nodosa caused by overuse of cosmetic treatment.

In some hair structural abnormalities such as monilethrix and pili torti, specific weathering patterns may be seen.

> **Some degree of weathering is present on all hair fibres**

Longitudinal ridging and grooving

One or several longitudinal grooves and ridges can occur along the hair shaft. The overlying cuticle is usually intact in the absence of severe weathering influences. It is a microscopic sign that may occur in many different forms in Marie–Unna syndrome, uncombable hair syndrome, the narrow internodes of monilethrix, and many other hereditary and congenital abnormalities, and may represent altered moulding of hair by misshapen internal root sheaths.

Bubble hair

This occurs when wet hair, after washing, is rapidly dried with a hot-air drier in which the thermostat is damaged. The water within the hair may thus boil, appearing like irregular bubbles in the hair shafts when examined microscopically.

TRAUMATIC ALOPECIA

This term is applied to alopecia induced by physical trauma. These cases fall into three main categories:

1. *Trichotillomania:* alopecia resulting from the deliberate, though at times unconscious, efforts of the patient, who is under tension or is psychologically disturbed. Within this type are the rarer patterns named trichoteiromania[11] and trichotemnomania.
2. *Cosmetic alopecia:* alopecia resulting from cosmetic procedures applied incorrectly or with misguided and excessive vigour or frequency.
3. *Accidental alopecia:* alopecia resulting from accidental trauma.

Trichotillomania

The term 'trichotillomania' (Figures 3.79–3.82) was first used more than 100 years ago to describe the compulsive habit of an individual repeatedly to pluck his or her own hair.[12] There are obvious objections to this overdramatic term for what is often a trivial problem. However, the term 'mania' was a more general term in the 19th century in contrast to the very specific modern psychiatric term, which is not relevant in this context.

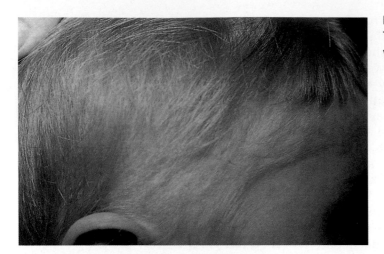

Figure 3.79
Trichotillomania – prepubertal type with good prognosis.

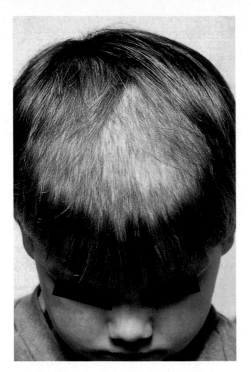

Figure 3.80
Another example of prepubertal trichotillomania.

Tonsure trichotillomania has a bad prognosis and may last for decades

Pathology

The histological changes vary according to the severity and duration of the hair-plucking. Numerous empty canals are the most consistent feature. Some follicles are severely damaged: there are clefts in the hair matrix, the follicular epithelium is separated from the connective tissue sheath, and there are intraepithelial and perifollicular haemorrhages and intrafollicular pigment casts. Injured follicles may form only soft, twisted hairs – a process which has been described as a separate entity under the name of trichomalacia. Many follicles are in catagen with very few or no follicles in telogen. Some dilated follicular infundibula contain horny plugs.

Aetiology and psychopathology

Trichotillomania occurs more than twice as frequently in females as in males, but below the age of 6 years boys outnumber girls in a ratio of 3 : 2, and the peak incidence in boys is in the 2–6 year age group. It is seven times more frequent in children than adults. The child develops the habit of twisting the

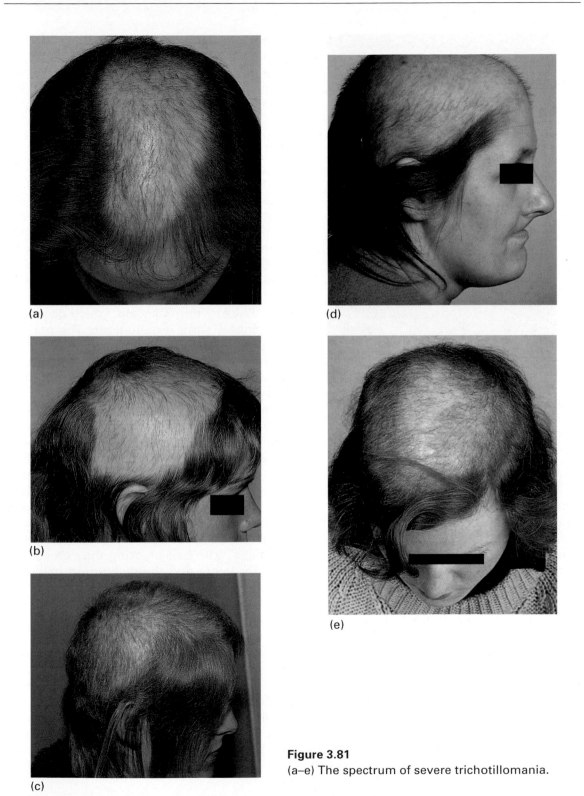

Figure 3.81
(a–e) The spectrum of severe trichotillomania.

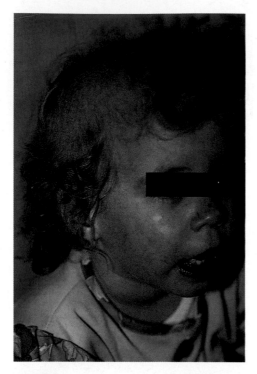

Figure 3.82
Trichotillomania caused by another individual in the classroom.

hair round the fingers and pulling it. The act is only partially conscious and may 'replace' the habit of thumb-sucking. Various psychiatric studies are not in complete agreement, but emotional deprivation in the maternal relationship is considered important in initiating the habit. The habit may become fully expressed following an apparently unrelated modification of lifestyle usually involving the loss of something or somebody important to the subject (for example, moving house or loss of contact with teachers or friends).

The more severe form (tonsure trichotillomania) occurs predominantly in females of any age from early adolescence onwards. Most patients are in the age range 11–40 years, with the peak incidence in females being between 11 and 17. The hair-pulling begins in a provocative social situation in a subject who is often greatly disturbed psychologically. Exceptionally severe forms may be seen in young patients and the minor forms in older patients.

Clinical features

In the younger patients the hair-pulling habit develops gradually and unconsciously, but is not usually denied by the patient. Hair is plucked most frequently from one frontoparietal region (Figures 3.79, 3.80). There results an ill-defined patch on which the hairs are twisted and broken at various, usually very short, distances from the clinically normal scalp, which occasionally shows some excoriations. The general outline of the area shows a geometrical shape, which contrasts with any natural balding process. The texture and colour of the broken hairs are unaffected.

In the more severe form the patient usually consistently denies that she is touching her hair. The patient presents with an extensive area of scalp on which the hair has been reduced to a coarse stubble uniformly 2.5–3 mm long (Figure 3.81). Most characteristically, the plucked area covers the entire scalp apart from the margin; hence the validity of the term 'tonsure alopecia'. The hair-plucking may be continued for years and the disfiguring baldness is held by the patient to be responsible for her psychological problems. A case is known of one young child who plucked the hairs of her contemporaries as well as her own (Figure 3.82). Occasionally, mother and daughter or two friends may be affected at the same time, as may the affected individual's doll!

Much more unusual is the habit of plucking the eyelashes, eyebrows and beard. Very exceptionally the patient may pluck hair also, or only, from other regions of the body, such as the mons pubis and perianal region.

A child may also suck and even eat the hair (trichophagy). In such cases examination of the mouth may reveal hairs, and enquiries should be made as to the presence of systemic symptoms related to the presence of a hair-ball, e.g. dysphagia, vomiting, anaemia, abdominal pain or constipation. This symptom is present in approximately 10% of children with trichotillomania.

Differential diagnosis

The minor form in young children is often confused with ringworm or with alopecia areata. In ringworm the texture of the infected hairs is abnormal and the scalp surface may be scaly. It is wise to examine all cases under Wood's light and also to examine broken hairs under the microscope. Alopecia areata may be difficult to exclude with certainty at the first examination, but the course of the condition soon establishes the correct diagnosis. Histology may be very useful in early lesions. We have known the hair-pulling tic to develop in a child recovering from typical alopecia areata.

Treatment and prognosis

The habit in young children is usually self-limiting, except in the mentally retarded. The child's problem should be discussed with the child and the parents. The diagnosis is often rejected by the parents, who have not observed the child pulling the hair and find it unacceptable to believe that the problem is self-inflicted. In some series, up to 50% have required psychiatric referral. Usually, support from the dermatologist is sufficient. Behaviour therapy has also been suggested to be helpful.

Trichoteiromania[12] due to compulsive rubbing of hair, and trichotemnomania due to compulsive cutting of hair occur in individuals with personality or psychiatric disorders similar to the adult forms of trichotillomania.

Tonsure trichotillomania is a very different proposition. Some patients recover, but many fail to do so, despite skilled psychiatric care, which may involve the use of major or minor tranquillizers and psychotherapy.[11] A significant proportion of patients with chronic trichotillomania have a depressive illness. A combined approach using behavioural modification, habit reversal or hypnotherapy can be used with selective serotonin reuptake inhibitors (SSRIs) such as venlafaxine, fluvoxamine and citalopram. Risperidone in addition to an SSRI may be useful in recalcitrant cases. Continuing destructive behaviour in adults may be helped by behavioural cognitive techniques with the aid of a clinical psychologist or psychiatrist.

Cosmetic traumatic alopecia

The dictates of religion, of custom and of fashion have imposed an immense variety of physical and chemical stresses on human hair[13] (Figures 3.83–3.89). The nomenclature of the resulting patterns of baldness inevitably lacks any consistency. It is possible only to list the clinical syndromes most widely reported; any new hairdressing technique may give rise to new patterns.

> **Patients do not like to admit to cosmetic 'abuse' of their hair!**

Pathology

Two processes are responsible for most of the pathological changes observed. Hair,

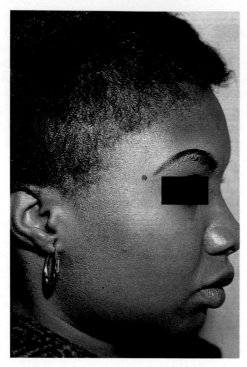

Figure 3.83
Cosmetic (hot-comb) alopecia – this may be permanent.

follicular inflammatory changes which may eventually lead to scarring. Traction alopecia is induced particularly readily in subjects with incipient common baldness, for the telogen hairs, which make up a higher proportion of the total, are more loosely attached and readily extracted than anagen hairs.

Traumatic and marginal alopecia

The essential changes in the many variants of this syndrome are the presence of short broken hairs, folliculitis and some scarring, circumscribed patches at the scalp margins (Figures 3.83–3.89).

In one form, which is caused by the tension imposed by procedures intended to straighten kinked hair, alopecia commonly begins in triangular areas in front of and above the ears; it may involve other parts of the scalp margin or even linear areas in other parts of the scalp. Itching and crusting may be pronounced. The so-called pony-tail hairstyle may cause similar changes in the frontal hair margin (Figure 3.89). Keratin cylinders – 'peripilar hair casts' – may surround many hairs just above the scalp surface.

sometimes already weakened by chemical applications, may be broken by friction or by traction. Prolonged tension may induce

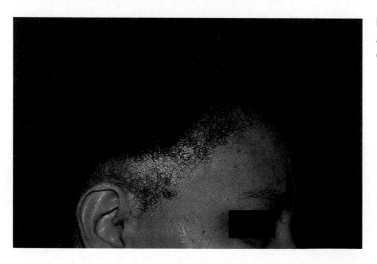

Figure 3.84
Another example of cosmetic (hot-comb) alopecia.

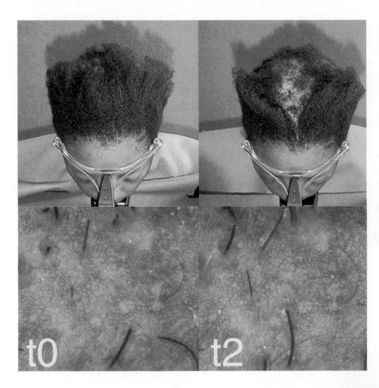

Figure 3.85
Follicular degeneration syndrome (FDS). Permanent hair loss in a patch on the top of the head. Close up view immediately after clipping (t0) and 48 h later (t2) shows almost 100% growth, indicating that the follicle is abruptly destroyed during anagen.
Reproduced with permission from: Van Neste D, Leroy T, de Ramecourt A, Hair removal and hair follicle targeting. In: *Hair Science and Technology*, pp 401–412.

Frontal and parietal traction alopecia may occur in young Sikh boys as a result of twisting their uncut hair tightly on top of the head. The Sudanese customs of tight braiding and the use of wooden combs produce traction alopecia. Frontal loss has been reported in Libyan women as a result of traction from a tight scarf.

Afro-Caribbean hairstyles with tight braiding of the hair into rows known variously as corn or cane rows or braids and Cain rows, may cause marginal alopecia and central alopecia with widening of the partings (Figure 3.86).

Brush-roller alopecia

Brush rollers, if applied frequently and with too much vigour, may cause irregular patches of more or less complete alopecia, surrounded by a zone of erythema with broken hairs.

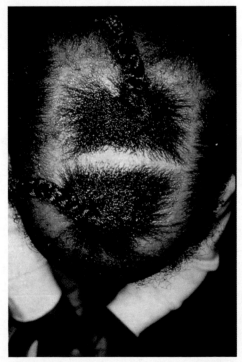

Figure 3.86
Traction alopecia.

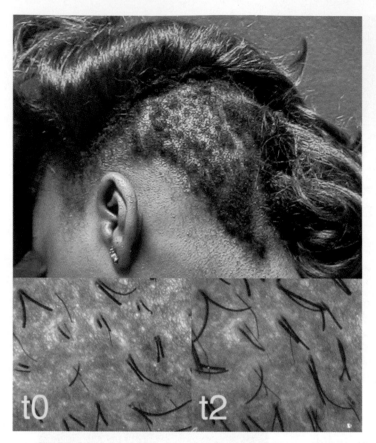

Figure 3.87
Traction alopecia. Traction results in reversible hair loss. Close-up view immediately after clipping (t0) and 48 h later (t2) shows some thin, regrowing hair. Few hair follicles are in telogen as the result of continuous exhaustive removal by traction. Reproduced with permission from: Van Neste D, Ceray T, de Ramecourt A, Hair removal and hair follicle targeting. In: *Hair Science and Technology*, pp 401–412.

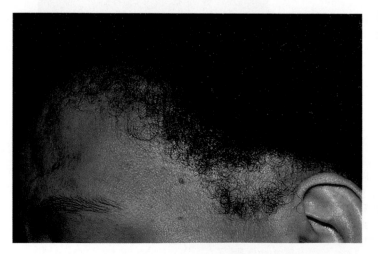

Figure 3.88
Cosmetic traumatic alopecia.

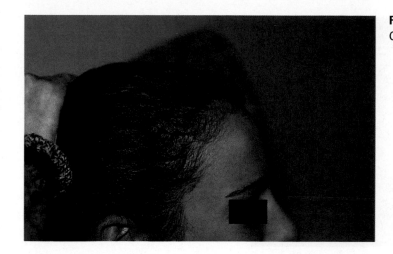

Figure 3.89
Cosmetic (traction) alopecia.

Hot-comb alopecia

Women with Negroid hair who use hot combs to straighten the hair may develop a progressive cicatricial alopecia, slowly extending centrifugally from the vertex (Figure 3.83). This procedure is now rarely carried out.

Massage alopecia

The overenthusiastic application of medication to the scalp, with firm massage, may cause baldness and excessive 'weathering' (trichorrhexis nodosa).

Brush alopecia

Vigorous brushing may cause significant damage to hair that is already fragile as the result of a developmental defect. Bristles with square or otherwise angular tips, present in some brushes made of synthetic fibres, may prove particularly traumatic.

Alopecia secondary to hair weaving

Patchy traction alopecia has been reported to result from the cosmetic procedure of weaving additional hair into persistent terminal hair in order to camouflage common baldness.

Deliberate alopecia

We have seen a family from Pakistan in which three sisters were subjected during childhood to tight plaiting and traction of the central V of the frontal hair. The resulting V alopecia was considered desirable. Similarly, in the Middle Ages, depilating the frontal hair line was fashionable as it increased the height of the forehead (front altier).

Diagnosis

The traumatic cosmetic alopecias do not present any diagnostic difficulties, provided

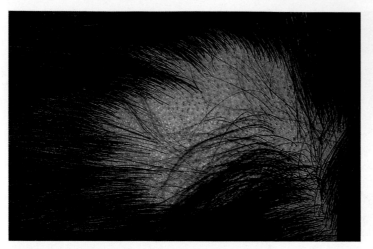

Figure 3.90
Accidental (hair pulled) traumatic
alopecia.

the possibility is considered. Their cause is rarely recognized by the patient and is often accepted with suspicion.

Accidental traumatic alopecia

Alopecia secondary to accidental mechanical trauma to the scalp is usually no diagnostic problem (Figure 3.90), but in some circumstances the trauma may be unperceived and the cause of the hair loss undetected.

Women who undergo prolonged pelvic operations in the Trendelenburg position have been found to develop a vertical patch of alopecia 12–26 days later, which is preceded by oedema, exudation and crusting. Pressure ischaemia during the operation is considered to be the cause of the alopecia (Figure 3.91). The hair loss may be permanent. Temporary alopecia may follow prolonged pressure on the scalp from a foam-rubber ring used to prevent such an occurrence. Chronic granulomatous inflammation and acute septic cellulitis of

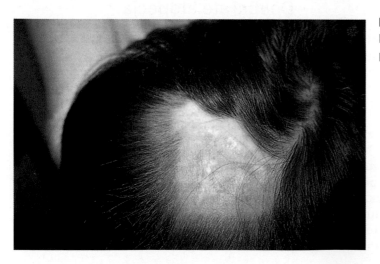

Figure 3.91
Pressure (ischaemic) alopecia after
prolonged anaesthesia.

the scalp secondary to the implantation in the dermis of artificial, or so-called natural, hair is responsible for loss of hair follicles that would or might have resisted the natural balding process. Therefore, creating a direct contact between the environment and the internal milieu (dermis and hypodemis) via an artificial implanted hair fibre should be considered a heretical practice and abandoned.

ANDROGENETIC ALOPECIA

Synonyms for this condition include common baldness, male pattern alopecia and androgen-dependent alopecia.

The human species is not the only primate species in which baldness is a natural phenomenon associated with sexual maturity. The orang-utan, the chimpanzee, the nakari and the stump-tailed macaque manifest it in varying forms. Studies in these animals have demonstrated clearly that common baldness is a physiological process in genetically predisposed individuals whether simian or human. Terminal follicles are progressively transformed into 'vellus' follicles; i.e. a 'miniaturization' process takes place.

The prevalence of common baldness in any population has not been accurately recorded, but it probably approaches 100% in the Caucasoid races. In other words, the replacement of some terminal follicles by vellus type follicles from puberty onwards is a universal phenomenon.

Until about 30 years ago it was thought by many authorities that androgenetic alopecia that had reached the stage of miniaturization was irreversible in man. Oral minoxidil used for hypertension led to some regrowth of miniaturized to obvious pigmented hair on the previously bald scalp.

Of great interest has been the recent finding that hair transplanted from balding

> **Androgenetic alopecia probably occurs to a degree in all adults some time after puberty – only being obvious in some women in old age**

and hairy androgenetic alopecia scalp regrows hair comparably well on immunodeficient nude mice.

Hair patterns

Hamilton produced the first useful grading scale after examining large numbers of adults (both sexes) of age 20–89 years.[14] This classification was modified by Norwood, who added grades IIIa, III vertex, IVa and Va.[15] The Norwood scoring system has been used extensively in clinical trials of regrowth, particularly with regard to topical minoxidil, and such tables are subject to continuous adaptation (Figure 3.92). Ludwig described the diffuse patterns of androgenetic alopecia particularly seen in women (Figure 3.93).[16]

Hamilton described the natural progression of the normal prepubertal scalp pattern (type I) in both sexes (Figures 3.94, 3.95) to type II in 96% of men and 79% of women after puberty. He also observed pattern types V to VIII in 58% of men aged over 50 years, with the extent of baldness tending to increase to the age of 70. About 25% of women developed type IV scalps by the age of 50 years, after which there was no further increase in balding. Indeed, after 50 years, some women who had developed type II at puberty, reverted to type I. Types V–VIII were not found in any women.

Although, as these figures show, androgenetic alopecia occurs in females with some frequency, androgenetic alopecia in

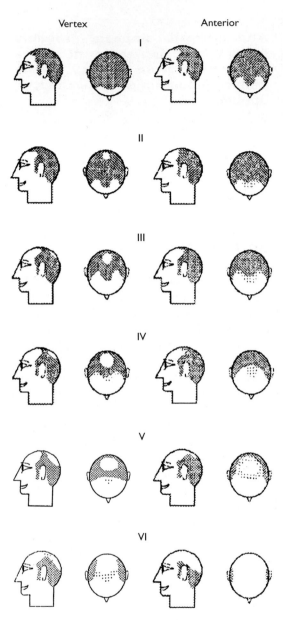

Figure 3.92
Androgenetic alopecia – changes in hair pattern over time (from I to VI), with either the vertex or the anterior being the most severely affected area in each case. (Reproduced with permission from H.A.I.R. Technology® [Skinterface, Tournai, Belgium].)

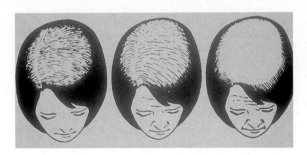

Figure 3.93
Androgenetic alopecia – Ludwig types.

women more often assumes a diffuse form (Figures 3.96–3.101).

A change of patterning has been shown to some degree in 100% of 564 Caucasian women over 20 years old.[17] In this study the investigators carefully wetted the vaultal hair, flattening the hair and removing any element of 'style', and observed from above. On analysis of the patients by decade, 87% of premenopausal women showed vaultal thinning of Ludwig patterns I–III and 13% had Hamilton types II–IV. Postmenopausal women showed an increased tendency to male patterning, with 63% showing Ludwig I–III and 37% showing Hamilton II–V, including some women with deep, M-shaped, bitemporal frontoparietal recession.

Other observations, much less accurately recorded, have tended to group together Hamilton types II, III and IV, and are therefore of interest only in confirming the great frequency of common baldness in other populations of Caucasoids.

It has been suggested that separating hair patterns into the eight Hamilton and three Ludwig types is only of use in defining a population for the purpose of clinical trial evaluation. The grades are imprecise measures of a continuum of hair patterns that are seen in adults of both sexes. The single consistent finding is a change from the prepubertal pattern in all adults. The magni-

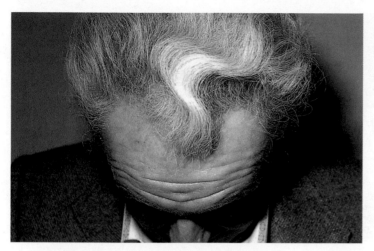

Figure 3.94
Androgenetic alopecia – Hamilton grade III/IV.

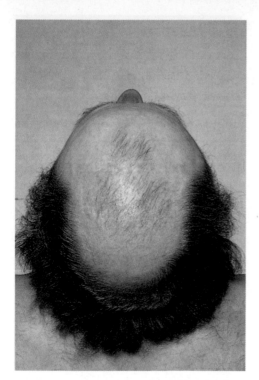

Figure 3.95
Androgenetic alopecia – Hamilton grade VIII.

level. The role played by nutritional status, stress and other causes of hair loss is difficult to measure, but may precipitate the progression of the balding process.

The Hamilton–Norwood and Ludwig patterns may be useful clinically in diagnosing androgenetic alopecia, and the traditional measurable assessments of hair density, etc., have helped in the study of human physiology. However, with the arrival of drugs that stem or even reverse the miniaturization of androgenetic alopecia, there has been a greater need for reliable, economical and minimally invasive means of measuring hair growth, and more specifically, response to therapy. The most valuable means of measurement at the present time are photography- and photogrichogram-based techniques (with digital image analysis) such as the 'trichoscan'. Subjective scoring systems are also of value in the overall assessment of response to therapy and these are currently underused and merit further refinements. Figure 3.102 shows one method, the scalp coverage score (SCS), as a measurement of the changes in androgenetic alopecia, whereas Chamberlain and Dawber[18] review in detail the invasive and non-invasive methods of evaluating hair growth.

tude and rate of that change are influenced by genetic predisposition and sex hormone levels in both sexes and evidently depend on androgen receptor status at follicular

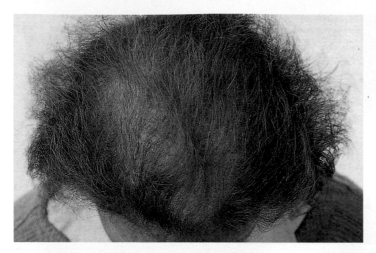

Figure 3.96
Androgenetic alopecia – Ludwig grade I.

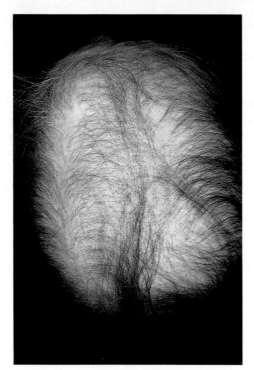

Figure 3.97
Androgenetic alopecia – Ludwig grade II/III.

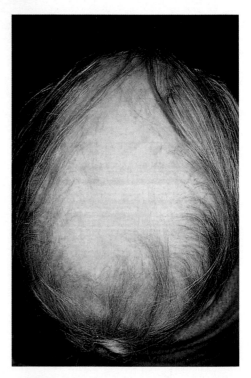

Figure 3.98
Androgenetic alopecia – Ludwig grade III.

Hamilton patterns can occur in normal women and the Ludwig variants in men

Aetiology

The very high frequency of common baldness has complicated the many attempts to establish its mode of inheritance. Moreover,

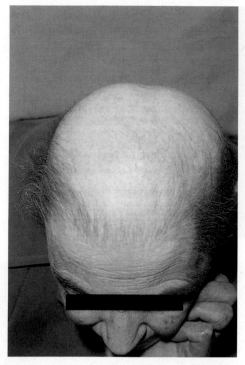

Figure 3.99
Androgenetic alopecia – severest Ludwig pattern (some frontal hair retained).

it is by no means clear that common baldness is genetically homogeneous, and some authorities differentiate between early onset (before the age of 30 years in men) and the same pattern 20 years later. It has been proposed that baldness is determined by a single pair of sex-influenced factors. Both gene frequency studies and family histories support this hypothesis.

Some authorities have suggested that baldness could develop in the heterozygous female as a result of dominant inheritance with increased penetrance in the male or multifactorial inheritance. The concept of multifactorial inheritance has been supported by others. It is still unclear whether early- and late-onset types of baldness are inherited separately. It is nevertheless certain that both are inherited and that both depend upon androgenic stimulation of susceptible follicles.

There is no association between baldness and dense hair patterns on the trunk and limbs; nor is there an association between hair loss and increased fertility or improved sexual behaviour.

Pathology

The earliest histological change is focal perivascular basophilic degeneration in the lower third of the connective tissue sheath of otherwise normal anagen follicles. This is followed by a perifollicular,

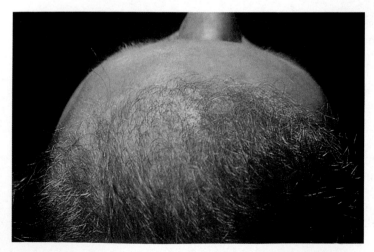

Figure 3.100
Androgenetic alopecia – Ludwig grade II.

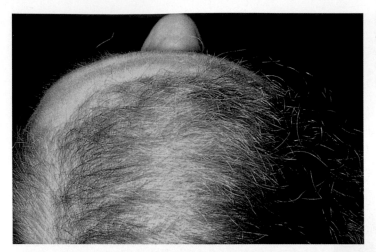

Figure 3.101
Androgenetic alopecia – same patient as Figure 3.100 after 6 months' treatment with oral antiandrogens.

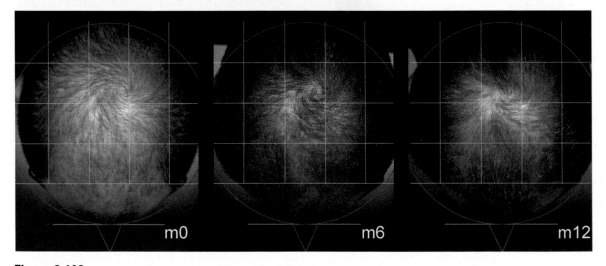

Figure 3.102
Androgenetic alopecia – SCS method. Scalp coverage scoring (SCS) as a measurement of the changes in androgenetic alopecia in man. A reference grid helps in separating clinically relevant scalp fields in these global photographs taken repeatedly over time (baseline = m0 and after 6 or 12 months; respectively m6 and m12). This patient complained of hair loss in a male pattern while on oral corticosteroid therapy for severe bronchial asthma. After steroids were withdrawn, clinically significant hair regrowth appreciated with the scalp coverage method (SCS, + 21%), occurred within less than 1 year after weaning of oral steroids.

lymphohistiocytic infiltrate at the level of the sebaceous duct. Hair-bearing, transitional, and alopecic scalp from males and females with progressive pattern alopecia has been examined.[19] Ultrastructural studies disclosed measurable thickening of the follicular adventitial sheaths of transitional and alopecic zones compared with those in the non-alopecic zones. This finding was associated with mast cell degranulation and fibroblast activation within the fibrous sheaths. Immunohistochemically, control biopsies were devoid of follicular inflammation, whereas transitional regions consistently showed the presence of activated T-cell infiltrates about the lower portions of follicular infundibula. These infiltrates were associated with the induction of class II antigens on the endothelial linings of venules within follicular adventitia and with apparent hyperplasia of follicular dendritic cells displaying the CD1 epitope. Inflammatory cells infiltrated the region of the follicular bulge, the putative source of stem cells in cycling follicles. The data suggest that progressive fibrosis of the perifollicular sheath occurs in lesions of pattern alopecia, and may begin with T-cell infiltration of follicular stem cell epithelium. Injury to follicular stem cell epithelium and/or thickening of adventitial sheaths may impair normal pilar cycling and result in hair loss. The basophilic sclerotic remains of the connective tissue sheath can be seen in the process as 'streamers'. The destruction of the connective tissue sheath may account for the irreversibility of hair loss. In about a third of biopsies, multinucleate giant cells are seen surrounding fragments of hair. The erector pili muscle decreases in size more slowly than the follicle. In the scalp which appears totally bald, most of the follicles are short and small with some quiescent terminal follicles.

The development of baldness is associated with shortening of the anagen phase of the hair cycle and consequently with an increase in the proportion of telogen hairs, which may be detected in trichograms of the frontovertical region before baldness is evident.

The reduction in the size of the affected follicles, which is the essential histological feature of ordinary baldness, necessarily results in a reduction in the diameter of the

hairs they produce together with a shorter anagen phase. This miniaturization and the degree to which it occurs can be best seen in horizontal sections of orientated scalp biopsies. Balding patients show a wide spread of hair shaft diameters with peaks at 0.04 and 0.06 mm, whereas non-bald subjects show a symmetrical distribution with a single peak at 0.08 mm. The linear growth rate of thinning hairs is also reduced. In total, the functional basis of the severity of the baldness is the consequence of a combination of shorter anagen duration, thinner hair, increased duration of the lag phase between two anagen phases and a decrease of the linear hair growth rate of thinning hairs.

Pathogenesis

Any unifying hypothesis for androgenetic alopecia has to explain the occurrence in both the human and simian species, strong autosomal inheritance, the involvement of both sexes, geographical patterning of hair loss on the scalp, and the coexistence of greasy skin, acne and hirsutism in some women.

Baldness does not develop in eunuchoids, men castrated at puberty and men castrated during adolescence. Following administration of testosterone, baldness develops in those who are genetically predisposed; when testosterone is discontinued the baldness does not progress, although it does not reverse. In further studies, it has been shown that the time interval between puberty and castration is crucial to the development of the beard in males. Castration before puberty prevents the development of a beard, between 16 and 20 years of age it partially prevents the full development of a beard, and after the age of 20 years it has no effect on beard development. Testosterone administration at any stage following castration allows full growth of beard. Very high doses of testosterone cause some virilization in relation to beard growth, but there is no record of change in the scalp hair pattern. It appears that the magnitude of the response of hair to androgens may be set permanently by modification of gene expression following puberty.

The discovery of the importance of exposure to androgens in the pathogenesis of baldness has led to claims of increased sexuality and androgens in balding males. Scientific support for this fanciful hypothesis is lacking. The ability to measure free and bound androgens has shown that normal male levels of androgen are sufficient to make manifest the degree of baldness determined genetically for the individual. The situation in women is different and it has become apparent that the degree of baldness may, in part, be related to circulating androgen levels. In addition, up to 50% of women presenting to an endocrine clinic with diffuse vertex alopecia may have evidence of polycystic ovarian disease.

All adult women show a change from the prepubertal hair pattern. The maximum and overt change in hair pattern occurs after the menopause when oestrogen levels decline and a more 'androgenic' environment exists. Androgens, in the normal female range, induce baldness only in premenopausal women with a strong genetic predisposition. In women with a less-strong genetic predisposition, baldness develops only when androgen production is increased, or drugs with androgen-like activity are taken – such as some progestogens in the oral contraceptive. In some women, even grossly abnormal levels of androgen cause no clinically significant baldness, although all such patients are necessarily hirsute.

The association of seborrhoea and common baldness led to the erroneous theories of the 19th century. The 'seborrhoea' probably has more to do with the refatting kinetics of fine hair than with any change in sebaceous gland activity, except in a few women. During the balding process the total number of sebaceous glands decreases significantly.

Sebaceous glands are under androgen control and in men seem to be under maximal stimulation from normal circulating androgen levels. In women, however, increased sebum production occurs following a small increase in circulating androgens. It is not surprising, therefore, that many young women with higher grades of baldness, who have demonstrable abnormalities in circulating androgens, also have greasier skin.

The weight of evidence strongly supports the opinion that the essential inherited factor responsible for ordinary baldness concerns the manner in which certain follicles in the frontovertical region of the scalp react to androgens. The ability of the pilosebaceous unit to metabolize a wide range of androgens has been established beyond doubt. The same androgens are responsible for the seborrhoea of acne, the conversion of vellus to terminal hair in the beard, pubic area and axillae, and, paradoxically, the opposite effect on hair in the balding process in both sexes. Sebaceous gland androgen metabolism has been studied extensively, but even with the pilosebaceous unit we cannot with certainty extrapolate results from the sebaceous gland to the hair follicle or vice versa. The presence of androgen receptors has been established in sebocytes of the hamster flank organ, but it has been much more difficult to localize androgen receptors or androgen-metabolizing enzyme systems in the hair follicle. The presence of androgen receptors on dermal papilla cells in culture and the ability of dermal papilla cells to metabolize a range of androgens suggest that this area holds much promise for further investigation. If individual variation in androgen metabolism is linked causally to hair loss or retention, it should be apparent in women and in young men before the onset of baldness.

In androgenetic alopecia, therefore, a change occurs in genetically prone follicles following exposure to androgens at puberty. From this time a 'genetic clock' is set running which eventually leads to the follicle undergoing cycles of decreasing length, producing stepwise finer and finer hair until full vellus change occurs.

In summary, in men, the development of androgenetic alopecia requires both genetic and hormonal factors to interact. The exact pattern of inheritance is not fully understood. It may be genetically heterogeneous: autosomal dominance with or without variable penetrance, sex linkage, and a polygenic or multifactorial aetiology have all been proposed. Clinical and recent biochemical data have confirmed the central role of androgens, especially the testosterone metabolite dihydrotestosterone (DHT) in the pathogenesis of androgenetic alopecia. After puberty androgens interact with the genetically determined androgen-sensitive hair follicles, resulting in a sequence of events that includes the progressive miniaturization of follicles, alteration of the hair growth cycle and, finally, a degree of thinning and loss of the hair. Distribution of androgen receptor and the androgen-converting enzymes, 5α-reductase type 1 and 2, and aromatase (17β-hydroxysteroid dehydrogenase) in the different portions of the scalp may influence pattern and severity of androgenetic alopecia. Androgen receptor levels vary between the frontal and the occipital region, with higher levels in the frontal than in the occipital region in men. The balance of androgen-converting enzymes at the target cells is important for the metabolism of hormones with different androgenic potential. The 5α-

reductase enzyme type 2 is responsible for the conversion of testosterone to DHT, which is responsible for the gradual miniaturization of the genetically programmed hair follicles by shortening the duration of the anagen phase and reducing the hair bulb matrix volume. High levels of the type 2 isoenzyme have been detected in the hair root sheath and in the dermal papilla. The central importance of type 2 5α-reductase in the development of androgenetic alopecia is shown by the fact that individuals with hereditary type 2 5α-reductase deficiency do not develop androgenetic alopecia. In men with androgenetic alopecia the scalp shows an increased conversion of testosterone to DHT. In women androgenetic alopecia is considered to be the same entity as in men. The differing clinical presentation may reflect the lower androgen levels in women together with lower levels of 5α-reductase (which converts testosterone to DHT), and higher levels of aromatase (which converts testosterone to oestradiol). In addition, the pattern of androgen-sensitive hair follicles differs in women as compared to men. Premenopausally, oestrogens indirectly act as antiandrogenic agents, and also lower free androgen levels by increasing sex hormone-binding globulin (SHBG).

Clinical features

The essential clinical feature of androgenetic alopecia in both sexes is the replacement of terminal hairs by progressively finer hairs, which are eventually short and virtually unpigmented. This process may begin at any age after puberty and may become clinically apparent by the age of 17 years in the normal male and by 25–30 years in the endocrinologically normal female. The reduction in the size of the follicles is accompanied by shortening of anagen and by increased shedding of telogen hairs.

Males

The replacement of terminal by smaller hairs occurs characteristically in a distinctive pattern which spares the posterior and lateral scalp margins, even in the most advanced cases, and even in old age. The sequence of patterns in the male is usually of the Hamilton type. Bitemporal recession is followed by balding of the vertex. Variations in the pattern are governed at least in part by genetic factors. The rate of progression is probably determined by heredity.

Females

The use of the term 'male pattern alopecia' must be held partly responsible for the frequent failure to appreciate that in its earlier stages androgenetic alopecia in women need not conform to the 'male pattern' (Figures 3.96–3.101). As in the male, increased shedding of telogen hairs accompanies the reduction of shaft diameter, but the follicles first affected are more widely distributed over the frontovertical region. As a result, many secondary vellus hairs are interspersed with hairs still normal and others only slightly reduced in diameter. Partial baldness is sometimes first apparent on the vertex, but the most frequent presentation of androgenetic alopecia in women is as diffuse alopecia, producing the distinctive clinical features of 'female pattern alopecia'. However, it has been shown that all women display a change of scalp hair pattern at some stage after puberty. The rate of change of patterning is very slow but accelerates during and after the menopause. It has also been shown that hair patterns of the classical 'male type' shown by Hamilton occur with increasing frequency after the menopause. The occurrence of Ludwig pattern III or Hamilton pattern V or greater in normal premenopausal women is

unlikely. A full medical history and examination are essential, and in many cases endocrinological investigation is desirable in all women with androgenetic alopecia of rapid onset, even if it be an isolated abnormality, and in women with baldness of gradual onset but accompanied by menstrual disturbance, hirsutism or recrudescence of acne. Hair loss of Hamilton type IV may occur in women without hirsutism, but more extensive baldness (types VI–VII) is always accompanied by hirsutism.

Management

People concerned about their androgenetic alopecia have four choices. They can do nothing, camouflage the hair loss either by topical agents or a wig, avail themselves of medical treatment or undergo surgery. Surgical treatment demands great skill and adverse results are not rare.

Androgenetic alopecia is a progressive condition to some degree in every case. Hairs decrease in number at a rate of approximately 5% per year. Despite this, for the vast majority of men to do nothing is the most appropriate option and they do not present to doctors. In addition many people seeking treatment will choose to do nothing when presented with the various options; for these individuals supportive counselling and reassurance may be of great assistance in helping them come to terms with their hair loss. Even when no treatment is recommended the physician can be of assistance to the patient by explaining the process of hair loss, the fact that it is common and the various available treatments. The great distress that hair loss causes for a minority of patients, particularly women, should not be underestimated, and doctors may inadvertently accentuate feelings of helplessness if they dismiss the problem too lightly.

The medical treatment of androgenetic alopecia in men is different to women. Androgen receptor antagonists are the mainstay of medical therapy in women, but are not suitable for men due to the risks of gynaecomastia, feminization and impotence.

> **All drug treatments of androgenetic alopecia are purely suppressive**

One problem in the routine management of patients on medical treatment is the difficulty of accurately monitoring the patient's response. In the absence of the sophisticated techniques used in trials, the patient's subjective assessment of progress is the mainstay of monitoring; however, the placebo response may be marked. The hair-pull test by which one determines the number of hairs that can be extracted by gentle traction is a semi-objective guide. Baseline photographs are helpful, but are unlikely to detect changes of less than 20% in hair density. A digital camera mounted on a stereotactic device identical to that used in recent therapeutic trials is an effective way to monitor treatment response and improve long-term patient treatment compliance.

While the pattern of the hair loss makes the diagnosis of male androgenetic alopecia and advanced female androgenetic alopecia straightforward, the diagnosis of early androgenetic alopecia in women is difficult. This is because female androgenetic alopecia may initially produce diffuse hair shedding without a discernible pattern to the loss. In such cases there are a number of differential diagnoses that should be considered. These women require further investigation to exclude nutritional, metabolic and iatrogenic causes of hair loss,[20,21] and iron studies, thyroid function tests and a drug history should be taken in all cases. It is also difficult to differentiate chronic diffuse hair loss in women as a prodrome to androgenetic alopecia from chronic telogen effluvium.[22] This is an entity that is self-limiting and does not respond to systemic antiandrogens. Classically, middle-aged women present with a profound increase in daily hair shedding often sufficient to block the shower drain or sink; it begins suddenly and continues for from 6 months to 6 or 7 years. In spite of reporting this massive loss, such women always seem to have a good head of hair.

The clinical features that favour the diagnosis of chronic telogen effluvium over androgenetic alopecia are diffuse shedding, bitemporal recession and absence of widening of the central hair parting; but these criteria are not absolute and androgenetic alopecia may closely mimic this presentation. In such cases differentiation of androgenetic alopecia from chronic telogen effluvium demands histology. As the prognosis and treatment of these two conditions are profoundly different, these women should have a scalp biopsy prior to commencing long-term antiandrogen therapy, the dose of which may spiral upwards in cases of chronic telogen effluvium in view of the poor clinical response. Optimal information is obtained with two 4 mm punch biopsies taken from the vertex of the scalp and processed horizontally and vertically. In chronic telogen effluvium the biopsy will be indistinguishable from normal scalp skin, whereas in androgenetic alopecia miniaturization will be evident by the increased number of vellus hairs.

Androgenetic alopecia in females may be a clue to systemic virilization, but further investigations looking for a source of systemic androgen excess are only required if the hair loss is associated with other features of virilization such as hirsutes, acne, menstrual irregularity or infertility. In such cases a single serum testosterone measurement is sufficient for the exclusion of enzyme deficiencies and virilizing tumours. While recession of the frontal and frontoparietal hairline was at one stage regarded as a marker for female virilization, a study of 564 healthy women showed this to be a 'subtle' normal finding in 13% of premenopausal women and 37% of postmenopausal women; it was not so obvious in women as in men.

Non-medical treatments

Many over-the-counter products are promoted for hair loss. Although their ingredients are generally safe for external use, they do not promote hair growth or prevent hair loss. In 1980 an advisory panel to the United States FDA evaluated a number of substances used in hair lotions and creams – including amino acids, aminobenzoic acid, ascorbic acid, benzoic acid, B vitamins, hormones, jojoba oil, lanolin, polysorbate 20 and 660, sulphanilimide, tetracaine hydrochloride, urea and wheat germ oil – and subsequently proposed they be removed from the market! Other ineffective remedies include scalp massage, dietary modification, frequent shampooing, electrical stimulation and Chinese herbal extracts.

Camouflage and wigs

Camouflage is the simplest, easiest and cheapest way of dealing with mild androgenetic alopecia. Balding becomes most noticeable when the scalp can be seen through the hair. Camouflage treatments dye the scalp the same colour as the hair, and give the illusion of thicker hair. Numerous brands are available in pressurized spray cans in a number of different colours and they are often combined with a 'holding' hairspray (and sunscreen). The hair is dried and styled before the dye that matches the patient's hair colour is sprayed onto the base of the hair. Although many of the newer agents are water resistant, problems may still arise in the rain if the hair gets wet and the dye runs. In addition patients should avoid touching their hair, as the dye will stain their hands. Towels and pillowcases may be stained. Patients are advised to remove the dye each night by shampooing and to reapply the dye each morning. Many affected individuals now use the 'spray on' fibrils that attach to hair and give a temporary sense of increased density.

Many men and women with diffuse alopecia prefer hairpieces or wigs to scalp surgery. Wigs can either be interwoven with existing hair or worn over the top of existing hair. Interwoven wigs tend to lift as the hair grows and require adjustment every few weeks. Wig hair is made from either synthetic acrylic fibre that withstands wear and tear very well or natural hair (usually Asian or European human hair). Natural hair wigs look better, are easier to style and last longer, but are considerably more expensive. Wigs can be styled and washed and modern wigs provide excellent coverage that looks natural. A disadvantage of wigs is that they may be uncomfortably hot in the summer, and some patients find them difficult to wear for this reason. Unfortunately, because the only wigs people see are the bad ones, they have a poor reputation. Excellent advice on wigs is usually available from the alopecia patient support groups that exist in the United Kingdom, United States and Australia. Clinicians are wise to familiarize themselves with the services that local organizations offer and the National Health Service programme that subsidizes wigs for patients with 'medical hair loss'.

Medical treatment of androgenetic alopecia in men

Currently, there are two treatments approved in most countries for the treatment of androgenetic alopecia in men – topical minoxidil and oral finasteride.

Minoxidil is available in both a 2% and 5% formulation. After observation of hypertrichosis in men treated for hypertension with oral minoxidil, a topical formulation was evolved that arrested progression of the hair loss and regrew some hair in about 40% of men, while 4% had a medium-to-dense regrowth of hair.[23] Much of the regrowth is of intermediate hairs rather than true terminal hairs and so the major benefit is to arrest progression of the balding process. On stopping treatment, there is a rapid correction with shedding of all minoxidil-dependent hairs. Side effects are few and include skin irritation and rare cases of contact allergic dermatitis.

Finasteride first received approval for the treatment of androgenetic alopecia in males in 1997 following completion of international, multicentre, double-blind, placebo-controlled phase III studies investigating the use of this potent 5α-reductase type 2 inhibitor. In the initial study, 933 men aged 18–41 with Hamilton stage III, IV and V hair loss were randomized to receive either finasteride 1 mg/day or placebo for 1 year. Evaluation of photographs by a 'blinded' panel of dermatologists revealed that in 1% of men the hair loss progressed, in 51% the hair loss stabilized and in 48% hair regrew. Hair regrowth was graded as slight in 30%, moderate in 16% and greatly increased in 2%. Long-term studies have shown good 'retention' of hair.[24,25]

While a response to finasteride may be seen within 3 months, patients should be encouraged to continue the treatment for at least 12 months and up to 24 months before evaluating it. If successful, the treatment should be continued indefinitely as the balding process continues on stopping of the treatment.

As the original phase III minoxidil studies were conducted on the vertex of the scalp, the licence of minoxidil for the treatment of androgenetic alopecia was limited to the vertex of the scalp. While there is no reason to believe that the pathogenesis of androgenetic alopecia differs on the frontal mid-scalp regions of the scalp, a precedent has been set for these areas to be studied independently. While finasteride is also efficacious on the frontal area, it is less so than on the vertex of the scalp, according to the hair count data and global photography. The mean hair count increase in a 1 inch circular area was 12 hairs on the frontal scalp and 107 on the vertex bald spot. These studies suggest either a lesser or delayed response of frontal hairs to treatment with finasteride. There are few side effects attributable to finasteride, and the only side effect of significance was loss of libido in 1.8% of men receiving finasteride versus 1.3% on placebo. This returned to normal on cessation of the medication in all cases and in many cases on continued treatment.

Management of androgenetic alopecia in women

Application of 2% topical minoxidil has been demonstrated either to arrest hair loss or induce hair regrowth in approximately 60% of women.[26] It may be used alone or in combination with oral antiandrogen therapy. On cessation of treatment there is a rapid correction, with shedding of all minoxidil-dependent hairs. The 5% minoxidil solution is not licensed in women because up to 4% of those using it developed 'distant' hypertrichosis;[27,28] any such hypertrichosis is reversible. Oral antiandrogen therapy with cyproterone acetate, spironolactone and flutamide is of benefit in arresting androgenetic alopecia in women.

Spironolactone is a synthetic steroid structurally related to aldosterone that acts by competitively blocking cytoplasmic receptors for dihydrotestosterone. Its principal use is as a diuretic and antihypertensive and many of its side effects and numerous drug interactions relate to this. Several studies have demonstrated the efficacy of spironolactone in the treatment of hirsutism, and some have found it also to be of benefit in androgenetic alopecia. Doses range from 100 to 200 mg per day. Side effects are dose related and include menstrual irregularities, postmenopausal bleeding, breast tenderness or enlargement, and fatigue. Spironolactone crosses the placenta and has the potential to feminize a male fetus. Women should not become pregnant while on spironolactone. Although it is not mandatory for women to take an oral contraceptive, concomitant use of oral contraceptives will reduce the hormonal side effects. The antialdosterone effect can result in an elevation of the serum potassium and a slight reduction in blood pressure, although this is rarely symptomatic in the absence of renal impairment.

Cyproterone acetate is an androgen receptor blocker and potent progestogen. It also has an antigonadotrophic effect. It has been in common usage for over 30 years. It has been shown to be of benefit in androgenetic alopecia and is widely used to treat it in women; however, to date, there have been no large, well-controlled studies of cyproterone acetate use in female androgenetic alopecia. While low-dose therapy with 2 mg daily of cyproterone acetate may be useful in hirsutes, higher doses of the order of 100 mg for 10 days of each menstrual cycle seem to be required in androgenetic alopecia. The side effects of cyproterone acetate are dose dependent and include lassitude, weight gain, breast tenderness, loss of libido and nausea. Rare cases of hepatocellular carcinoma and hepatitis have been reported, but with substantially higher doses. Feminization of a male fetus may occur and so patients should be advised to cease the medication before conception. The combination of cyproterone acetate and oral oestrogen therapy will both provide effective contraception and stabilize any menstrual irregularities.

For postmenopausal women cyproterone acetate may be used continuously and with or without oestrogens. The average dose required is 50 mg daily.

Flutamide is a non-steroidal antiandrogen that acts by inhibiting androgen uptake and by inhibiting nuclear binding of androgen within the target tissue. While some studies have suggested that flutamide is superior to cyproterone acetate and spironolactone in the treatment of hirsutes, there are no large, well-controlled studies examining this in androgenetic alopecia.

Finasteride has only been tested in postmenopausal women and there was unfortunately no significant benefit.

Scalp surgery

Scalp surgery using excision of bald scalp with or without tissue expansion, scalp flaps and hair transplantation has been used in the treatment of advanced androgenetic alopecia for a number of years and is constantly undergoing revision and improvement (Figure 3.103). While artificial fibre implantation has been used for androgenetic alopecia when donor fibres are unavailable, great caution is advised as foreign body reactions and infections are potentially serious complications. In general, scalp surgery is less useful for the diffuse thinning over the vertex seen in women with Ludwig II pattern androgenetic alopecia, and its use is limited to those women

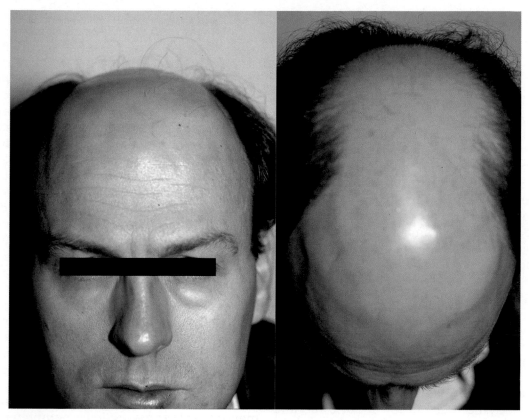

Figure 3.103
Scalp surgery. Surgical interventions may be proposed that do not modify the scalp hairiness; as such, they may be classified as malpractice!
Reproduced with permission from: Van Neste D, My management plan of the male patient with androgenetic alopecia. In: *Hair Science and Technology*, pp 301–309.

with a completely bald area over the vertex of the scalp.

The possibility of gene therapy for androgenetic alopecia has been advanced by the development of a topical cream containing liposomes to deliver entrapped DNA selectively to hair follicles in mice. While the development of a cream that could permanently downregulate androgen receptor expression within the hair follicle is many years away, identification of markers such as keratin 15, for the stem cell population in the hair bulge, may enable these cells to be targeted. In this way any genetic modification would be immortalized in that follicle and expressed with each subsequent hair cycle.

> **Women with androgen-dependent alopecia have more psychosocial problems than those who perceive their hair as 'normal'**
>
> **Men have to accept their overt hair patterns and generally do – but those who do not or cannot may have profound mental disturbance**

DISTURBANCES OF HAIR CYCLE: TELOGEN EFFLUVIUM

In the normal young adult scalp, 80–90% of follicles are in the anagen phase of hair cycle, although there is some variation with site and age. The term 'telogen effluvium (acute)' was introduced to describe the shedding of normal club hairs which follows the premature precipitation of anagen follicles into telogen, a process which may be regarded as the common response of the follicles to many different types of stress. Fever, prolonged and difficult childbirth, surgical operations, haemorrhage (including blood donation), sudden severe reduction of food intake ('crash' dieting) and emotional stress, including perhaps that of prolonged jet flights, may all induce this response. The proportion of follicles affected, and hence the severity of the subsequent alopecia, depend partly on the duration and severity of the stress and partly on unexplained individual variation in susceptibility. The club hairs may be retained for about 3 months until the affected follicles are well advanced in a new anagen or may be shed prematurely. The most frequent form, postpartum effluvium, is probably due to the withdrawal of factors which have prevented normal entry to catagen during later pregnancy. It is universal in some degree and often subclinical. A similar, though more subtle, state of affairs prevails when the contraceptive pill is discontinued after it has been taken continuously for some time.

> **Telogen effluvium affects the whole scalp, not just the vertex**

Clinical features

Diffuse shedding of hairs is the only symptom. The patient may be aware of increased loss on the brush or comb or during shampooing. The daily loss ranges from under 100 to over 1000 hairs. If the lower rates of shedding are continued for only a short period there may be no obvious baldness in the previously normal scalp, since a loss of over 25% of the total complement of hairs is never attained.

In a patient of either sex with previously inconspicuous, androgenetic alopecia, the added diffuse loss may reveal it, or a previously recognized slight baldness may become more conspicuous. If shedding occurs at higher rates, or is long continued, obvious diffuse baldness is produced (Figure 3.104). Unless the 'stress' is repeated, spontaneous complete regrowth takes place almost invariably within a few months. More frequently, female subjects complain that the length of the hair never equals that present before the pregnancy. This must be considered as a step in the progression of natural balding, with shorter anagen follicles being initiated. Exceptionally, prolonged or high fevers, such as typhoid, may destroy some follicles completely so that only partial recovery is possible. If postpartum effluvium is severe and recurs after

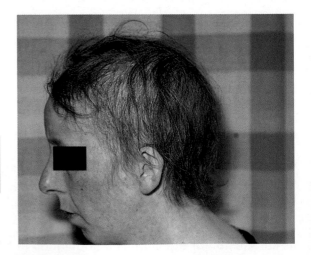

Figure 3.104
Telogen effluvium.

successive pregnancies, regrowth may ultimately be incomplete.

Diagnosis

The diagnosis is usually simple: increased shedding of hair is clearly related to the stressful episode which preceded it by a few weeks or up to a few months. Plucked hairs show a large proportion of normal clubs until the shedding is complete. The alopecia induced by heparin is very similar, but the time interval is often shorter. Alopecia areata of very rapid onset is usually patchy at first but may become total within a week. Telogen effluvium is always diffuse and never total. Acute syphilitic alopecia is patchy. Increased shedding of club hairs is of course a variable, but often very obvious, symptom of early androgenetic alopecia.

Chronic telogen is a relatively recently defined entity.[22] It is particularly seen in middle-aged women. Excessive hair shedding occurs with no overt baldness and no other general or laboratory abnormality found. It resolves spontaneously within a few years and may be helped by 2% minoxidil.

DIFFUSE ALOPECIA OF ENDOCRINE ORIGIN

Diffuse alopecia occurs in many endocrine syndromes, but the mechanisms have not been fully investigated in humans. In many case reports the criteria for the diagnosis of the endocrine disorder have been inadequate.

Hypopituitary states

A hypopituitary dwarf is usually totally hairless. In pituitary deficiency beginning after puberty, as in Sheehan's syndrome, the scalp hair becomes very thin, and pubic and axillary hair is totally lost. The skin is yellowish and dry and lacks turgidity.

Hypothyroidism

Diffuse loss of scalp hair (Figure 3.105), and later of body hair, is frequent in hypothyroidism. Sparsity of the eyebrows, especially in their outer half, may be conspicuous, and a decrease in axillary hair is evident in about 50% of cases. The trichogram shows the proportion of roots in telogen to be abnormally high, suggesting either prolonged telogen or premature catagen or both. Regrowth is usual when the hypothyroidism is controlled, but may be incomplete. Reports to the contrary probably apply to the association of androgenetic alopecia, possibly owing to more 'free'

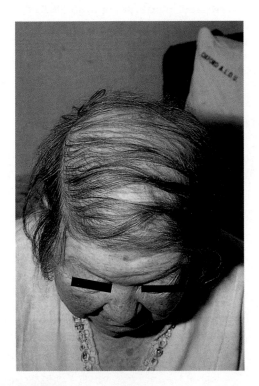

Figure 3.105
Diffuse alopecia in severe hypothyroidism.

androgen due to decreased SHBG. Diffuse alopecia may be the only clinical manifestation of hypothyroidism. The diagnosis of hypothyroidism must be based on critical clinical assessment, together with estimation of the thyroxin level and thyroid-stimulating hormone (TSH). In case of minor changes, dynamic exploration is desirable (stimulation with TRH).

Hyperthyroidism

In hyperthyroidism, diffuse alopecia develops in 40–50% of cases, but is rarely severe. It is reversible. Alopecia areata and vitiligo occur with increased frequency.

Hypoparathyroidism

The scalp hair is coarse, sparse and dry. It is easily shed with slight trauma and the alopecia may appear irregularly patchy. Similar changes have been reported in pseudohypoparathyroidism.

Diabetes mellitus

In poorly controlled diabetes, diffuse alopecia may occur, usually of telogen effluvium type.

Oral contraceptives

Diffuse alopecia has been attributed to oral contraceptives, but the evidence is conflicting. Studies of anagen–telogen counts have shown variable response, some women showing a temporary, some a more prolonged increase in telogen ratio, and others no change. In general, no clinically significant changes are induced, but in some women diffuse hair shedding follows 3–4 weeks after the contraceptive is discontinued and, as after pregnancy, recovery occurs spontaneously. It is possible that some follicles react to a change of the cyclic variations when the hormone therapy is first installed as well as when it is discontinued or modified.

ALOPECIA OF CHEMICAL ORIGIN

Many chemicals which are capable of inducing alopecia are in frequent use therapeutically. Humans are only rarely and accidentally exposed to other types of chemicals. Taken together, therapeutic chemicals account for a small but increasing proportion of cases of diffuse alopecia. In many instances their mode of action is uncertain and a logical classification is therefore impracticable (Figure 3.106).

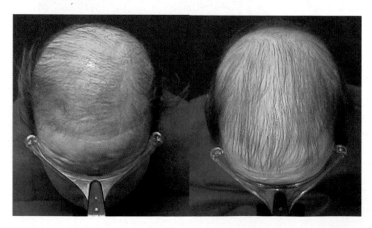

Figure 3.106
Effect of Aromasin (exemestane). Lack of recovery after chemotherapy induced hair loss.
    Chemotherapy with docetaxel for relapsing breast cancer and maintenance therapy with exemestane, an aromatase inhibitor, resulted in severe hair loss. No recovery was observed either spontaneously or after a 6 months' trial of topical minoxidil (5% solution, once a day) in combination with finasteride (1 mg/day).

Table 3.3 Drugs/chemicals causing hair loss

Therapeutic class	Chemical name
Analgesics/anti-inflammatories	ibuprofen indometacin
Antibiotics/anthelmetics	paraminosalicylates benzimidazoles (albendazole, mebendazole) chloramphenicol ethambutol gentamicin nitrofurantoin sulfasalazine
Anticoagulants	coumarins heparin phenindione pentosane polysulphate
Antiepileptics/CNS drugs/psychotrophic drugs	amfetamines carbamazepine desipramine dixyrazine fluoxetine hydantoins imipramine levodope (L-DOPA) lithium methysergide oxcarbamazepine sodium valproate trimethadione triparanol
Cytotoxic drugs/immunosuppressants	actinomycin-D amsacrine azathioprine bleomycin chlorambucil (rare) cyclophosphamide cytarabine dacarbazine daunorubicin doxorubicin (Adriamycin) etoposide

Table 3.3 Continued

Therapeutic class	Chemical name
Cytotoxic drugs/immunosuppressants	floxuridine
	fludarabine
	fluorouracil
	hexamethylmelamine
	hydroxycarbamide
	hydroxyurea
	ifosfamide
	lomustine
	melphalan
	methotrexate
	mitomycin
	mitozantrone
	nitrogen mustard
	nitrosureas
	procarbazine
	docetaxel
	thiotepa
	vinblastine
	vincristine
Cardiovascular drugs/ACE inhibitors	amiodarone
	captopril
	enalapril
	methyldopa
	metoprolol
	nadolol
	potassium thiocynate
	propranolol
Drugs used in rheumatic diseases	allopurinol
	antimalarials (chloroquine, mepacrine)
	colchicine
	penicillamine (left-stereoisomers only)
Endocrine drugs	bromocriptine
	carbimazole
	danazol
	thiouracil
Immunostimulants/interferons	immunoglobulin IV
	interferon alpha
	interferon gamma

Table 3.3 Continued

Therapeutic class	Chemical name
Lipid-lowering drugs	clofibrate fenofibrate triparanol
Retinoids	13-*cis*-retinoic acid acitretin etretinate vitamin A (large doses)
Miscellaneous	butyrophenones cantharidine cimetidine metyrapone pyridostigmine bromide terfenadine
Miscellaneous (antiseptics)	boric acid salts
Miscellaneous (heavy metals)	mercury bismuth, lithium, gold, thallium, arsenic, copper, cadmium

Miscellaneous (plants)	*Astragalus pectinatus* (contains
	   selenocystathionine)
	Lecythis olaria (coco de mono
	   seeds contain
	   selenocystathionine)
	Leucaena glauca (seeds contain
	   leucenine, also known as
	   leucenol or mimosine)
	Stanleya pinnata (contains
	   selenocystathionine)

See: Dubertret L, *Thérapeutique Dermatologique* (Paris, Flammarion, 1991); Rook A, Dawber RPR (eds), *Diseases of the Hair and Scalp* (Oxford, Blackwell Scientific Publications, 1997); and Olsen E (ed), *Disorders of Hair Growth* (New York, McGraw-Hill, 1994).

Table 3.3 shows a list of such chemicals compiled from three recently published text-books.

Thallium

Thallium salts are no longer prescribed in the UK for the depilation of the scalp infected with ringworm, and are not contained in any preparation on sale to the public. In many other countries they are still used as pesticides, and serious outbreaks of poisoning have followed the contamination of grain stores and other food. Thallium salts are tasteless and have been used in homicide and suicide. Thallium is rapidly taken up by anagen follicles and disturbs keratinization. Many hairs break within the follicle. Irregularity of the air-filled keratogenous zone and air bubbles within the shaft near the tapered tip give a distinctive appearance. Many other follicles enter catagen prematurely. Surface keratinization is also disturbed. Alopecia is the most constant symptom. The loss of hair begins after approximately 10 days of diffuse shedding of abnormal anagen hairs. It may rapidly become complete or, with lower doses, may be followed by the gradual shedding of club hairs over a period of 3 or 4 months. In severe poisoning, death may result from acute cerebral and renal damage before hair loss can occur. In less severe cases, the associated symptoms are very variable: ataxia, weakness, somnolence, tremor, headache, nausea and vomiting are among the most constant. In mild poisoning, alopecia may be the only symptom. In all cases the hair regrows completely within 6 months, but there may be persistent signs of residual cerebral damage. The diagnosis may be suspected on clinical grounds but can be confirmed only by the detection of the thallium in the urine and faeces, in which it may continue to be excreted for 4 or 5 months. There is no specific treatment.

Thyroid antagonists

Some patients with thyrotoxicosis treated with thiouracil or carbimazole develop diffuse alopecia. Long-continued administration of iodides has been shown to induce hypothyroid alopecia.

Anticoagulants

All the anticoagulant drugs (heparin, heparinoids and coumarins) induce alopecia. Coumarins such as warfarin are widely used as rodent poisons and are sometimes acci-

dentally ingested by children. The dose, and not the duration of the exposure, determines the degree of hair loss. Apparently normal club hairs are shed some 2–3 months after the effective blood level is achieved. There is often moderately increased shedding without obvious alopecia, but with high doses moderate or severe alopecia may occur. Full recovery follows withdrawal of the drug.

> **Chronic anticoagulation, not the drugs, causes hair loss**

Cytostatic agents

Many cytostatic agents employed therapeutically or given with criminal intent can cause hair loss, mainly of anagen effluvium type. Experimental and clinical studies with cyclophosphamide have shown that some anagen follicles enter catagen prematurely or that the inhibition of mitosis in the matrix results in a constriction in the shaft (Figures 3.107, 3.108) or a complete break. A similar

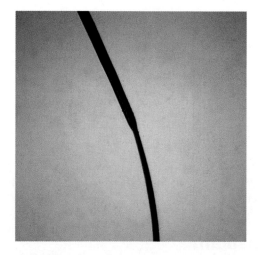

Figure 3.107
Hair-narrowing due to cytotoxic drug therapy.

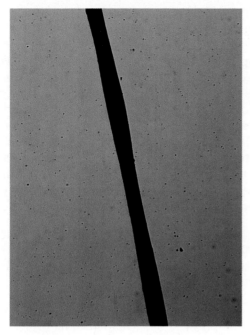

Figure 3.108
Hair 'nodes' similar to those in monilethrix due to intermittent cytotoxic drug therapy.

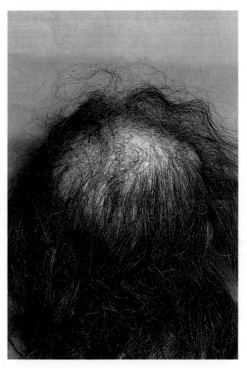

Figure 3.109
Diffuse alopecia due to X-ray epilation treatment.

constriction is produced by aminopterin. Clinically, alopecia is frequently observed after cyclophosphamide therapy. It has also been reported after therapeutic doses of colchicine, after an abortifacient dose of aminopterin and after cantharidin. Hairs with broken constricted shafts may be shed diffusely as early as 4–6 days after the first effective dose, and shedding of apparently normal telogen hairs may continue for some months.

When cytostatic drugs are indicated, the loss of hair can be minimized by scalp hypothermia, e.g. by applying ice packs to the scalp for 30 minutes before the drug is injected. X-radiation may cause similar hair loss (Figure 3.109).

Triparanol

Triparanol and the chemically unrelated, antipsychotic drug fluorobutyrophenone disturb keratinization by inhibiting cholesterol synthesis. Scalp and body hair becomes dry and sparse, and light in colour. The skin is generally dry and ichthyotic. Cataracts develop later in some cases.

Hypervitaminosis A

Excessive consumption of vitamin A gives rise to a variable syndrome in which the principal features are dryness, irritability and sometimes pigmentation of the skin, and slowly progressive thinning of scalp and body hairs, eyebrows and eyelashes. Loss of weight, fatigue, anaemia and bone pain are frequent, and the liver and spleen are sometimes enlarged. The symptoms develop insidiously after doses in excess of 50 000 units daily – usually very much higher – have been ingested for many months. The mode of action of vitamin A on hair growth is unknown. Diagnosis is established by estimation of the fasting blood level of the vitamin. Slow recovery takes place when the vitamin A is discontinued. The alopecia associated with oral retinoids has a similar mechanism but is clearly much less severe.

Boric acid

Occupational exposure to sodium borate has caused diffuse alopecia. Boric acid mouthwashes have caused a similar pattern of hair loss and result in elevated serum boric acid levels. Boric acid taken with suicidal intent has been shown to cause total alopecia after 10 days.

Other chemicals

Reversible alopecia is occasionally induced by other chemicals: potassium thiocyanate, formerly prescribed for hypertension; trimethadione, employed in the control of epilepsy; bismuth, after prolonged overdosage; and cyclic condensation products of monomeric chloroprene, after exposure during the manufacture of rubber. Other drugs reported as inducing hair loss include lithium carbonate, pyridostigmine, dixyrazine and etretinate.

Propanolol, metoprolol, levodopa, cimetidine and ibuprofen have all been suspected of causing diffuse alopecia after several months of administration.

The amino acid mimosine from leguminous plants including *Leucaena glauca* and a toxic substance in the nut *Lecythis*, which appears to be selenocystathionine, have also caused alopecia. Seleniferous plants are a well-known cause of hair loss in cattle, and there are occasional reports of a similar effect in humans.

There are many anecdotal and unsubstantiated cases of alopecia thought to be related to specific drugs – amiodarone, cimetidine, danazol, gentamicin, itraconazole, metyrapone, sulfasalazine and terfenadine.

> **Cytotoxic drugs can induce telogen shedding – more subtle than anagen loss**

ALOPECIA OF NUTRITIONAL AND METABOLIC ORIGIN

Hair is affected early in protein deficiency. Since the needs of the hair follicle 'fuel supply' are enormous, the tissue is highly sensitive to protein starvation. There is no proof for any specific mechanism in the organism to deprive specifically the hair follicle of protein and to conserve it for more essential purposes. The same holds true for iron supply. Malnutrition influences the structure of the hair shaft and, sometimes, the colour of the hair. Short-term experimental protein deprivation causes atrophy of the bulb and loss of internal and external root sheaths but no changes in the anagen-to-telogen ratio, although these would probably develop if the protein deprivation were continued.

Marasmus is the result of protein calorie deficiency, usually in the first year of life. The hair is fine and dry, the diameter of the hair bulbs is reduced to a third of normal and almost all follicles are in telogen. Kwashiorkor occurs during the second year of life in children suddenly weaned to a diet very low in protein and high in carbohydrate. The hair changes are similar to those in marasmus, but there are more anagen follicles although most are atrophic. The differences between the findings in these two states of malnutrition may be related to the degree and rapidity of protein deprivation. In both states the hair is brittle and easily shed, and partial or complete alopecia may occur; the hair is lustreless and if normally black, may assume a reddish tinge. Many hair shafts may show constrictions which increase their vulnerability to trauma. The amino acid composition of such hairs very much resembles that of trichothiodystrophy. The data suggest that regulation of high-sulphur protein is involved in the constitutive weakness of the hair shaft in malnutrition syndromes.

Iron deficiency is occasionally associated with diffuse alopecia (Figure 3.110), even in the absence of anaemia, for the same reasons as protein deficiency; however, the idea that a serum ferritin of less than the mean level in men (70 ng/ml) can itself cause diffuse hair loss in women remains controversial. A decrease in iron supply in females is not proven, but there is chronic elimination of iron due to blood loss in the menses. Therefore, controlling iron metabolism is a prerequisite, especially in women, before starting any treatment. The association is often difficult to prove because it is not always easy to evaluate other possibly associated factors.

Zinc deficiency resulting from a failure in absorption gives rise to alopecia (Figures 3.111, 3.112) and cutaneous changes in acrodermatitis enteropathia. Zinc deficiency

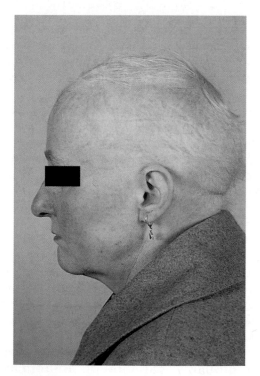

Figure 3.110
Alopecia due to chronic iron-deficiency anaemia.

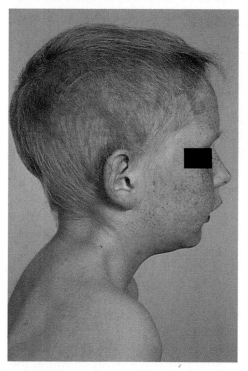

Figure 3.111
Alopecia in zinc deficiency.

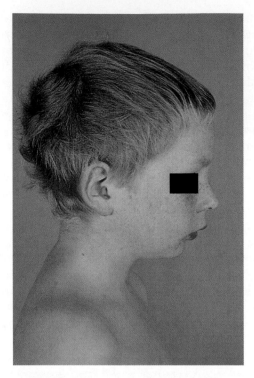

Figure 3.112
Alopecia in zinc deficiency, 4 months after oral zinc therapy.

may result from prolonged parenteral alimentation with erythema, scaling, bullae and hair loss. Parenteral alimentation may also cause deficiency of essential fatty acids. This results in erythema, scaling of the scalp and eyebrows, and diffuse alopecia. The remaining hair is dry and unruly, but this may be reversed by the topical application of safflower oil. Both defects influence the growth of hair because they are essential co-factors to cellular metabolism.

Defects of hair growth occur in certain metabolic disorders. For example, changes resembling trichorrhexis nodosa have been reliably related to arginosuccinic aciduria. In homocysteinuria, an inborn error in the metabolic pathways of methionine, the hair is sparse, fine and fair. It appears normal on microscopy but shows an orange-red fluorescence when stained with acridine orange and examined under ultraviolet light. Affected children are mentally retarded, have a shuffling duck-like gait, a malar flush and a wide variety of skeletal defects. In hereditary orotic aciduria, a rare inborn error of pyrimidine metabolism characterized by retarded physical and mental development and macrocytic anaemia, the hair is fine, short and sparse. A genetically determined defect in the incorporation of histidine, tyrosine and arginine into hair keratin has been found in a syndrome in which dry, lustreless, tightly curled hair is associated with flat, fragile dystrophic nails and enamel hypoplasia of the teeth.

CHRONIC DIFFUSE ALOPECIA

> After androgenetic alopecia and causes of acute telogen shedding have been excluded, there are still many women with cryptogenic diffuse alopecia – what is the cause of this?

More or less evenly distributed loss of hair occurring continuously, but sometimes fluctuating in severity, is common in both sexes. It is seen more frequently in women over the age of 35 years, either because certain forms occur more often in women or because women are more eager to seek advice.

'Chronic diffuse alopecia' is not an ideal diagnostic category. This clinical state may be brought about by a number of different factors, singly or in combination. In many cases no fully convincing cause can be established, but the majority of cases are probably variants of androgenetic alopecia.

A factor which is usually ignored, but which probably makes a significant though small contribution in many cases, is the diffuse reduction in follicle density which may occur from the third decade onwards.

Other factors which must be carefully assessed in each case are as follows:

1. *Androgenetic alopecia.* Endocrine investigations, notably the estimation of plasma testosterone levels (free and total) have shown that androgenetic alopecia is common in women. The diagnosis has tended to be overlooked when, as is usually the case, the pattern of loss is a diffuse, frontovertical thinning differing from the typical more sharply bitemporal and vertical alopecia seen in men. In our experience the great majority of women presenting with chronic diffuse alopecia have androgenetic alopecia as the principal or only defect.

2. *Other endocrine factors.* Hypothyroidism is a relatively frequent factor in some series of cases, but there are regional variations, in its prevalence and it is often diagnosed on inadequate evidence. Hyperthyroidism, hypopituitarism and, perhaps, diabetes mellitus are occasionally implicated. Diffuse hair loss has appeared to be related to oophorectomy, though there is no evidence that it follows a normal menopause (compare androgenetic alopecia).

3. *Telogen effluvium.* Acute telogen effluvium following 3 or 4 months after a clearly defined episode such as childbirth or severe stress is not a diagnostic problem, but it is uncertain whether prolonged emotional stress can maintain an increased rate of hair loss by the regular precipitation of small numbers of follicles prematurely into telogen. A high telogen count alone does not establish this diagnosis, for high counts may be found in hypothyroidism, protein deficiency and other conditions, including androgenetic alopecia. Chronic telogen effluvium of unknown cause has been shown to be relatively common in adult women; it is most easily identifiable by histological studies and is a temporary phenomenon.

4. *Nutritional deficiency* (as described before).

5. *Impaired liver function.* In many patients with impaired liver function from hepatitis or cirrhosis the telogen ratio is increased and in some there is clinically evident alopecia. Disturbed amino acid metabolism has been postulated as its cause.

6. *Severe chronic illness.* Neoplastic disease may result in mild or moderate alopecia, the severity of which cannot as yet be related to such factors as the degree of anaemia, or of cachexia, and which may prove to be determined by secondary endocrine effects. Occasionally, alopecia may be a presenting symptom of neoplasia, e.g. Hodgkin's disease, either owing to increased telogen shedding, or to specific tumour infiltration, i.e. alopecia neoplastica.

When all these factors have been excluded, many cases remain unexplained, the majority of them in women in the age range 30–50 years.[21] This group of unexplained cases does not represent a single uniform entity, though some have chronic telogen effluvium. In some patients the alopecia fluctuates in severity over months or years but eventually recovers more or less completely. In other patients, notably those in whom the hair is becoming finer, the alopecia tends to be progressive, though often progressing extremely slowly. The alopecia, which has been shown not to be androgen dependent, is markedly accentuated on the vertex, rather than in the whole frontovertical region as in androgenetic alopecia.

Some women who are deeply distressed about 'loss of hair' show no evidence of alopecia or at least show no greater thinning of hair than their uncomplaining contemporaries: this is known as a dysmorphophobic state. Some of such women are often clinically depressed. The psychiatric diagnosis of dysmorphophobia must always be considered – this is important because suicide may be a sequela.

ALOPECIA IN CENTRAL NERVOUS SYSTEM DISORDERS

Alopecia has been described in association with a number of diseases of the central nervous system, but in many instances the association is probably coincidental. There are four forms of hair loss in which the association appears to be valid, although the mechanisms are unknown:

- Total and permanent alopecia has accompanied lesions of the mid-brain and brainstem: for example, a glioma in the region of the hypothalamus or post-encephalitic damage to the mid-brain.
- Temporary diffuse alopecia may follow head injuries, particularly in children, and may be associated with reversible hirsutism.
- Total loss of hair has been reported to occur at about annual intervals for 20 years in a patient with syringomyelia and syringobulbia.
- Androgenetic baldness occurs early in myotonic dystrophy.[29] A genetic linkage rather than a direct effect of the neurological changes is probably concerned. Other superficial androgen-dependent changes may be seen despite often lower than average androgen levels.

CICATRICIAL ALOPECIA

Cicatricial alopecia is the general term applied to alopecia that accompanies or follows the destruction of hair follicles, whether by a disease affecting the follicles themselves or by some process external to them. The follicles may be absent as the result of a developmental defect or may be irretrievably injured by trauma, as in the burns of radiodermatitis. They may be destroyed by a specific and identifiable infection – for example, favus, tuberculosis or syphilis – or by the encroachment of a tumour. In other cases their destruction can be reliably attributed to a named disease process such as lichen planus or lupus erythematosus (LE). When all the clinically and histologically acceptable causes have been eliminated, two named syndromes of cutaneous origin remain: pseudopelade and the less well-defined folliculitis decalvans. Once these two have been excluded, there still remain cases in which any greater precision of diagnosis than 'cicatricial alopecia' may be unwarranted. Once the preliminary diagnosis of cicatricial alopecia has been made, the scalp should be searched for other changes – folliculitis, follicular plugging or broken hairs – and hairs, even if grossly normal in appearance, should be extracted from the edge of the bald area for fungal microscopy and culture. If no firm diagnosis is achieved, then general skin examination and systemic studies should be carried out where appropriate.

If the decision is made to take a biopsy, its site must be carefully selected and an

> **Patchy, focal, non-pustular alopecia of the scalp is usually within the diagnostic triad of pseudopelade, lupus erythematosus and lichen planus**

early lesion is preferred. Several punch biopsies are preferable to a single elliptical biopsy because the biopsies can be orientated along follicles and different stages of the disease process can be investigated.

Classification

The causes of cicatricial alopecia can be classified into the broad groups shown in Table 3.4. The commoner causes are

Table 3.4 Classification of cicatricial alopecia

Developmental defects and hereditary disorders
Aplasia cutis
Facial hemiatrophy (Rombert's syndrome)
Epidermal naevi
Hair follicle hamartoma
Incontinentia pigmenti
Focal dermal hypoplasia of Goltz
Porokeratosis of Mibelli
Scarring follicular keratosis
Ichthyosis
Darier's disease
Epidermolysis bullosa
Polyostotic fibrous dysplasia
Conradi's syndrome (chondrodystrophia punctata)

Physical injuries
Mechanical trauma
Scalp necrosis after immobilization surgery
Burns
Radiodermatitis

Medicaments

Fungal infections
Kerion
Trichophyton violaceum
Trichophyton sulphureum
Favus

Bacterial infections
Tuberculosis
Syphilis

Pyogenic infections
Carbuncle
Furuncle
Folliculitis
Acne necrotica

Protozoal infections
Leishmaniasis

AIDS – secondary infections (various)

Virus infections
Herpes zoster

Tumours
Basal cell epithelioma
Squamous cell epithelioma
Syringoma
Other metastatic tumours
Reticuloses
Adnexal tumours

Dermatoses of uncertain aetiology
Lichen planus
Graham Little syndrome
Frontal fibrosing alopecia in a patterned distribution
Follicular degeneration syndrome (syn. central centrifugal alopecia)
Dermatomyositis
Lupus erythematosus
Sclerodermal morphoea
Necrobiosis lipoidica
Pyoderma gangrenosum
Lichen sclerosus
Mastocytosis
Sarcoidosis
Cicatricial pemphigoid
Follicular mucinosis
Temporal arteritis
Erosive pustular dermatosis
Eosinophilic cellulitis

Clinical syndromes
Dissecting cellulitis of the scalp
Pseudopelade
Folliculitis decalvans and tufted folliculitis
Alopecia parvimacularis

considered in greater detail in the following section. For details of the many rare entities, the reader is referred to more detailed texts.

Clinical syndromes

In the 19th century and earlier, there were descriptions of cases of cicatricial alopecia probably conforming to these clinical syndromes. Pseudopelade was described more than a century ago and is now regarded as a syndrome in which destruction of follicles leading to permanent patchy baldness is not accompanied by any clinically evident inflammatory pathology – probably a specific entity, possibly autoimmune.

A form of scarring alopecia in which pustular folliculitis of the advancing margin is a conspicuous feature has been delineated. To this condition the term 'folliculitis decalvans' is now commonly applied.

Alopecia parvimacularis is a questionable entity. It has been regarded as pseudopelade occurring in childhood, but it differs from that syndrome in several respects; it may represent scarring lichen planus.

Lupus erythematosus (LE)

Systemic LE does not generally cause scarring alopecia. More typically, it causes diffuse shedding of hair as in telogen effluvium, often during active unstable phases of the disease.

Discoid LE very frequently affects the scalp. It may produce red, spreading, centrally scarring lesions similar to discoid LE at other body sites. However, in the absence of lesions elsewhere, it may be difficult to differentiate from pseudopelade or lichen planus, even with appropriate histological and immunofluorescent studies (Figures 3.113–3.115).

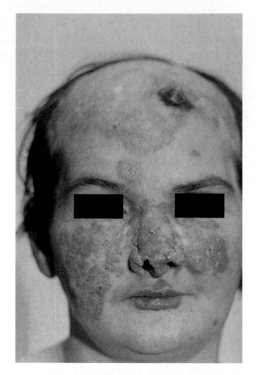

Figure 3.113
Severe chronic discoid lupus erythematosus – face and scalp.

Pseudopelade

The term 'pseudopelade' is used here to designate a slowly progressive cicatricial alopecia, without clinically evident folliculitis and with no marked inflammation. There is no doubt that lichen planus can produce a very similar clinical picture and there are some authorities who maintain on the basis of associated skin lesions and histopathological findings that 90% of cases of 'pseudopelade' are caused by lichen planus. At a later stage, LE can also cause similar changes. However, some patients with pseudopelade never show any clinical or histological evidence of lichen planus. Pseudopelade is therefore generally regarded as a clinical syndrome which may be the end

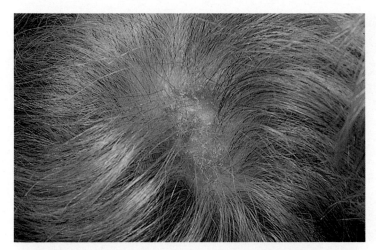

Figure 3.114
Discoid lupus erythematosus – early lesions.

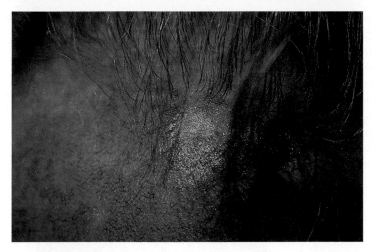

Figure 3.115
Discoid lupus erythematosus at the scalp margin.

result of any one of a number of different pathological processes (known and unknown), though a specific clinically uninflamed type has always been recognized.

Pathology
In clinically normal scalp at the edge of a plaque of pseudopelade, numerous lymphocytes can be found around the upper third of the follicles. Later the follicles are destroyed, and the epidermis becomes thin and atrophic, and the dermis densely sclerotic. Follicular 'ghosts' without inflammatory changes are seen.

> **Pseudopelade may be a primary autoimmune atrophy of hair follicles**

Clinical features
Although both sexes may be affected, and the condition may occur in childhood, the patient is usually a woman and usually over the age of 40 years. She may complain of slight irritation at first, but more often a small bald patch or patches, discovered by chance by the patient or by her hairdresser, are the first evidence of the disease. The

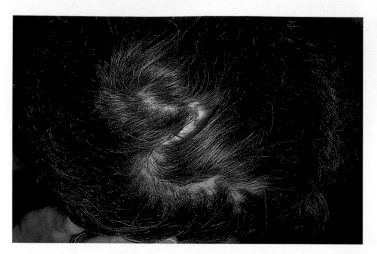

Figure 3.116
Pseudopelade – early multiple lesions.

initial patch is most often on the vertex, but may occur anywhere on the scalp. The course thereafter is extremely variable. In a majority of cases extension of the process takes place only very slowly; indeed, after 15 or 20 years the patient may still be able to arrange her hair to conceal the patches effectively. In some cases extension occurs more rapidly, and exceptionally there may be almost total baldness after 2 or 3 years (Figures 3.116, 3.117).

On examination, the affected patches are smooth, soft and slightly depressed. At an early stage in the development of any individual patch, there may be some erythema. The patches tend to be small and round or oval, but irregular bald patches may be formed by the confluence of many lesions. The hair in uninvolved scalp is normal, but if the process is active the hairs at the edges of each patch are very easily extracted. Detailed clinical, histological and immunohistochemical examination strongly supports the idea that pseudopelade is a distinct entity with the following diagnostic criteria:

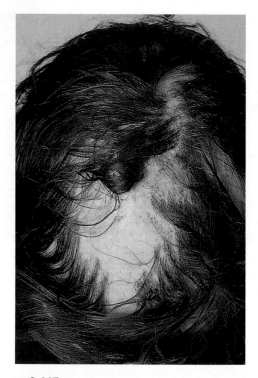

Figure 3.117
Pseudopelade – late stage.

• Clinical criteria:
  Irregularly defined and confluent patches of alopecia
  Moderate atrophy (late stage)

  Mild perifollicular erythema (early stage)
  Female : male = 3 : 1
  Long course (more than 2 years)

Slow progression with spontaneous termination possible
- Direct immunofluorescence:
  Negative, or at least only IgM
- Histological criteria:
  Absence of marked inflammation
  Absence of widespread scarring
  Absence of significant follicular plugging
  Absence, or at least decrease, of sebaceous glands
  Presence of normal epidermis (only occasionally atrophy)
  Fibrotic streams into subcutis.

Treatment

If the scarring alopecia can be shown to be secondary to lichen planus or LE, then the treatment appropriate for these conditions may be prescribed. However, whether the baldness is of known or unknown origin, it is irreversible. If the disfigurement is considerable and no active inflammatory changes are present, autografting from unaffected to scarred scalp, or surgical 'expansion' techniques in severe cases, may be considered.

The intradermal injection of corticosteroids does not seem to influence the extension of the disease process in cases of unknown origin.

Dissecting cellulitis

Dissecting cellulitis is a rare progressive inflammatory disease of the scalp seen mainly in black African men. It may occur in association with hidradenitis suppurativa and acne conglobata. Much of the often massive purulent inflammation is subcutaneous with interconnecting sinuses. Treatment is predominantly by systemic antibiotics related to swabs for bacterial cultures.

Folliculitis decalvans and tufted folliculitis

Under the general term 'folliculitis decalvans'[30,31] we group together the various syndromes in which clinically evident chronic folliculitis leads to progressive scarring (Figure 3.118).

The cause of folliculitis decalvans is still uncertain, but *Staphylococcus aureus* may be grown from the pustules. Some

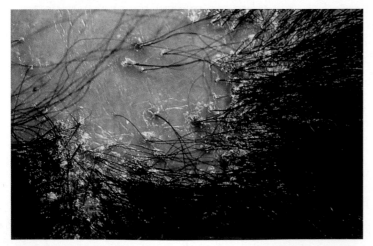

Figure 3.118
Folliculitis decalvans.

abnormality of the host must be postulated. Some authors have emphasized the possible role of the seborrhoeic state and some use the term 'cicatrizing seborrhoeic eczema', but folliculitis decalvans is rare and the seborrhoeic state is common, so the association probably has no special significance.

It is possible that a local failure in the immune response or in leucocyte function may be the essential abnormality in most cases, but no specific defect has yet been found.[30,31] Folliculitis decalvans of the scalp occurs in both sexes. It typically affects women aged 30–60 years, and men from adolescence onwards.

> **Folliculitis decalvans is most likely an abnormal 'host response' to various common bacteria**

Pathology
Follicular 'abscesses' with a polymorphonuclear infiltrate are directly succeeded by scarring, or there may be a prolonged intermediate stage of granulomatous folliculitis with numerous lymphocytes, and some plasma cells and giant cells; i.e. the inflammatory reaction proceeds from an acute to a chronic phase.

Clinical features
Any or all hairy regions may be involved, and in the syndrome sometimes referred to as 'atrophic folliculitis in seborrhoeic dermatitis' the beard, pubes, axillae and inner thighs may be involved, and less often the scalp as well. The severity of the inflammatory changes fluctuates, but the course is prolonged.

The scalp alone may be involved or the scalp together with pubes and axillae. There are multiple rounded or oval patches, each surrounded by crops of follicular pustules. There may be no other changes, but successive crops of pustules, each followed by destruction of the affected follicles, produce slow extension of the alopecia.

Tufted folliculitis may be a variant of this entity in which an upper follicular acute inflammatory polymorphonuclear infiltrate is clinically associated with close groupings or 'tufting' of hairs.

Treatment
All patients should be investigated for underlying defects of immune response and of leucocyte function as a possible guide to effective treatment. Systemic antibiotics will often prevent further extension of the disease, but only for as long as they are administered.

It has been clearly shown that a good and even curative response can be obtained by oral rifampicin 300 mg twice daily and clindamycin 300 mg twice daily, both for 10 weeks. This is evidently antibacterial but also modulates the immune overreactivity.[31]

Lichen planus

Lichen planus is a disease or, more probably, a 'reaction pattern' of unknown origin but belonging to the autoimmune group of conditions. It occurs throughout the world, but there are marked regional variations in its incidence and in its clinical manifestations. These variations probably result from relative differences in the importance of various aetiological agents.

Pathology
The initial abnormality is in the epidermis. Fibrillar changes in the basal cells lead to the formation of colloid bodies, and, at an early stage, these and macrophages containing pigment may be seen in the dermis. By immunofluorescence, fibrin and IgM may be detected in the upper dermis, and various components of complement in the

basement membrane zone. The 'wounded' basal cells are the equivalent of apoptotic bodies and are continually replaced by the migration of cells from neighbouring normal epidermis. In the established lesion the horny layer and granular layer are thickened and there is irregular acanthosis. Flattening of the rete pegs gives rise to a sawtooth configuration. There is liquefaction degeneration of the basal cells. Close up against the epidermis is a dense infiltrate of lymphocytes and some histiocytes. In many sections some colloid bodies can be seen. If the process involves hair follicles, the infiltrate extends around them, especially affecting the bulge area, and the hairs after being lost are replaced by keratin plugs. As the stem cell population appears to be affected, the hair follicles may ultimately be totally destroyed.

Clinical features

Lichen planus occurs at any age, but in over 80% of cases the onset is between the ages of 30 and 70 years. Significant involvement of the scalp is relatively infrequent – only 10 of 807 patients in one series – but the incidence is probably rather higher than such figures suggest (Figures 3.119–3.123) since they tend to

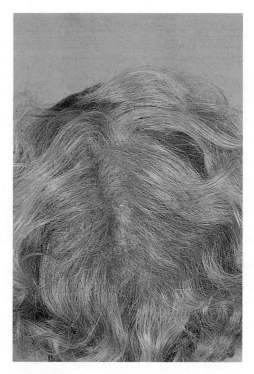

Figure 3.119
Lichen planus of scalp – early stage.

exclude those patients in whom alopecia, classified as pseudopelade, is the only manifestation of the disease. Scalp involvement occurs in over 40% of patients

Figure 3.120
Lichen planus – severe scarring alopecia.

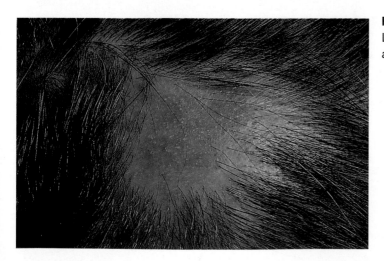

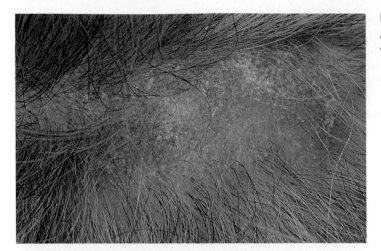

Figure 3.121
Another example of lichen planus
with severe scarring alopecia.

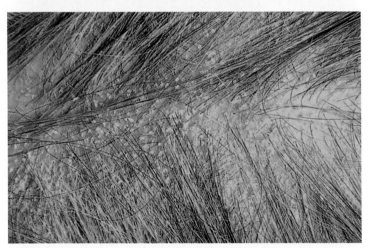

Figure 3.122
Lichen planus showing prominent
follicular keratotic 'plugging'.

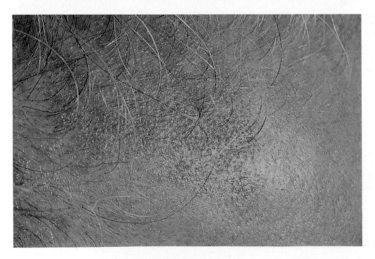

Figure 3.123
Another example of lichen planus
showing prominent follicular
keratotic 'plugging'.

with either of two unusual variants of lichen planus, the bullous or erosive form and lichen planopilaris. Most patients seen with scalp lesions are middle-aged women.

Recent scalp lesions may show violaceous papules, erythema and scaling (Figures 3.119, 3.121). Eventually, follicular plugs become conspicuous and scarring replaces all other changes (Figures 3.120, 3.121). The plugs are subsequently shed from the scarred areas, which remain white and smooth. If the patch is extending, horny plugs may still be present in follicles around its margins.

More often the scalp lesions are well established by the time the patient attends hospital and the irregular white patches are not clinically diagnostic, and may indeed not show any distinctive histological features. This is the clinical picture known as pseudopelade. The diagnosis of lichen planus can be made only in the presence of unquestionable lesions elsewhere and lichen planus histology. These may take the form of bullous lichen planus with shedding of nails, of bullous lesions associated with typical lichen planus of the skin and mucous membranes, or of lichen planus of very limited extent involving, for example, only the nails or vulva.

In a clinical syndrome which has caused much controversy (Graham Little syndrome), groups of horny follicular papules on the trunk and limbs either precede or follow the development of scarring alopecia. The evidence that this syndrome is at least in many cases a manifestation of lichen planus is based on its occasional association with typical lichen planus and the presence in early lesions of histological changes acceptable as lichen planus.

Prognosis
In some patients the course of lichen planus of the scalp is slow and only a few inconspicuous patches are present after many years. However, particularly if the skin lesions are of bullous or planopilaris type, they may rapidly result in extensive and permanent baldness. The rare childhood cicatricial lichen planus has a very poor prognosis.

Treatment
In some cases a short course of systemic treatment with a corticosteroid may be desirable. In other cases intralesional corticosteroids are helpful but only at a stage when active inflammatory changes are still present. Potent topical steroids such as clobetasol propionate in scalp application twice daily may slightly inhibit the process. The oral intake of griseofulvin still has its advocates, but its mechanism of action is not known and its efficacy has never been established in controlled trials. The dosage is approximately 10 mg/kg per day, i.e. 4 × 125 mg per day.

Graham Little syndrome (follicular lichen planus)

Whether this syndrome is or is not a form of lichen planus is still unresolved, although the immunofluorescent findings in typical cases strongly suggest lichen planus. However, whatever its cause or causes, the syndrome is distinctive. It is known eponymously and variously as the Graham Little, Lassueur–Graham Little or Piccardi–Lassueur–Little syndrome.

> **Scalp follicular lichen planus looks a bit like keratosis pilaris with inflammation and hair loss**

Pathology
In the scalp, the mouths of affected follicles are filled by horny plugs. The underlying

follicle is progressively destroyed and eventually an atrophic epidermis covers sclerotic dermis. In the axillae and pubic region the follicles are likewise destroyed, although the skin does not appear clinically to be atrophic.

Clinical features

Most patients are women between the ages of 30 and 70 years. The essential features are progressively cicatricial alopecia of the scalp, loss of pubic and axillary hair without clinically evident scarring and the development of follicular keratosis (Figures 3.122, 3.123).

In most patients the earliest change is patchy cicatricial alopecia of the scalp. In general, the scalp alopecia precedes the widespread keratotic follicular lesions by months or years. In some patients the alopecia and the keratotic follicular lesions appear to develop more or less simultaneously, or the keratotic follicular lesions precede the discovery of the alopecia.

Keratosis pilaris is referred to in early case reports of lichen spinulosus, which emphasizes that the horny papules are prolonged into conspicuous spines. In most cases they have developed aggressively over a period of weeks or months and have been grouped into plaques, often on the trunk, or the trunk and limbs, but occasionally involving the eyebrows and the sides of the face. Thinning and ultimately total loss of pubic and axillary hair have been noted in many cases.

Treatment

None is known. Surgical treatment may be considered as in other cicatricial alopecias.

Fibrosing alopecias

The majority of cicatricial (scarring) alopecias fall within the groups already described, such as LE, lichen planus and pseudopelade – those with a primary destruction of the follicular epithelium, follicular-destructive alopecias that may also affect the adjacent skin. There is another group in which more subtle focal chronic perifolliculitis leads to ultimate loss of follicles: these include frontal fibrosing alopecia in a pattern distribution (FFAPD) most commonly seen in Caucasian women and other patterns seen in African or Afro-American women – hot-comb alopecia (probably a misnomer; 105), central centripetal alopecia (CCA) and follicular degeneration syndrome (FDS). It has been suggested that these are all 'patterned-variants' of essentially the same condition – cause unknown!

Circumscribed scleroderma

Circumscribed scleroderma is rare in the scalp, but may occur there as single or multiple lesions. The early stages of morphoea are rarely seen in the scalp unless a bald area is affected. Morphoea tends to regress spontaneously after 3–5 years, but the plaque may continue to enlarge for much longer periods. The hair is shed at an early stage to leave a cicatricial alopecia. The diagnosis must be confirmed histologically. Linear circumscribed morphoea may extend into the scalp area (Figure 3.124). It has been associated with hereditary deficiency of complement fraction C2.

Development defects and hereditary disorders

Scarring follicular keratosis

Numerous syndromes have been described and elaborately named, characterized by keratosis pilaris, associated with some

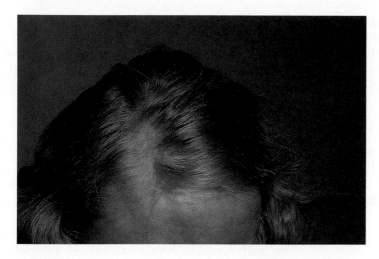

Figure 3.124
Scalp morphoea (localized scleroderma), linear type ('en coup de sabre').

degree of inflammatory change leading to destruction of the affected follicles. Only detailed clinical and genetic studies can provide the essential facts to allow reliable differentiation of syndromes which some authorities regard as forms or degrees of a single state and others regard as distinct entities. The reported cases can be conveniently classified in three groups, and, in addition, certain apparently well-defined entities can be recognized:

1. Atrophoderma vermiculata (acne vermiculata, folliculitis ulerythematosa reticulata). There is honeycomb atrophy of the cheeks. Scarring alopecia may occur, but rarely.
2. Keratosis pilaris atrophicans faciei (ulerythema oophryogenes). The process is more or less confined to the eyebrow region.
3. Keratosis pilaris decalvans (keratosis follicularis spinulosa decalvans, follicular ichthyosis). Keratosis pilaris of variable extent is associated with cicatricial alopecia.

All these conditions are assumed to be genetically determined, although many cases occur sporadically. Such genetic data as are available are considered under the individual forms.

The follicles are initially distended by horny plugs, the dermis is oedematous and there is some lymphocytic infiltration around follicles and vessels. Later the follicles are destroyed. Small epithelial cysts may be numerous, particularly in keratosis pilaris atrophicans faciei.

Clinical features
Atrophoderma vermiculata usually begins in childhood. Follicular plugs, often in the preauricular regions, are gradually shed to leave reticulate atrophy. On the face, the extent of the process is variable.

Keratosis pilaris atrophicans faciei (ulerythema oophryogenes) is present from early infancy. Erythema and horny plugs begin in the outer halves of the eyebrows, which they eventually destroy, and then advance medially and to a variable extent on the cheeks. Involvement of the scalp has apparently not been reported in cases in which the eyebrows are predominantly involved.

Keratosis pilaris decalvans is also such a variable syndrome that several genotypes must be considered. Keratosis pilaris begins in infancy or childhood, often on the face. Its ultimate extent may be confined to the face or to the face and limbs, or may be more or less universal. It is often succeeded by atrophy on the face, but rarely on the limbs or trunk. Cicatricial alopecia is noted from early childhood or later, and may be localized or extensive.

Treatment

Only symptomatic measures are available. Retinotic acid deserves a trial. The status of oral retinoids remains controversial, although there are anecdotal reports of its effectiveness.

Porokeratosis of Mibelli

This is a rare disorder of keratinization characterized by extending plaques of hyperkeratosis succeeded by atrophy. A report of the rapid extension of a previously minimal lesion in a patient receiving immunosuppressive agents suggests that in porokeratosis there is a mutant clone of cells in the epidermis, the proliferation of which is normally controlled by immune processes.

Porokeratosis of Mibelli commonly begins in childhood, but may first appear at any age. It is most frequent on the limbs, particularly the hands and feet, the neck, the shoulders and the face, but may occur anywhere including the scalp.

The initial lesion is a crateriform horny papule which gradually extends to form a circinate or irregular atrophic plaque with a raised horny margin which may be surmounted by a furrow from which the lamina of horn projects. In the scalp there is loss of hair in the atrophic phase.

Incontinentia pigmenti

This rare syndrome occurs almost exclusively in females; its inheritance is probably determined by an X-linked gene, usually lethal in the male.

Cicatricial alopecia has been present in at least 25% of reported cases. It appears in early infancy and ceases to extend after a variable period of up to 2 years, but the loss of hair is permanent. Other hair defects present in some cases are hypoplasia of the eyebrows and eyelashes and woolly hair naevus of the scalp.

Epidermolysis bullosa

The term 'epidermolysis bullosa' is applied to a group of distinct, genetically determined disorders characterized by the formation of bullae and erosions in the skin, and often also in the mucous membranes, in response to trauma or spontaneously. Only one of these diseases is consistently accompanied by abnormalities of scalp or hair – recessive dystrophic epidermolysis bullosa. Alopecia may also occur in junctional epidermolysis bullosa. Bullae form at the dermoepidermal junction and fragments of dermis may adhere to the roof.

The inexorable blistering of skin and mucous membranes dominates the picture. The blisters are followed by atrophic scarring. This may give rise to extensive cicatricial alopecia of the scalp.

Cleft lip–palate, ectodermal dysplasia and syndactyly

This rare, or rarely recognized, syndrome is probably hereditary, and determined by an autosomal recessive gene.

The constant features of the syndrome are mental retardation, cleft palate, genital hypoplasia, cicatricial alopecia, defective teeth and syndactyly.

Cicatricial pemphigoid (benign mucosal pemphigoid/ocular pemphigus)

Cicatricial pemphigoid affects predominantly the elderly, and women more than men.

Bullae are formed at the dermoepidermal junction. Linear deposits of IgG, C3 and C4 may be found in the basement membrane zone, but circulating basement membrane zone antibodies (IgG or IgA) are not always demonstrable.

The skin is involved in 40–50% of cases, and the disease affects predominantly the ocular and/or genital mucous membrane. However, the skin lesions may precede the mucosal lesions by months or years. The skin lesions repeatedly recur and leave dense scars. The favoured sites are the face, and in particular the scalp. Skin lesions, predominantly on the head and neck, are the major feature of the Brunsting–Perry variant (Figure 3.125).

Management is often dictated by the need to control the mucosal lesions. If recurrent bullae in a localized area of skin are troublesome, excision and grafting may be successful. Whether to prescribe oral corticosteroids or immunosuppressive drugs for skin lesions alone is controversial, but topical clobetasol propionate cream may inhibit the process to some degree.

> **Cicatricial pemphigoid may occur on the scalp alone – always biopsy scarring alopecia and perform direct immunofluorescence study**

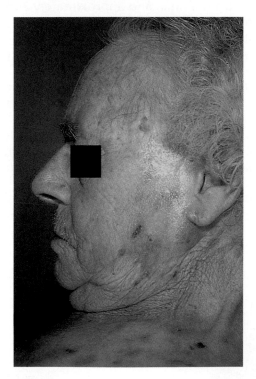

Figure 3.125
Cicatricial pemphigoid.

Erosive pustular dermatosis of the scalp

This clinical entity particularly affects balding men from middle age onwards. Its cause is unknown, but local trauma and sun damage are particularly important.

Histological examination shows areas of epidermal erosion; a chronic inflammatory infiltration in the dermis, consisting predominantly of lymphocytes and plasma cells; and sometimes small foci of foreign body giant cells where hair follicles have been destroyed.

Initially, a small area of scalp becomes red, crusted and irritating. Crusting and superficial pustulation overlie a moist eroded surface (Figure 3.126). As the condition extends, areas of activity coexist with areas of cicatricial alopecia. Squamous carcinoma may develop in the scars.

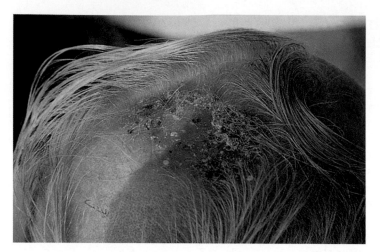

Figure 3.126
Erosive pustular dermatosis of the scalp.

Differential diagnosis
Pyogenic and yeast infection is excluded by microbiological examination and the lack of response to antibacterial or antifungal agents. Biopsy may be necessary to exclude pustular psoriasis, cicatricial pemphigoid, 'irritated' solar keratosis or squamous cell carcinoma.

Treatment
The stronger topical corticosteroids such as 0.05% clobetasol propionate, if necessary with occlusion, will suppress the inflammatory changes. Oral zinc sulphate can be curative in some cases.

Necrobiosis lipoidica

Necrobiosis occurs in 0.2–0.3% of cases of diabetes mellitus, and approximately 70% of patients with necrobiosis have diabetes. The diabetic cases begin in childhood or early adult life, and the non-diabetic cases rather later and usually in women.

Oval atrophic plaques classically occur on the shins but may be seen in other parts of the body including the scalp (Figures 3.127, 3.128). The patches are glazed and yellowish, often with conspicuous telangiectasia. Scarring may be dense. The clinical features

Figure 3.127
Necrobiosis lipoidica visible at the scalp margin.

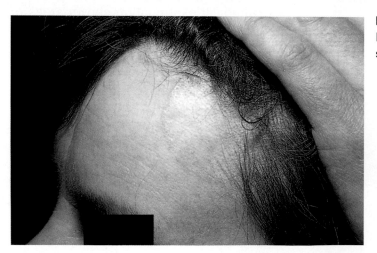

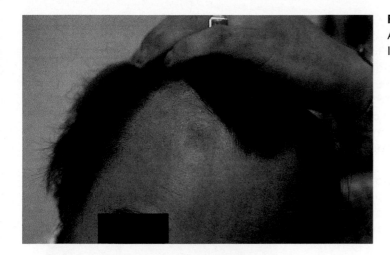

Figure 3.128
Another example of necrobiosis lipoidica.

in the scalp vary from large plaques of cicatricial alopecia to multiple small areas of scarring.

An atrophic form affecting predominantly the forehead and the scalp has been described. In general the differential diagnosis is from sarcoidosis.

Lichen sclerosis et atrophicus

This relatively uncommon disease affects females 10 times more often than males. Lichen sclerosis of the scalp appears to be rare. There may also be lesions of the trunk and of the vulva, which are diagnostic.

Physical trauma

The diagnosis and treatment of the consequences of physical injuries to the scalp will seldom confront dermatologists, but they may be consulted as to the cause of an apparent physical injury: for example, aplasia cutis may be falsely attributed to a forceps injury at childbirth. The attachment of an electrode to the scalp for monitoring the fetal heartbeat during labour may occasionally cause some superficial damage to the scalp and this may be followed by a small scar. Aplasia cutis has sometimes been mistaken for such a lesion.

Exceptionally, self-inflicted injuries may involve the scalp and leave scars.

Halo scalp ring

A type of alopecia that may be temporary or permanent is an area of scalp hair loss due to prolonged pressure on the vertex by the uterine cervix during or prior to delivery, resulting in a haemorrhagic form of caput succedaneum.

Scalp necrosis after surgical embolization

Ischaemic necrosis of the occipital scalp may occur following embolization and surgery for large meningiomata.

Chronic radiodermatitis

Roentgen discovered X-rays in 1895. The X-ray epilation of the face for hirsutism was frequently employed during the first two decades of the 20th century. X-ray epilation for the treatment of scalp ringworm was introduced in Paris in 1904. The discovery of griseofulvin in 1958 gradually made X-ray epilation unnecessary, but it has been estimated that between 1904 and 1959 some 300 000 children throughout the world were treated with X-rays for ringworm of the scalp. Correct dosage did not cause toxicity; however, technical errors were frequent from the use of inadequate and poorly calibrated apparatus. Scarring alopecia due to this may be seen in older age groups who will not always remember the cause. The treatment produced complete epilation in about 3 weeks and regrowth after 2 months. The follow-up of patients treated in childhood showed a higher incidence of cancer in the patients than in a control group. Radiodermatitis of the scalp may also occur as an unavoidable consequence of skin damage during the treatment of both internal malignant disease and malignant disease of the skin.

The use of X-rays for epilation depends on the high susceptibility of anagen hairs to radiation. Epilating and sub-epilating doses produce dystrophic changes in human hairs as early as the fourth day after exposure. Chronic radiodermatitis may follow acute

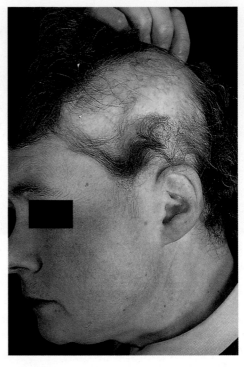

Figure 3.129
Cicatricial alopecia – chronic change following X-radiation.

radiodermatitis but may develop only slowly as degenerative changes induced by sun exposure and ageing become super-

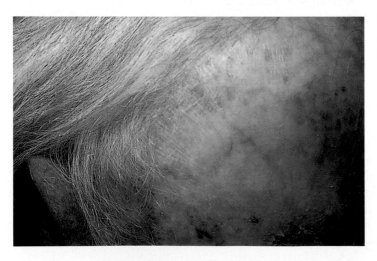

Figure 3.130
Another example of cicatricial alopecia following X-radiation.

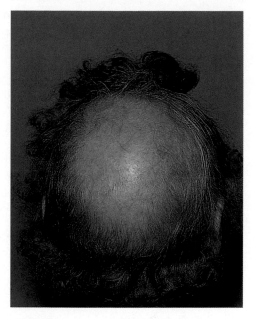

Figure 3.131
A further example of cicatricial alopecia
following X-radiation.

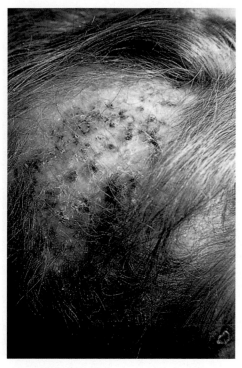

Figure 3.132
Basal cell carcinoma due to scalp X-radiation.

imposed. In chronic radiodermatitis the epidermis is generally atrophic with loss of hair follicles and sebaceous glands, but there are also irregular areas of acanthosis. Degenerative changes and nuclear abnormalities are frequent in the epidermis. Dermal collagen stains irregularly. Superficial small vessels are telangiectatic, but deeper vessels are partially or completely occluded by fibrosis (Figures 3.129–3.131).

Clinical features
The development of a basal cell carcinoma in middle age or later in a still hairy area of the scalp should lead the dermatologist to enquire about X-ray epilation for ringworm in childhood (Figures 3.132, 3.133). In other cases the patient complains of ordinary baldness which is apparently accentuated in certain areas, and these areas are found to

show both common baldness and reduction of follicle population as a result of the earlier radiation.

Chronic radiodermatitis produced by radiation therapy of a malignant tumour of the scalp presents a circumscribed area of cicatricial alopecia. Radiation necrosis may simulate a recurrence of carcinoma, but the edges of the necrotic ulcer are not raised. The diagnosis should be confirmed by a biopsy. Superficial X-radiation of the Grenz ray type does not penetrate deeply enough to damage scalp follicles; but such wavelengths used in the past for psoriasis and lichen simplex may lead to basal and squamous cell carcinomas many years later – without alopecia. Malignant tumours arising in radiodermatitis should be excised, though cryosurgery may be useful for some cases, after diagnostic biopsy.

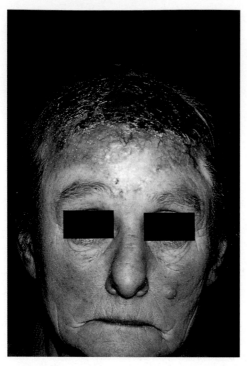

Figure 3.133
Another example of basal cell carcinoma due to
scalp X-radiation.

REFERENCES

1. Sinclair R, Banfield CC, Dawber RPR (1999)
   Handbook of diseases of the hair and scalp
   (Oxford, Blackwell Science), pp 136–138.
2. Salmon T (1981) Hypotrichosis and alopecia
   in cases of genodermatosis. In: *Hair research
   status and future aspects*, eds Orfanos CE,
   Montagna W, Stuttgen G (Berlin, Springer
   Verlag), pp 396–407.
3. Sinclair R, De Berker D (1997) Hereditary and
   congenital alopecia: In: *Diseases of the
   hair and scalp*, ed. Dawber RPR (Oxford,
   Blackwell Science), pp 151–203.
4. Misciali C, Tosti A, Fanta PA, Borrello P,
   Piraccini BM (1992) Atrichia with papular
   lesions: report of a case, *Dermatology* **185:**
   284–288.
5. Ahmad W, Abdul Haque MF, Brancolini V,
   Tsou HC (1998) Alopecia universalis associated with a mutation in the human hairless
   gene, *Science* **279:** 720–724.
6. Ziotogorski A, Panteleyev AA, Aita VM,
   Christiano AM (2002) Clinical and molecular
   diagnostic criteria of congenital atrichia with
   papular lesions, *J Invest Dermatol* **118:**
   887–890.
7. Klein I, Bergman R, Indelman M, Sprecher E
   (2002) A novel missence mutation affecting
   the human hairless thyroid receptor interact-
   ing domain 2 causes congenital alopecia,
   J Invest Dermatol **119:** 920–922.
8. Der Berker D, Dawber RPR (1990) Monilethrix treated with oral retinoids, *Clin Exp
   Dermatol* **16:** 226–228.
9. Auerbach AD, Verlander PC (1997). Disorders
   of DNA replication and repair, *Curr Opin
   Paediatr* **9:** 600–616.
10. Li VW, Baden HP, Kvedar JC (1997) Loose
    anagen syndrome and loose anagen hair,
    Dermatol Clin **14:** 745–751.
11. Freyschmidt-Paul P, Hoffman R, Happle R
    (2001) Trichoteiromania, *Eur J Dermatol* **11:**
    369–371.
12. Hautmann G, Hercogova J, Lotti T (2002)
    Trichotillomania, *J Am Acad Dermatol* **46:**
    807–821.
13. Cray J, Dawber R, Whiting D (1997) *The hair
    shaft – aesthetics, disease and damage*
    (London, Royal Society of Medicine Press),
    pp 13–30.
14. Hamilton JB (1951) Patterned loss of hair in
    man; types and incidence, *Ann N Y Acad Sci*
    53: 708–728.
15. Norwood OT (1975) Male-pattern baldness:
    classification and incidence, *South Med J*
    68: 1359–1370.
16. Ludwig E (1977) Classification of the types of
    androgenic alopecia (common baldness)
    arising in the female sex, *Br J Dermatol* **97:**
    249–256.
17. Venning VA, Dawber RPR (1998) Patterned
    androgenetic alopecia, *J Am Acad Dermatol*
    18: 1073–1078.

18. Chamberlain AJ, Dawber RPR (2003) Methods of evaluating hair growth, *Austr J Dermatol* **44:** 10–18.

19. Jaworsky C, Kligman AM, Murphy GF (1992) Characterisation of inflammatory infiltrate in male pattern alopecia: implications for pathogenesis, *Br J Dermatol* **127:** 239–246.

20. Whiting DA (1993) Diagnostic and predictive value of horizontal sections of scalp biopsy specimens in androgenetic alopecia, *J Am Acad Dermatol* **28:** 755–763.

21. Van Neste DJ, Rushton DH (1997) Hair problems in women, *Clin Dermatol* **15:** 113–125.

22. Whiting D (1996) Chronic telogen effluvium, *Dermatol Clin* **14:** 697–711.

23. Savin RC (1987) Use of topical minoxidil in the treatment of male pattern alopecia, *J Am Acad Dermatol* **16:** 696–704.

24. Kaufman KD (2002) Long-term (5 yr) multinational experience with finasteride 1 mg in the treatment of men with androgenetic alopecia, *Eur J Dermatol* **12:** 38–49.

25. Price VH, Menefee E, Sanchez M, Ruane P, Kaufman KD (2002) Changes in hair weight and hair count in men with androgenetic alopecia after treatment with finasteride 1 mg daily, *J Am Acad Dermatol* **46:** 517–523.

26. Devillez RL, Jacobs JP, Szpunar MPH (1994) Androgenetic alopecia in the female. Treatment with 2% minoxidil solution, *Arch Dermatol* **130:** 303–307.

27. Dawber RPR, Rundegren J (2003) Hypertrichosis in females applying minoxidil topical solution and in normal controls, *J Eur Acad Dermatol* **17:** 271–275.

28. Dawber RPR (2000) Update on minoxidil treatment of hair loss. In: *Hair and its disorders*, eds Camacho FM, Randall VA, Price VH (London, Martin Dunitz), pp 167–176.

29. Cooper SM, Dawber RPR, Hilton-Jones D (2003) Three cases of androgen-dependent disease associated with myotonic dystrophy, *J Eur Acad Dermatol* **17:** 56–58.

30. Loo WJ, Dawber RPR (2002) Dissecting cellulitis of the scalp. In: *Treatment of skin diseases*, eds Lebwohl MG, Heymann WR, Berth-Jones J, Coulson I (London, Mosby), pp 169–171.

31. Powell JJ, Dawber RPR, Gatter K (1999) Folliculitis decalvans including tufted folliculitis: clinical, histological and therapeutic findings, *Br J Dermatol* **140:** 328–333.

4   Excess hair growth

Growth of hair on any given site which is coarser, longer or more profuse than is normal for the age, sex and race of the individual is regarded as excessive. It is clear that the perception of hairiness is much influenced by the social environment. A few hairs can appear to be unacceptable when people of a given genetic background migrate to another cultural environment. The terms 'hirsutism' and 'hypertrichosis' are often applied interchangeably and indiscriminately to excessive hair growth of any type in any distribution. On phylogenetic grounds, and on the basis of its specific androgenic induction, the growth in the female of coarse terminal hair, in the 'male' adult sexual pattern, should be differentiated clearly from the numerous other forms of excessive hair growth of widely varying aetiology. The term 'hirsutism' will be restricted to androgen-dependent hair patterns, and the term 'hypertrichosis' will be applied to other patterns of excessive hair growth.

This section does not aim to be a comprehensive text on congenital, hereditary and endocrine causes of excess hair growth – it is more a description of conditions that an interested skin physician may sometimes see in clinical practice. Details of the rarer entities are listed in Tables 4.1–4.5.[1]

HYPERTRICHOSIS

Hypertrichosis lanuginosa

In congenital hypertrichosis the fetal pelage is not replaced by vellus and terminal hair but persists, grows excessively and is constantly renewed throughout life. In the acquired form the previously normal follicles of all types revert at any age to the production of hair with lanugo characteristics.

Table 4.1 Types of congenital localized hypertrichosis

Congenital melanocytic naevus
Congenital scalp dermoid cyst
Becker naevus
Smooth muscle hamartoma
Nevoid hypertrichosis
Underlying neurofibroma
Hypertrichosis cubiti (hairy elbows syndrome)
Hemihypertrophy
Hairy palms and soles
Hairy pinnae
Spinal dysraphism – lumbosacral hypertrichosis (faun-tail naevus)
Cervical hypertrichosis – anterior posterior

Table 4.2 Congenital hereditary syndromes associated with hypertrichosis

Byars–Jarkiewicz syndrome	Winchester syndrome
Brachmann–de Lange syndrome	Cornelia de Lange syndrome
Cowden disease	Congenital porphyrias:
Fetal exposures:	Erythropoietic porphyria
Fetal hydantoin syndrome	Erythropoietic protoporphyria
Fetal alcohol syndrome	Porphyria cutanea tarda
Krabbe's disease	Hereditary coporphyria
Lipoatrophic diabetes:	Variegate porphyria
Berardinelli–Seip syndrome	Rubinstein–Taybi syndrome
Donohue syndrome	Schinzel-Giedion syndrome
Leprechaunism	Trisomy 18
Mucopolysaccharidoses:	Barber–Say syndrome
Hurler's syndrome	Coffin–Siris syndrome
Hunter's syndrome	Hemimaxillofacial dysplasia
Sanfilippo's syndrome	Craniofacial dysostosis
Congenital macrogingivae	Hypomelanosis of Ito
Stiff-skin syndrome	MELAS syndrome
Epidermolysis bullosa	

Table 4.3 Causes of localized, acquired hypertrichosis

'Acquired' Becker's naevus	Venous malformations, venous thrombosis
Chemicals	Osteomyelitis
Iodine	Edge of burns
Psoralens/PUVA	Vaccination sites
Orthopaedic casts and splints	Pretibia myxoedema
Fractures	Hairy pinnae
Friction	Hypertrichosis singularis
Sack bearers and costaleros	Trichomegaly
Lichen simplex	HIV/AIDS
Habitual skin biting	Systemic lupus erythematosus
Chronic insect bite reactions	Latanoprost
Atopic eczema	Linear scleroderma

Congenital hypertrichosis lanuginosa

Only about 60 cases of this rare syndrome have been described. Traditionally, the cases have been classified into two groups – 'dog-faced', and 'simian' – but it has been suggested that there may be only a single genotype, with considerable interfamily variation in the phenotype. With one exception, the published pedigrees suggest autosomal dominant inheritance (chromosome site Xq24–q27.1).

Clinical features
The child is usually noticed to be excessively hairy at birth. The hair gradually lengthens until by early childhood the entire

Table 4.4 Causes of widespread acquired hypertrichosis

Cerebral disturbances
Acrodynia
Infection
Malnutrition
Dermatomyositis
Thyroid abnormalities
Lawrence–Seip syndrome
Acquired porphyrias
Acquired hypertrichosis lanuginosa
POEMS (Crow–Fukase) syndrome

Table 4.5 Pharmacological causes of hypertrichosis

Diphenylhydantoin
Acetazolamide
Streptomycin
Glucocorticoids
Anabolic steroids
Latanoprost
Ciclosporin
Psoralen/PUVA
Diazoxide
Minoxidil
Penicillamine
Benoxaprofen

skin, apart from the palms and soles, is covered by silky hair which may be 10 cm or more in length. Long eyelashes and thick eyebrows are conspicuous features. Some affected individuals are normal at birth and sometimes for the first few years of life, before the universal replacement of other hair by the lanugo type. Once established, the hypertrichosis is permanent, but some diminution of hairiness of trunk and limbs may be noted in later childhood. At puberty, axillary, pubic and beard hairs retain their downy character. Hypodontia or anodontia and deformities of the external ear are apparently associated in some families, but the physical and mental development of most patients is usually normal. In a Mexican family, hypertrichosis was associated with osteochondral dysplasia.

The status of the apparently recessive form is still uncertain. Three children of a normal mother were densely hairy at birth and died within a week. Neonatal shaving was of cosmetic benefit in one rare case.

Acquired hypertrichosis lanuginosa

In its severe form this syndrome is rare. It usually accompanies a serious and often fatal illness. Fine, downy hair grows over a large area of the body, replacing normal hair and primary and secondary vellus hair (Figures 4.1–4.4). Many cases have been reported and all except a very small minority (less than 2%) were suffering from malignant disease of the gastrointestinal tract, bronchus, breast, gall bladder, uterus, bladder or other organs. Rarely, lymphoma or lymphatic leukaemia occurs with acquired ichthyosis as well as hypertrichosis. The hypertrichosis may precede the diagnosis of a malignancy by several years.

Pathologically, one may see the lanugo follicles almost parallel to the surface.

Clinical features
In the milder forms ('malignant down'), hair is confined to the face, where it attracts attention by its appearance on the nose and eyelids and other sites which are normally clinically hairless. As the growth of hair continues it may eventually involve the entire body, except for the palms and soles. Existing terminal hair of scalp, beard and pubes may not be replaced and may contrast in colour and texture with the very fine, white or blond lanugo. Such hair may grow abundantly even on a previously bald scalp. The hair may grow exceedingly rapidly, and may be more than 10 cm long.

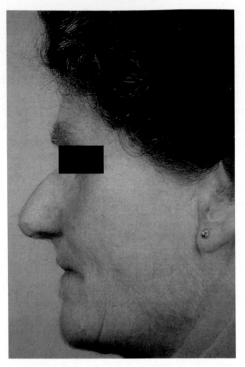

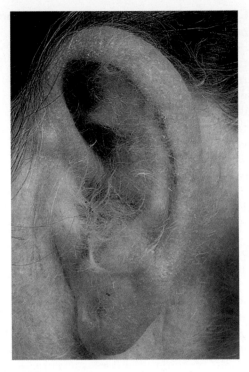

Figure 4.1
Acquired hypertrichosis lanuginosa on the face.
(Courtesy of Dr M Price, Brighton, UK.)

Figure 4.2
Acquired hypertrichosis lanuginosa on the ear.
(Courtesy of Dr M Price, Brighton, UK.)

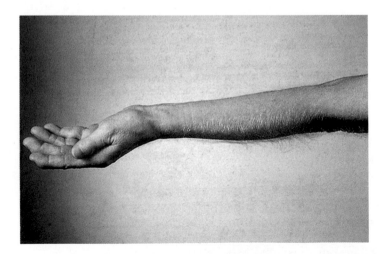

Figure 4.3
Acquired hypertrichosis
lanuginosa on the arm. (Courtesy
of Dr M Price, Brighton, UK.)

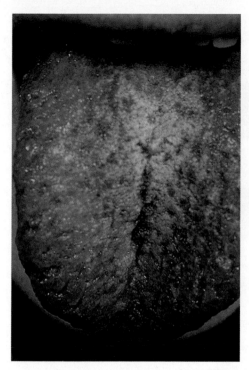

Figure 4.4
Acquired hypertrichosis lanuginosa – tongue changes. (Courtesy of Dr M Price, Brighton, UK.)

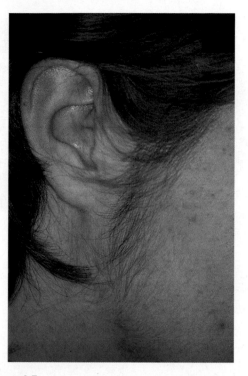

Figure 4.5
Normal hair – adolescent girl of Pakistani origin.

> **Malignant 'down' may precede tumour diagnosis by many years**

Universal hypertrichosis

This term describes a condition in which the hair pattern is normal, but in any site the hairs are larger and coarser than usual. The eyebrows may be double (two per side or very thick).

Inheritance is determined by an autosomal dominant gene. The condition is not very rare, and modern fashions exposing more of the traditionally covered areas are bringing to hospital patients who would previously have been content to keep their bodies covered (Figure 4.5).

The condition is most often seen in dark-skinned Caucasians of the Mediterranean area and Middle East (Figure 4.6).

Naevoid hypertrichosis

The growth of hair abnormal for the site and the age of the patient in its length, shaft diameter and colour may occur as a circumscribed developmental defect, either isolated or associated with other naevoid abnormalities (Figures 4.7–4.11).

Melanocytic naevi may be accompanied by vigorous growth of coarse hair, and this is putatively due to an androgen-dependent mechanism as increased numbers of androgen receptors are present in melanocytic naevi (Figures 4.9, 4.10). The hair may be present from infancy or may develop at puberty.

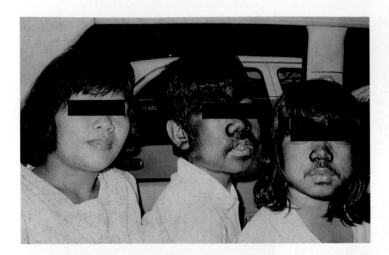

Figure 4.6
Severe congenital (familial) hypertrichosis.

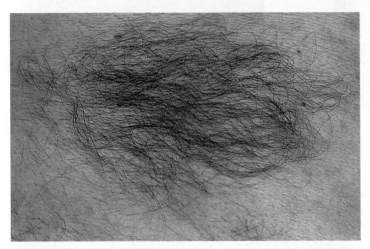

Figure 4.7
Hair follicle naevus.

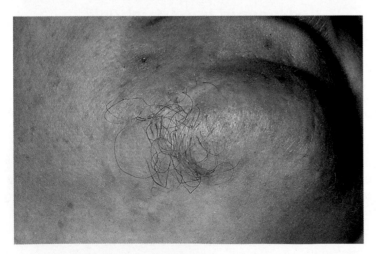

Figure 4.8
Hair follicle naevus.

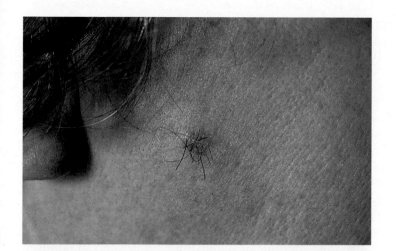

Figure 4.9
Hairy pigmented naevus.

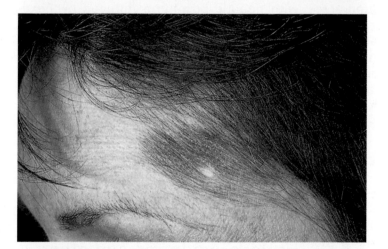

Figure 4.10
Hairy congenital pigmented naevus.

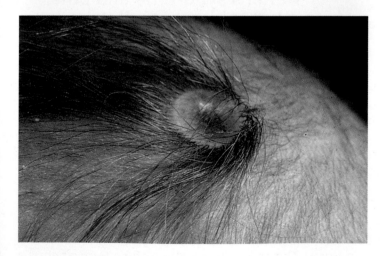

Figure 4.11
Congenital dermoid cyst with hypertrichosis. (Courtesy of Dr C Darley, Brighton, UK.)

Less often, circumscribed hypertrichosis may occur as the only clinical abnormality. Histologically the epidermis is acanthotic and the follicles are large, but there is no excess of melanocytes (Figures 4.7, 4.8).

Hypertrichosis is a characteristic feature of Becker's naevus (Figure 4.12). The coarse hairs develop in the same body regions as the pigmentation, usually the thoracic or pelvic girdle in a mainly unilateral segmented pattern, but pigmentation and hypertrichosis are not always co-extensive. It has been suggested that this naevus is a functional one, being androgen dependent; acne may occur in the affected area, and the increasing hairiness of the pigmented area tends to increase progressively after puberty.

A tuft of hair in the lumbosacral region, the so-called faun-tail naevus, is often associated with diastematomyelia. Radiographs (or other imaging methods where appropriate) are mandatory in all cases with faun-tail naevus (Figures 4.13, 4.14).

Symptomatic hypertrichosis

Hypertrichosis, symmetrical and usually widespread, occurs as a sequela to or manifestation of a wide variety of pathological states. In none is the pathogenesis of the hair growth fully understood. In some an endocrine mechanism can be assumed (Figure 4.15). In others, an abnormality of dermal connective tissue, including the hair papilla, provoked by some biochemical agent can be postulated with some degree of probability. In the remaining conditions the pathogenesis of the hypertrichosis is even more obscure.

Hereditary disorders

Porphyria

Hypertrichosis of exposed skin is a common feature of the very rare erythropoietic por-

phyria (chromosome site 10q25.2–q26.3). Appearing first on the forehead, it later extends to the cheeks and chin, and, to a lesser degree, to other exposed areas. It is also present in many cases of erythropoietic protoporphyria (chromosome site 18q21.3).

In porphyria cutanea tarda, hypertrichosis is an inconstant finding, but may accompany the pigmentation, blistering and scleroderma-like changes on exposed skin and is well marked in some children with the disease. In Negroid individuals, hypertrichosis and pigmentation may be present without blistering. The most extreme degree of hypertrichosis is seen in children with hepatic porphyria induced by hexachlorobenzene or other chemicals. Hypertrichosis is frequent in porphyria variegata. The temples, forehead and cheeks are covered with downy hair. There is also increased pigmentation.

Epidermolysis bullosa

Gross hypertrichosis of the face and limbs has been recorded in association with epidermolysis bullosa of the dystrophic type.

Hurler's syndrome and other mucopolysaccharidoses

Hypertrichosis is usually present from early infancy or early childhood on the face, trunk and limbs and may be a conspicuous feature. The eyebrows are often bushy and confluent. In abortive forms, the hair growth may first appear after puberty and be more limited in extent.

Congenital macrogingivae

Exuberant overgrowth of the gingivae as an isolated congenital defect is not uncommon. The association with profuse hypertrichosis

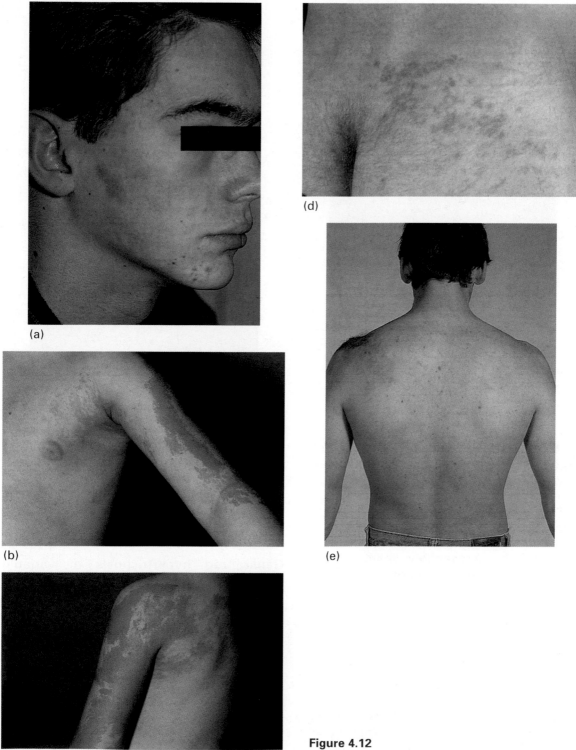

Figure 4.12
(a–e) The spectrum of Becker's naevus.

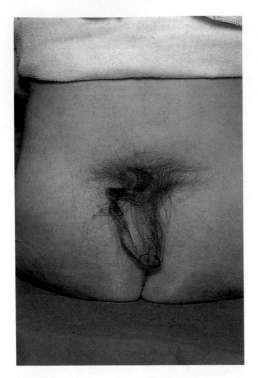

Figure 4.13
Faun-tail naevus (lumbosacral hypertrichosis).

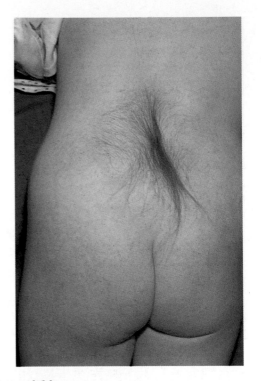

Figure 4.14
Another example of faun-tail naevus.

of trunk, limbs and lower face has been reported on several occasions. Some patients have markedly acromegaloid features.

Cornelia de Lange syndrome

These mildly microcephalic, mentally defective children have a low hairline and profuse overgrowth of the eyebrows. The forehead is covered with long, fine hair. Hypertrichosis is usually also conspicuous on the lower back and may be generalized.

Winchester syndrome

This rare hereditary disorder is characterized by dwarfism, joint destruction and corneal opacities. The skin in many parts of the body becomes thickened, hyperpigmented and hypertrichotic.

Trisomy 18

Generalized hypertrichosis of variable degree is present in these patients.

Endocrine disturbances

Hypothyroidism

A profuse growth of hair on the back and the extensor aspects of the limbs develops in some children with hypothyroidism.

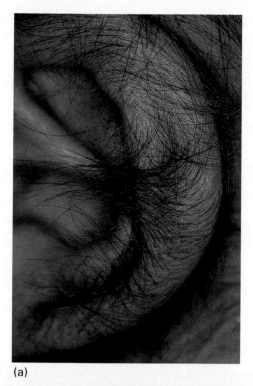

(a)

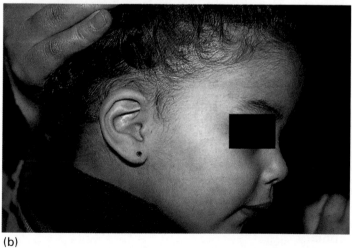

(b)

Figure 4.15
(a) Congenital ear hypertrichosis –
child of diabetic mother. (b) No
hypertrichosis remaining several
months later.

Hyperthyroidism

Coarse hair often grows over the plaques of
pretibial myxoedema.

Berardinelli's syndrome

From early life, growth and maturation are
accelerated and there is lipodystrophy with

muscular hypertrophy. An enlarged liver and hyperlipidaemia are other constant features. The skin is coarse and often hypertrichotic.

Possible diencephalic or pituitary mechanisms

Severe generalized hypertrichosis has been reported in young children after encephalitis and after mumps followed by the sudden onset of obesity. A diencephalic disturbance is postulated. Generalized hypertrichosis may occur after traumatic shock and remit in approximately 6 months. There are many reports of hypertrichosis after head injuries, especially in children. The hair growth is first noticed 4–12 weeks after the injury, which seems to be of no consistent type, and appears as fine, silky hair on the forehead, cheeks, back, arms and legs and may be asymmetrical. It is sometimes shed after a few months, but may persist.

Krabbe's disease

Hypertrichosis occurs in the rare, hereditary globoid leucodystrophy, Krabbe's disease. Most patients die in infancy.

Teratogenic syndromes

Fetal alcohol syndrome

Mental and physical retardation affects the infants of many mothers with chronic alcoholism. The cutaneous changes include hypertrichosis and capillary haemangiomatosis.

Other conditions

Malnutrition

Gross malnutrition, which may be primary or occur in coeliac disease or other malab-

sorption states or in severe infections, may cause profuse generalized hypertrichosis in children.

Anorexia nervosa

An increased growth of fine, downy hair on face, trunk and arms, sometimes of severe degree, has been reported in up to 20% of cases. The visible pattern may be in a subtle hirsute form.

> **In hair terms, anorexia nervosa skin may look like subtle hirsutism in contrast to hypopituitarism, which shows widespread hair loss**

Acrodynia

Some increased growth of hair on the limbs is common. In severe cases the hypertrichosis may be very conspicuous on the face, trunk and limbs and occasionally appear 'monkey-like'.

Dermatomyositis

Excessive hair growth has been noted mainly in children and principally on the forearms, legs and temples; it may rarely be more extensive.

Drug-induced hypertrichosis

In drug-induced hypertrichosis, there is a uniform growth of fine hair increased over extensive areas of the trunk, hands and face, i.e. unrelated to androgen-dependent hair growth (Figures 4.16–4.27).

The mode of action of the offending drugs on hair follicles is not known; the same mechanism is not involved in all cases.

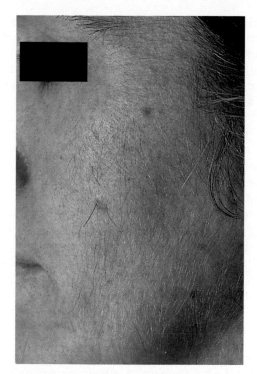

Figure 4.16
Hypertrichosis on the face due to oral diazoxide.

dency of sunlight to induce this temporary change. The stimulation of hair growth on sun-exposed sites by benoxaprofen may have a similar mechanism. Existing vellus hairs increase in length and less so in diameter. The hairs are seldom more than 3 cm in length and are considerably finer than terminal hair.

Diphenylhydantoin induces hypertrichosis after 2–3 months of treatment. It affects the extensor aspects of the limbs, and then the face and trunk and clears within a year of cessation of therapy.

Diazoxide produces hypertrichosis in all those treated, but it seems to cause a cosmetic problem in only about 50%. In adults, the anagen phase may last longer (Figures 4.16–4.18). There are no associated changes in the sebaceous glands.

Oral minoxidil commonly induces hypertrichosis (in up to 80% of patients). It is apparent after a few weeks of therapy (Figures 4.19–4.22). Topical minoxidil applied in excess to vellus hair sites may also enhance hair growth (Figure 4.23).

Hypertrichosis of some degree develops in 80% of patients treated with ciclosporin (Figures 4.24–4.26). A condition evocative of keratosis pilaris may occur in 21% of patients preceding the appearance of thick, pigmented hair on the face, trunk and limbs.

Corticosteroids, diphenylhydantoin and penicillamine are all known to affect collagen, but in different ways. Psoralens presumably induce hypertrichosis in predisposed subjects by accentuating the ten-

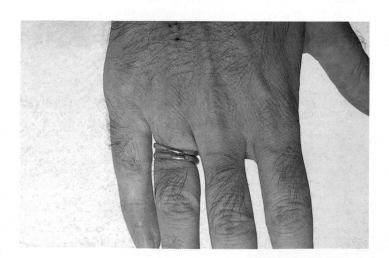

Figure 4.17
Hypertrichosis on the back of the hand and fingers due to oral diazoxide.

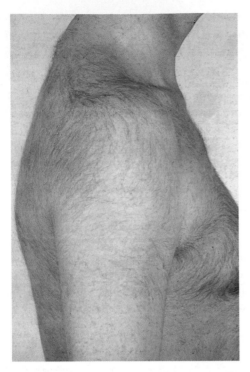

Figure 4.18
Hypertrichosis on the upper torso due to oral diazoxide.

Involvement of other parts of the pilosebaceous unit may occur: sebaceous hyperplasia (10%) and acne (15%).

Benoxaprofen induces a fine, downy growth of hair on the face and exposed extremities after only a few weeks.

Streptomycin has been reported to cause hypertrichosis in over 80% of children who had received 1 g daily for miliary tuberculous meningitis. Hypertrichosis occurs in about 66% of cases of meningitis so treated; it is possible that the streptomycin does not act directly on the follicles.

Prolonged administration of oral corticosteroids may induce hypertrichosis, most marked on the forehead, the temples and the sides of the cheeks, but also on the back and the extensor aspects of the limbs.

Penicillamine appears to cause lengthening and coarsening of hair on the trunk and limbs.

Psoralens, used in the treatment of vitiligo and psoriasis, may induce temporary hypertrichosis of light-exposed skin; whether the UVA treatment used with the drug (PUVA) contributes to the hair growth is not known.

> **Oral ciclosporin A gives prominent hypertrichosis in over 80% of those treated**

Acquired circumscribed hypertrichosis

Cutting or shaving the hair has not been shown to influence either the rate of growth

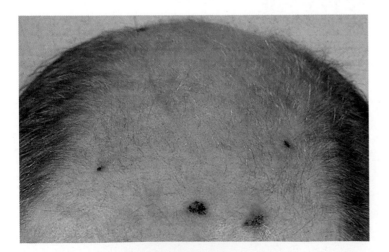

Figure 4.19
Hypertrichosis on the bald part of the head due to oral minoxidil.

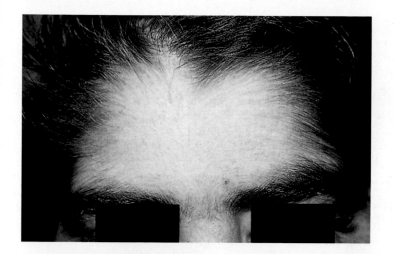

Figure 4.20
Hypertrichosis on the forehead and eyebrows due to oral minoxidil.

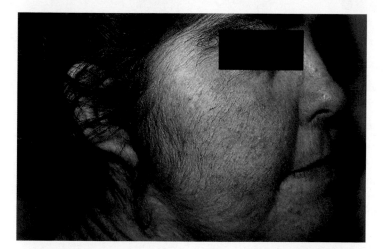

Figure 4.21
Hypertrichosis on the face due to oral minoxidil.

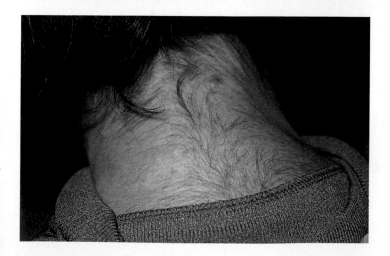

Figure 4.22
Hypertrichosis on the back of the neck due to oral minoxidil.

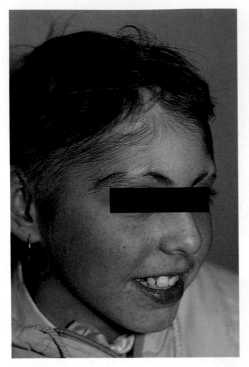

Figure 4.23
Focal hypertrichosis due to topical minoxidil.

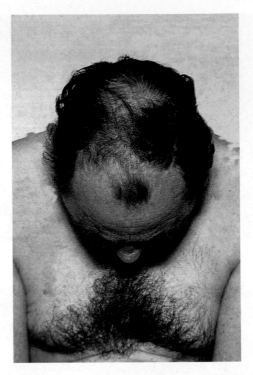

Figure 4.25
Another example of hypertrichosis due to oral
ciclosporin A.

or the diameter of the hair shaft. However,
repeated or long-continued inflammatory
changes involving the dermis, whether or
not clinically evident scarring is produced,

may result in the growth of long and coarse
hair at the site. The cause of the hair growth
is usually obvious, but may be overlooked

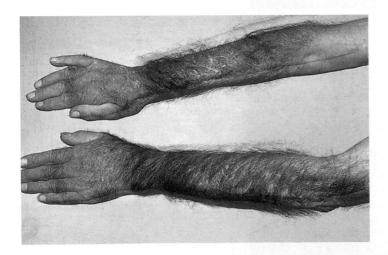

Figure 4.24
Hypertrichosis due to oral
ciclosporin A.

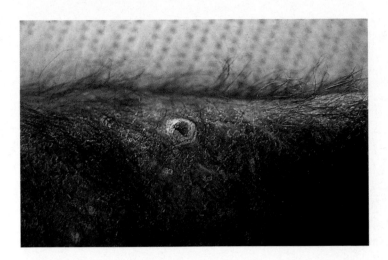

Figure 4.26
Associated drug-induced squamous carcinoma in a case of hypertrichosis due to ciclosporin A.

when the trauma is occupational; for example, circumscribed patches of hypertrichosis on the left shoulder in men frequently carrying heavy sacks. A patch of hypertrichosis on one forearm is sometimes seen in mentally subnormal individuals who have acquired the habit of chewing this site.

Sometimes hypertrichosis, which may involve too few follicles to have attracted the patient's attention, develops at the site of an accidental wound or a vaccination scar. It has been seen on the back of the hand and fingers 3 months after the excision of warts. It has been reported also in irregular pattern on the legs in chronic venous insufficiency, around the edges of a burn, and at the site of multiple clusters or excoriated insect bites. Hypertrichosis of this type may occur near inflamed joints and has been reported particularly in association with gonococcal arthritis and in the skin overlying chronic osteomyelitis of the tibia.

Very exceptionally, inflammatory dermatoses, especially in children, may induce a temporary overgrowth of hair, e.g. after eczema or varicella. A linear pattern of hypertrichosis on the leg has been described after recurrent thrombophlebitis which persisted for a year. Hypertrichosis may occur

in the indurated skin in melorheostotic scleroderma; the diagnosis is established by radiological examination when the skin has completely healed. The damaged skin in epidermolysis bullosa may also become hypertrichotic. Children have developed itching eczema and local hypertrichosis at the site of injection of diphtheria–tetanus vaccine adsorbed on aluminium chloride.

Hypertrichosis of one leg, one arm or the back of a hand after a prolonged (6 weeks) period of occlusion by plaster of Paris (especially after shaving and surgery) is a phenome-non well-known to orthopaedic surgeons (Figure 4.27). It occurs mainly in children. The hypertrichosis may possibly be attributed either to protection of the skin by the plaster from normal weathering or to increased skin temperature. Cosmetic procedures such as bleaching with hydrogen peroxide to clear the hairs may be necessary. The hair returns to normal within a few weeks of removal of the plaster.

HIRSUTISM[2,3]

Perception of hirsuties is by definition subjective and women present with a wide variation in severity. Both the severity of the

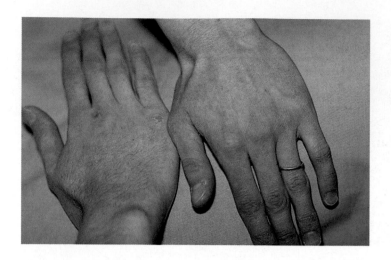

Figure 4.27
Hypertrichosis following fracture immobilization by plaster of Paris.

hirsuties and the degree of acceptance is dependent on racial, cultural and social factors. Even the criteria for the definition of hirsuties used by physicians vary widely. In order to solve this issue, different groups have evolved different grading schemes for hair growth. The grading of Ferriman and Gallwey, which has become the standard grading system, has defined hirsuties purely on quantitative grounds (Figure 4.28). Other physicians have examined women complaining of hirsuties and compared them with controls; they have demonstrated that there is a considerable overlap in the grades of hirsuties between those women who consider themselves to be hirsute and control women. Hair on the face, chest or upper back is a good discriminating factor between hirsute women and controls with similar hair growth scores (Figures 4.29, 4.30).

Hair is second only to the skin as a feature of racial difference. Facial and body hair is less commonly seen in the Mongoloid, Negroid and Native American races than on Caucasians. Even among Caucasians there are differences; hair growth is heavier on people of Mediterranean than of Nordic ancestry. The pattern of hair growth in

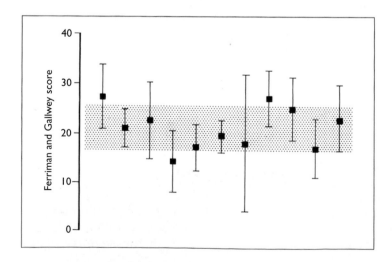

Figure 4.28
Diagram showing wide variety of Ferriman and Gallwey scores in different studies. (Courtesy of Dr J Barth, Leeds, UK.)

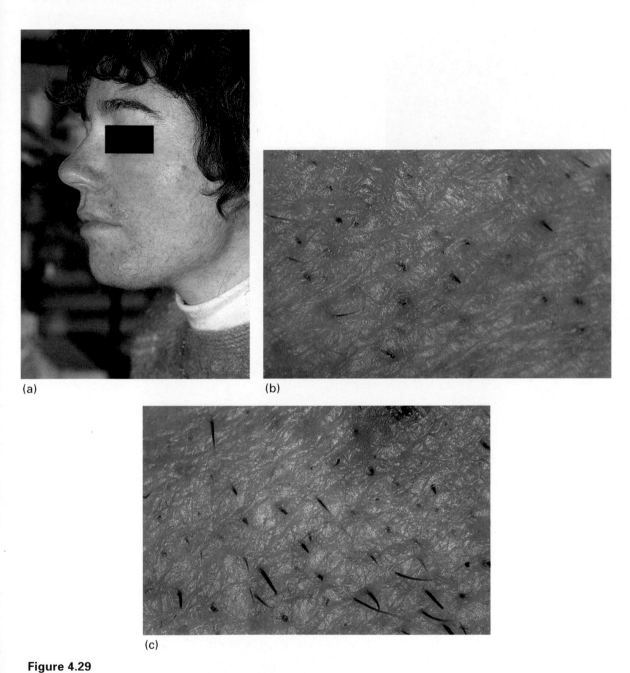

(a)

(b)

(c)

Figure 4.29
(a) Hirsutism of the face. (b) A shaved area of the same face. (c) Same area photographed 2 days later, showing rapid regrowth.

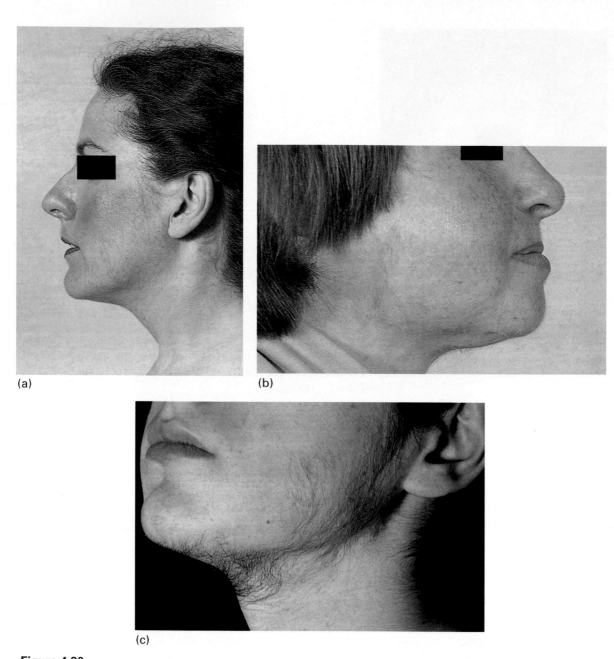

(a)

(b)

(c)

Figure 4.30
(a–e) The spectrum of facial hirsutism.

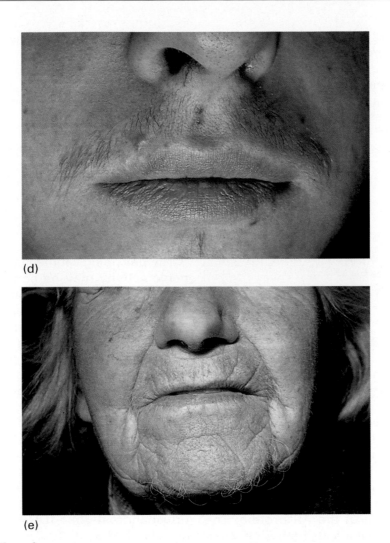

(d)

(e)

Figure 4.30 Continued

hirsuties within different racial groups is identical; however, different criteria have made the determination of the comparative incidence and severity within these groups difficult to assess. It is important to the definition of hirsuties that a sizeable proportion of normal women have some terminal hairs on their faces, breasts or lower abdomen. This tendency to familial clustering in hirsutism is well recognized since many of the underlying disorders which result in hyperandrogenism may have a familial basis; for example, congenital adrenal hyperplasia is linked to the major histocompatibility complex and a very strong family relationship has been reported in the polycystic ovary syndrome (PCOS).

In conditions like hirsutism, society determines the threshold level for 'normality', and this is now highly influenced by the media. Women receive a barrage of advertisements for cosmetics which are based on the premise that only a woman with a hairless body can be normal, healthy and happy! We are all influenced by advertising!

There have been few studies on the psychological status of hirsute women. Some have noted anxiety and reactive psychic disturbances, while other control studies have detected proven associated mental states. Many eminent authorities have stated their conviction that 'stress' often predates hirsutism.

> **If an adult woman thinks she is hirsute, she is!**

Androgens and hirsutism

Androgenic hormones are diverse in nature, but it is believed that their effect is mediated via the protein products of a single androgen receptor gene encoded on the X chromosome. The AR (androgen receptor) contains a highly polymorphic trinucleotide repeat (CAGn) in the region of exon 1, coding for a variable length of polyglutamine chain in the amino terminal, the transactivation domain of the AR protein. The length of this repeat affects both AR expression and function. The number of CAG repeats is inversely correlated with androgen levels and has been associated with various conditions, including hirsutism, acne, PCOS and male baldness.

Many attempts have been made to correlate hair growth in women with plasma androgen levels, but these have yielded very conflicting results – from considerable variability between hair growth scores and free testosterone but no significant relationship, to a correlation with hair growth when a complex formula is used:

Testosterone/sex hormone-binding globulin

\+

androstenedione/100

\+

dehydroepiandrosterone sulphate/100

This correlates with hair growth only in women with idiopathic hirsuties! A relationship has been implied between hair growth and salivary testosterone levels. These relationships are clearly unsatisfactory since they cannot explain the differential response to androgens by hair follicles at different sites on the body.

The physiological mechanisms for androgenic activity may be considered in three stages: (1) production of androgens by the adrenal glands and ovaries; (2) their transport in the blood on carrier proteins, principally sex hormone-binding globulin (SHBG); and (3) their intracellular modification and binding to the AR.

The first sign of androgen production in women occurs 2–3 years before puberty, due to adrenal secretion. The signal for this development is unknown; there may be increased activity of C17–20-lyase, which redirects glucocorticoid precursors towards the androgen pathway; or there may be a reduced forward metabolism of dehydroisoandrosterone (DHA) due to reduced activity of Δ^5-3β-hydroxysteroid dehydrogenase. This process represents a maturation of the adrenal zona reticularis. The major androgens secreted by the adrenal glands are androstenedione, DHA and DHA sulphate (DHAS). Their control during post-pubertal life is unknown, but it is thought that androstenedione and DHA may be controlled by adrenocorticotrophic hormone (ACTH) as their serum levels mirror those of cortisol.

Ovarian androgen production begins under the influence of the pubertal secretion of luteinizing hormone (LH) and takes place in the theca cells. The androgen secreted by the ovaries is androstenedione during the reproductive years, and testosterone after the menopause. Androgen secretion continues throughout the menstrual cycle but peaks at the middle of an ovulatory cycle.

In normal women the majority of testosterone production (50–70%) is derived from peripheral conversion of androstenedione in skin and other extra-splanchnic sites. The remaining proportion is secreted directly by the adrenal glands and ovaries. The relative proportion estimated from each gland varies between reported studies from 5% to 20% from the ovary and from 0% to 30% from the adrenal glands. DHA is the source of less than 10% of circulating androstenedione and 1% of circulating testosterone.

> **Systemic circulating androgen 'faults' are more common in hirsutism than androgenetic alopecia**

Androgen transport proteins

In non-pregnant women, the majority of circulating androgens are bound to the high-affinity β-globulin, SHBG. A further 20–25% is transported loosely bound to albumin, and about 1% circulates freely. The free steroid is believed to be active and the binding protein is therefore of paramount importance. The affinity of the androgens for SHBG is proportional to their biological activity.

The function of SHBG is unknown. It is probable that its main role is to buffer acute changes in unbound androgen levels and to protect androgens from degradation. It may act as a biological 'modifier'. High oestrogen levels increase SHBG and therefore reduce available androgen; high androgen levels reduce SHBG and increase available free androgen.

Androgen pathophysiology in hirsuties

Hirsuties is a response of the hair follicles to androgenic stimulation and increased hair growth is therefore often seen in endocrine disorders characterized by hyperandrogenism. These disorders may be due to abnormalities of either the ovaries or adrenal glands. It is likely that the majority of hirsute women have underlying PCOS (Table 4.6). A small proportion of hirsute women have no detectable hormonal abnormality and are usually classified as 'idiopathic' hirsuties.

This subgroup is gradually becoming smaller as diagnostic techniques become more refined, and is probably due to more subtle forms of ovarian or adrenal hypersecretion alterations in serum androgen-binding proteins or in the cutaneous metabolism of androgens. Although many hirsute women are obese, the role of this is undefined, but it is important to recognize that weight loss by obese hirsute women with menstrual irregularities results in regulation of menses and a reduction in body hair.

> **Obesity may be associated with, or produce, hirsutism and other 'virilization' signs**

Polycystic ovary syndrome (PCOS)[4,5]
The perception of PCOS has changed dramatically since it was first described as Stein–Leventhal syndrome 60 years ago.

Table 4.6 Causes of hirsutism

Idiopathic
Ovarian:
   Polycystic ovary syndrome (PCOS)
   Ovarian androgen-secreting tumours
   Thecal tumour
   Leydig cell tumour
   Arrhenoblastoma
   Menopause
Adrenal:
Congenital adrenal hyperplasia
   21-hydroxylase deficiency
   11β-hydroxylase deficiency
   3β-hydroxysteroid dehydrogenase
     deficiency
   Late-onset congenital adrenal hyperplasia
   Cushing's syndrome

Benign adrenal adenoma
Adrenal carcinoma
Pituitary:
   Cushing's disease
   Prolactinoma
   Acromegaly
Drugs:
   For example, glucocorticoids, anabolic
     steroids, progestins
Other causes:
   Hyperandrogenism, insulin resistance
     and acanthosis nigricans (HAIR-AN)
     syndrome
   Seborrhoea, acne, hirsutism and
     androgenetic alopecia (SAHA)
     syndrome

The syndrome consists of obesity, amenorrhoea, hirsutism and infertility associated with enlarged polycystic ovaries. This disorder has been a controversial diagnosis as it was defined by the macroscopic appearance of organs that were difficult to visualize. This has led to the use of multiple diagnostic formulations based on clinical and biochemical abnormalities. A more fundamental issue has been raised by modern imaging techniques, which have revealed the frequent presence of polycystic ovaries in apparently normal women. Ideas concerning the pathogenesis of PCOS have been as controversial as the diagnosis, and different authorities embrace the belief that it is primarily due to either an ovarian abnormality, inappropriate gonadotrophin secretion, a disorder of the adrenal glands or increased peripheral aromatase activity resulting in hyperoestrogenaemia. Whether the increased androgen is of adrenal or ovarian origin still remains controversial.

The pattern of clinical features of patients with PCOS depends to an extent on the diagnostic definition of the disorder and upon the presenting symptom, be it dermatological, endocrine or gynaecological. Using ultrasound visualization of polycystic ovaries as the diagnostic criterion, many studies have found the following clinical features in PCOS: hirsuties, acne, alopecia, acanthosis nigricans, obesity, menorrhagia, oligomenorrhoea, amenorrhoea and infertility. However, those patients who present to dermatologists will invariably have acne, hirsuties and/or androgenetic alopecia.

Laboratory investigations in PCOS usually reveal an elevated level of LH, often with an increased luteinizing/follicle-stimulating hormone ratio, and elevated levels of testosterone, androstenedione and oestradiol. The demonstration by ultrasound examination of multiple peripheral ovarian cysts around a dense central core will depend on the expertise of the operator.

Ovarian tumours
Hirsuties is almost universally present in virilizing ovarian tumours; however, functioning tumours which cause virilization represent only approximately 1% of ovarian

tumours. Amenorrhoea or oligomenorrhoea develop in all premenopausal patients and alopecia, clitoromegaly, deepening of the voice and a male habitus develop in about 50% of the patients. The majority of those with virilization ovarian tumours have raised plasma testosterone levels.

Hirsutism in pregnancy

Hirsutism has only rarely been reported to develop during pregnancy. It may be due to the development of PCOS or a virilizing tumour after initiation of the pregnancy. A good historical example of this is the painting by Ribera of the bearded woman breastfeeding her child. Such a sudden development was most probably due to a thecoma tumour developing during pregnancy. PCOS may present with virilization during the first or third trimester and regress postpartum. Androgens freely cross the placenta and virilization of a female fetus can occur.

Congenital adrenal hyperplasia

Cholesterol is metabolized in the adrenal cortex by a complex pathway into aldosterone, cortisol, androgens and oestrogens. A defect in a pathway leads to a reduction of the product of the pathway involved with a redistribution of the precursors to other pathways, which results in overproduction of the other hormones. Total absence of a particular enzyme may be incompatible with life and severe reduction in enzyme activity is usually apparent at birth or during early childhood due to dehydration with a salt-losing state and/or virilization.

Partial reduction in enzyme activity may present after childhood and recently a small proportion of women presenting with postpubertal hirsuties have been shown to have subtle forms of 'late-onset' congenital adrenal hyperplasia (CAH). The diagnosis cannot be made clinically and dynamic endocrine investigations are required to differentiate between PCOS and 'idiopathic' hirsuties. Women with late-onset CAH may have normal menstrual cycles, even though approximately 80% have polycystic ovaries.

The commonest defect associated with late-onset CAH is 21-hydroxylase deficiency. As many as 3–6% of women presenting with hirsuties may be affected by this type. It is an allelic variant of the classic childhood salt-wasting type; the classic form is associated with HLA-Bw-47 and the late-onset form with HLA-B14. Of women with this abnormality, 75% will present with hirsutism with or without menstrual irregularities.

Less common in CAH are 3β- and 11β-hydroxysteroid dehydrogenase deficiencies and these are thus less frequently found in hirsute women.

> **Congenital adrenal hyperplasia may be diagnosed for the first time in adults who present with quite mild hirsutism and/or vertex hair loss and acne**

Acquired adrenocortical disease

Patients with adrenal carcinomata usually present with abdominal swelling or pain. However, 10% of both adenomata and carcinomata may present with isolated virilization. The combination of virilization and Cushing's syndrome strongly suggests the presence of a carcinoma. The testosterone level is usually markedly raised in the latter.

Patients with Cushing's syndrome may have hypertrichosis, a generalized diffuse growth of fine hair due to hypercortisolaemia, and androgen-induced coarse hair in the usual male pattern.

Gonadal dysgenesis

All patients with 46,XY gonadal dysgenesis have unambiguously female genitalia but male skeletal characteristics (wide span, broad shoulders and chest); other findings include hirsuties, temporal recession and a deep voice. Cases with this entity may present with slowly progressive hirsuties and secondary amenorrhoea.

Hyperprolactinaemia

The exact relationship between prolactin and hirsuties still remains uncertain. Hirsuties occurs in the amenorrhoea–galactorrhoea syndrome in 22–60% of patients. This may be due to a direct effect of prolactin on adrenal androgen production or to PCOS, with which it is frequently associated.

Prolactin is thought to attenuate cutaneous 5α-reductase activity both in vivo and in vitro.

Idiopathic hirsuties

Idiopathic hirsuties is the diagnostic category given to those hirsute women in whom no specific underlying pathological endocrine disorder can be detected. There are a number of subtle dynamic alterations in the androgen metabolism of hirsute women compared with non-hirsute women. In hirsute women, daily testosterone production is increased 3.5–5-fold and most of the androgen is secreted as testosterone (hirsute 75% vs normal <40%) rather than as androstenedione. Increased androgens in hirsute women are associated with lower levels of SHBG, which binds less testosterone and increases its free level. More free testosterone is, therefore, available for peripheral metabolism and clearance. Free testosterone is a more sensitive measure of testosterone status and there is approximately three times more in hirsute than in non-hirsute women.

Normal values for total testosterone are found in 25–60% of hirsute women and in 80% of those with regular menstrual cycles. This may be due to the effect of SHBG or to the wide fluctuations in plasma testosterone seen in hirsute women. Therefore, multiple measurements are often required to detect the increased levels. Some women, however, do not demonstrate elevations of testosterone despite exhaustive investigation. Paradoxically, in these women, the growth of hair by their skin is the only, and most sensitive, androgen bioassay.

Cutaneous virilism

Alterations in the cutaneous sensitivity to androgens is the reason cited for the existence of hirsutism in the presence of normal serum androgens and the lack of hirsuties in women with raised androgens. However, there has been no systematic study of hyperandrogenized non-hirsute women to determine whether or not they have other cutaneous features of androgen excess. Furthermore, it would be necessary to define the specific cell population that should react on androgen stimulation and this has not yet been achieved. Indeed, the skin is a complex structure containing many different tissues, and it is now recognized that all the structures within the skin are modified by androgens, and they may also be modifiers of androgen metabolism. The eccrine and sebaceous glands are more active and the skin is thicker and contains more collagen in men than in women. Inflammation of the apocrine glands in hidradenitis suppurativa is associated with hyperandrogenism, as is occlusion of the follicular duct both in vellus and terminal hairs. It is possible, therefore, that the skin of non-hirsute hyperandrogenized women does respond to androgens, but not by the development of terminal hairs.

It has been proposed that, in some individuals, the genetically determined level of cutaneous enzymes is sufficiently active to produce a negative feedback on the ovaries and adrenals, so enhancing androgen production, and thus giving a primary role to the skin. Many investigators have provided data for a primary increase in cutaneous androgen metabolism. It has been noted, for example, that the only androgen abnormality in women who have a very short history of hirsuties (less than 1 year) is an increase in the cutaneous androgen products dihydrotestosterone (DHT) and 3α-androstanediol. The metabolic activity of skin in hirsuties is increased both in direct incubation assays of skin and by measurements in vivo, for example, of 3α-androstanediol glucuronide. Whole skin homogenates from genital and pubic skin of hirsute women have been shown to express increased conversion of testosterone to DHT. However, isolated hair follicles from hirsute women do not appear to have different enzyme activities to those from controls. As the pilosebaceous units contain considerable androgen-metabolizing ability, the increased conversion of testosterone by whole skin homogenates may merely reflect the increased mass of pilosebaceous tissue in hirsute women.

3α-Androstanediol glucuronide has been suggested to be a specific marker of cutaneous androgen metabolism. Early studies have suggested that it is raised only in hirsute women with polycystic ovaries, but not in controls or non-hirsute women with polycystic ovaries, but more recent investigations have cast doubt on its infallibility.

Hirsute women have a number of metabolic and systemic abnormalities, which suggests that hirsuties is not only a cosmetic disability but also may have a more significant prognosis. Hirsute women in general have body shapes that tend towards the 'male' shape and, with this, they have altered lipid profiles that would suggest an increased risk of cardiovascular disease. A relationship between diabetes and hyperandrogenism in women, or 'diabetes of bearded women', has been recognized for many years. However, it has now been established that the disordered carbohydrate metabolism is due to insulin resistance (IR). Furthermore, acanthosis nigricans (AN) acts as a cutaneous marker for IR. The combination of AN and IR occurs in 5% of women with hyperandrogenism (HA) and in 7% of women presenting with hirsuties. Women with HAIR-AN have very obvious features of virilism: that is a muscular physique, acne, alopecia and hidradenitis suppurativa.

Insulin may have an important role in the pathogenesis of hyperandrogenism. Studies in vitro have demonstrated that insulin exerts a stimulatory effect on ovarian androgen production and that it inhibits the synthesis of SHBG by the liver. Its mode of action may be through the receptors for insulin-like growth factors which are present both on the ovaries and in the skin. Stimulation of the latter may result in acanthosis nigricans. It is, however, unknown whether the hyperinsulinaemia and IR are primary or secondary.

> **Cutaneous virilism is a useful clinical term for patients with skin 'end-organ' androgen signs and no measurable circulating endocrine abnormality**

Diagnostic approach to the hirsute woman

Many hirsute women have been aware of excess hair since puberty. Some will give a shorter history, but it will still be in the order of years. Some women are so expert at cosmetic procedures that they do not appear hirsute at all. It is important to obtain facts from the history regarding patterns of hirsuties and alopecia or other features of cutaneous virilism and evidence for PCOS, for example, irregular menses or infertility. A family history of childhood dehydration or precocious puberty in a brother might be a feature of congenital adrenal hyperplasia. A drug history may point to an ingested source of androgens, for example, glucocorticoid or anabolic steroids. The progestogenic components of many oral contraceptive preparations are relatively androgenic and this is often cited as a cause of hirsuties (Table 4.7).

The cutaneous examination should include the pattern and severity of hair growth and the associated presence of acne, androgenic alopecia and AN. Features suggestive of systemic virilization include a deepening of the voice, increased muscle bulk and loss of smooth skin contours, hypertension, striae distensae and clitoromegaly. This last feature, cliteromegaly, is probably the most important physical sign pointing towards systemic virilization. The cause of systemic virilization, especially where there is a history of less than 1 year, could well be a tumour. It is thus quite different from 'cutaneous virilism'.

The extent to which it is necessary for hirsute women to be investigated is highly debatable. The main reason for the depth of investigation of hirsute women is the inability to differentiate between idiopathic hirsuties, PCOS and CAH on clinical grounds and it is out of this quagmire that the standard of over-investigation has arisen. The therapeutic tools available at present are too clumsy to achieve such diagnostic definition.

Therapy[2,3]

Most women will be satisfied with the assurance that they are not 'turning into men' and may not require any medical help or may only need advice about local destructive measures; however, many women will already have tried these methods before presenting to a doctor.

Cosmetic and physical measures

Methods for removing or 'masking' unwanted hair vary from simple, inexpensive means of home treatment, such as bleaching, shaving, plucking and depilatories, to the more expensive and time-consuming means used by nurses, medical practitioners and trained technical experts, i.e. electrolysis, lasers and (rarely) X-rays. All these methods have a context in which they may be the treatment of choice in specific individuals, at particular sites, depending on the degree of hirsutism. The terms 'epilation' and 'depilation' have varied in their definitions over the years. It is therefore better to define the exact process used, or the principle behind it, under the general term 'hair removers'. No method is entirely satisfactory, and the one adopted will often depend on personal preference.

Bleaching
This is very widely used for hair, particularly on the upper lip and the arms. It is painless (but when frequently repeated can inflict sufficient damage to cause hair breakage). However, bleached hair can look very obvious against dark skin. Some individuals develop an irritant reaction to bleach; and it is therefore advisable to carry out a

Table 4.7 Investigations for hirsutism

Investigations	Suspected condition	Comments
Stage 1 Testosterone • Dehydroepiandrosterone sulphate • Sex hormone-binding globulin • 17-alpha-hydroxyprogesterone	• Late-onset congenital adrenal hyperplasia • Congenital adrenal hyperplasia (21-hydroxylase deficiency)	Take tests at the follicular phase of the menstrual cycle (different tests are required for rarer forms of congenital adrenal hyperplasia)
Stage 2 • Luteinizing hormone/follicle stimulating hormone ratio • Pelvis ultrasound or transvaginal ultrasound • Lipid profile • Glucose tolerance	• Polycystic ovary syndrome (PCOS)	Luteinizing hormone/follicle stimulating hormone ratio of more than 3 is found in approximately two-thirds of PCOS cases
• Prolactin	• Prolactinoma	('Prolactin'?) may be raised in PCOS also
• Serum cortisol or 24-hour urinary free cortisol • Dexamenthasone suppression	• Cushing's syndrome • Adrenal pathology	0900 hours serum level is best Clear suppression of testosterone makes a neoplastic cause less likely
• Pelvis MRI or CT scan • Pituitary fossa CT scan or MRI	• Tumour or malignancy • Pituitary pathology	A glucose tolerance test with growth hormone assay is required for acromegaly

Note: *If there are features strongly suggesting a particular diagnosis, stage 2 investigations can be done at the initial visit.*
CT, computed tomography; MRI, magnetic resonance imaging.

preliminary test – if irritation occurs within 30–60 minutes, the peroxide strength and duration of application should be reduced.

Shaving

This is unacceptable to some women as being too 'masculine'; however, the majority are happy to shave axillary and leg hair. Modern bathing costumes are very brief, and require wearers to shave their inner thighs and even part of the pubic region. In these sites it is common to experience folliculitis during regrowth, sometimes also due to infection with *Staphylococcus aureus*.

In some experimental mice shaving triggers a switch from telogen to anagen, but not in humans. But shaving does remove the tapered tip of an uncut hair and leaves a coarse, 'blunt' tip as it grows away from the scalp: however, the kinetics of hair growth are not altered.

Waxing

This is one of the oldest methods known. Typically, the wax is preheated, applied to the area to be treated, allowed to cool, and then stripped off, taking the embedded hair with it. Some 'cold' waxes are available that act in the same way. Glucose and zinc oxide waxing has the advantage of lasting up to several weeks before a repeat is required. Only relatively long hair can be treated in this way. Some women find it painful and irritating. It is more often used by beauticians than in the home. The process known as sugaring works on similar principles.

Plucking

This is really satisfactory only for individual or small groups of scattered coarse hairs. It is useful for sparse nipple or abdominal hair. It is usually done with tweezers. As with waxing, it requires to be repeated only every few weeks. The widely advertised electronic or radiofrequency tweezers are little more

than 'sophisticated' ways of plucking. Side effects of plucking include hypopigmentation, folliculitis and even scarring.

Chemical hair removers

These are now widely used for superfluous hair removal from most sites, including the face, although their use there is limited by their irritancy potential. Sulphides and stannites, widely used in the past, have now been largely superseded by substituted mercaptans. Sulphides are unsatisfactory – both because of skin irritancy and because of their odour (due to hydrogen sulphide), generated particularly when the preparation is washed off; however, strontium sulphide preparations are still available. Substituted thiols (mercaptans) form the basis of virtually all modern chemical depilatory preparations. They are slower in action than the sulphides, but are safe enough for facial use if necessary. Thioglycolates are used in a concentration of 2–4% and typically act within 5–15 minutes. Of the thioglycolates, the calcium salt is most favoured, since it is the least irritant – the pH is maintained by an excess of calcium hydroxide, which also acts to prevent the excess alkalinity known to irritate the skin. Attempts to formulate products that accelerate the rather slow thioglycolate action have not been particularly successful. Modern preparations are available in foam, cream, liquid and aerosol forms, the one chosen depending on personal preference. Since thioglycolates attack keratin, not specifically hair, they may have adverse effects on the epidermis if manufacturers' recommendations are not adhered to; it is generally suggested that a small test site should first be treated in order to prevent more extensive irritant reactions in susceptible individuals.

Electrolysis[6]

All the above methods are temporary; the only practical permanent treatment before the advent of lasers was 'electrolysis'. This involves passing a fine wire needle into the hair follicle and destroying the bulb with an electric current passed along it – the hair is loosened and plucked from each treated follicle. Disposable needles should be used to prevent transmission of infection. Either a galvanic or modified high-frequency electric current is used. Galvanic electrolysis is slower, but destroys more follicles in one treatment. High-frequency current (electro-coagulation) is quicker, but more regrowth is seen with this method. Relatively cheap, battery-operated machines have been developed for home use. These have all the disadvantages and potential hazards of those used by electrolysists, with the added problem of an amateur operator.

The limitations of electrolysis in skilled hands are those of cost and time; even the best operators can only deal with 25–100 hairs per sitting and hair regrows in up to 40% of the follicles treated. Shaving, a few days prior to electrolysis, increases the number of hairs in anagen and these are more easily destroyed. In general, electrolysis is mostly used for localized, coarse facial hair, and alternative methods are employed for excess hair on other body sites. Apart from regrowth of hair, the problems that can occur with this mode of hair removal include discomfort during treatment, perifollicular inflammation and scarring, punctate hyperpigmentation and, rarely, bacterial infection.

In a controlled investigation carried out to compare the results of electrolysis with those of diathermy, permanent destruction of the hairs could be achieved by either method, and the time required for the total destruction of all hair roots in a given area was the same; but the diameter of hairs regrowing after diathermy was greater than that of hairs regrowing after electrolysis. The results of depilation depend on the skill and dexterity of the operator. In the United Kingdom, in which a Diploma in Medical Electrolysis exists, patients should wherever possible be referred to technicians who have obtained this certification of their proficiency. In the United States, the American Electrolysis Association regulates professional standards.

Lasers[7]

Several different lasers have become available for hair removal (Table 4.8). They vary in the active medium and thus in the wavelength of monochromatic light produced.[2,5–7]

The absorption of the laser light by a specific chromatophore, regardless of the active medium, transforms the energy into heat, the rate and extent of the heating being determined by the power density (power output/effective spot size) and the length of exposure. The thermal damage resulting leads to denaturization or coagulation of the target proteins. The principle of selective thermolysis predicts that this damage will be entirely limited to the given target, if this site gives sufficient selective absorption of light. Thus, because with many lasers, melanin is the target, only pigmented hair follicles will respond.

Up to the present, no follow-up study of laser-treated hair sites has given permanence of hair removal.

To try to increase the number of hairs in anagen, in order to increase hairs 'available' for laser epilation, Liew et al carried out wax epilation 2 weeks before alexandrite laser treatment.[7] The cosmetic improvement at 1 month showed increased cosmetic outcome.

Eflornithine hydrochloride cream (Vaniqa)[8]

Ornithine decarboxylase (ODC) is a key enzyme involved in the synthesis of new hair. Inhibition of this enzyme inhibits cell

Table 4.8 Characteristics of different types of laser

	Energy (nm)	Spot size (mm)	Target
Ruby laser	694	Up to 10	Melanin
Diode	800	9 × 9	Melanin
Alexandrite	755	Up to 12.5	Melanin
Neodymium YAG	1064	10	Topical chromophore

division in the hair bulb and synthetic functions which affect hair growth. Eflornithine is an inhibitor of ODC, and Vaniqa (eflornithine) cream, 11.5%, has also been shown to reduce the rate of hair growth in preclinical studies. Twenty-four weeks of twice daily application led to 70% of subjects showing improvement or better. These studies were only carried out on lower facial and chin hair. Within 8 weeks of the treatment being stopped, the hair growth returned to pretreatment levels.

Systemic antiandrogen therapy

Since hirsutism is a condition mediated by androgens, attempts have been made to ameliorate the growth of hair using drugs with antiandrogenic properties.[3,9] The complete spectrum of therapeutic agents evaluated in the treatment of hirsutism is described below. It is, however, common practice to use cyproterone acetate and spironolactone as first-line therapy for those women whose hirsuties is so severe as to warrant systemic therapy.

It is important that hirsute women are carefully selected prior to initiating therapy for the following reasons. First, the effect on hair growth takes several months to become apparent, and only partial improvements may be expected. Secondly, antiandrogens feminize male fetuses, and it is essential that the women do not become pregnant. Thirdly, these drugs only have a suppressive, and not a curative, effect,

which wears off a few months after cessation of therapy, and so therapy may need to be taken indefinitely if a favourable improvement occurs. Finally, the long-term safety of these drugs is unknown, and tumours in laboratory animals have been reported with several of the following agents.

Cyproterone acetate
Cyproterone acetate (CPA) is both an antiandrogen and an inhibitor of gonadotrophin secretion. It reduces androgen production, increases the metabolic clearance of testosterone and binds to the AR; in addition, long-term therapy is associated with a reduction in cutaneous 5α-reductase activity. CPA is a potent progestogen, but does not reliably inhibit ovulation. It is usually administered with cyclical oestrogens in order to maintain regular menstruation and to prevent conception in view of the risk of feminizing a male fetus.

Several dose regimens have been advocated. Low-dose therapy (Dianette, Schering Health) is an oral contraceptive containing 35 μg ethinylestradiol and 2 mg CPA, taken daily for 21 days in every 28. However, all of the dose-ranging and efficacy studies have been performed using the preparation containing 50 μg ethinylestradiol – this may be relevant, since only the higher dose of oestrogen increases SHBG. Current dosage recommendations for CPA usually advise that 50 or 100 mg CPA should be administered for 10 days/cycle. However, there have now been many dose-ranging studies suggesting that there is no dose effect. Objective studies comparing Dianette with and without extra CPA found no difference, either in the reduction of the overall hirsuties grade or in the reduction in hair shaft diameter.

Side effects of CPA include weight gain, fatigue, loss of libido, mastodynia, nausea, headaches and depression. All of these are more frequent with a higher dose. Contraindications to its use are the same as for the contraceptive pill, and include cigarette smoking, age, obesity and hypertension.

Spironolactone

Spironolactone has several antiandrogenic pharmacological properties. It reduces the bioavailability of testosterone by interfering with its production, and increases its metabolic clearance. It binds to the AR, and like CPA, long-term therapy is associated with a reduction in cutaneous 5α-reductase activity. It was an act of serendipity that demonstrated its therapeutic advantage in hirsutism. A 19-year-old hirsute woman with PCOS was treated with spironolactone (200 mg daily) for concurrent hypertension, and she noted after 3 months that she needed to shave less frequently. This report was soon followed by studies demonstrating that spironolactone reduced testosterone production and subjectively reduced hair growth in hirsute women. Different dose schedules of spironolactone have been studied, varying between 50 and 200 mg taken either daily or cyclically (daily for 3 weeks in every 4). Within this dose range, the one chosen will depend on the severity of the hirsuties.

> **Cyproterone acetate and spironolactone are fairly equal in suppressing hirsutism**

Corticosteroids

These are first-line therapy for congenital adrenal hyperplasia, and were the first endocrine therapies to be employed in the treatment of hirsuties with the rationale of suppressing the production of adrenal androgens. Corticosteroids are effective in reducing plasma androgen levels, but there are contradictory reports regarding their therapeutic effect on hair growth.

Medroxyprogesterone acetate

Medroxyprogesterone acetate (MPA) is a synthetic progestogen that was introduced as an anovulatory agent because of its ability to block gonadotrophin secretion. It reduces androgen levels by reducing the production of testosterone and increasing its metabolic clearance.

A comparison of topical (0.2% ointment) with systemic therapy either by intramuscular injection (150 mg every 6 weeks) or by subcutaneous injection (100 mg every 6 weeks) of MPA gave a beneficial response in most patients. MPA given alone may result in menorrhagia.

Desogestrel

This is the progestogen used in the Marvelon contraceptive pill (Organon Ltd), which contains 30 μg ethinylestradiol and 150 mg desogestrel. All the studies undertaken have reported subjective and/or objective reductions in hair growth of 20–25% after 6–9 months of therapy, with a high degree of patient satisfaction.

Ketoconazole

This is a potent inhibitor of adrenal and ovarian steroid synthesis. There have been only isolated reports of its use in hirsuties, but these have demonstrated a marked reduction in hair growth after 6 months. However, this treatment cannot be recommended, in view of the risks of hepatic toxicity during long-term therapy.

Gonadotrophin-releasing hormone agonists

Gonadotrophin-releasing hormone (GnRH) agonists inhibit LH production and this results in profound suppression of androgen production. These agents are presently under investigation, but preliminary studies suggest that they effectively reduce hair growth and acne in women with PCOS.

Cimetidine

This is a weak antiandrogen as mediated by AR-binding studies. A study of patients with idiopathic hirsuties demonstrated a marked reduction in hair growth, using hair weight, whereas no such effect was seen in controls given only a placebo.

Bromocriptine

This is a dopamine agonist, and long-term therapy with it regulates menstrual cycle length, but 12 months, therapy produced no measurable effect on linear hair growth in women with polycystic ovaries.

Finasteride

Finasteride blocks enzyme 5α-reductase type 2, thereby preventing the conversion of testosterone to the more potent DHT. It has been found to be beneficial in the treatment of hirsutism and is well tolerated. Using 5 mg of finasteride daily has shown a reduction in hair within 3–6 months and was as effective as flutamide and CPA in early studies; however, when used with oral contraceptives, it can increase levels of cholesterol.[10]

Flutamide

Flutamide acts as a pure antiandrogen and works by blocking the androgen P450 receptor. Treatment with 250 mg of flutamide twice weekly for a year has shown a reduction in Ferriman–Gallwey score to what is considered normal. Liver toxicity is a side effect and monitoring is required.

Metformin

Insulin-lowering drugs, such as metformin, have been used successfully to treat hirsutism related to PCOS. Metformin has been shown to reduce insulin resistance, reduce free testosterone levels, increase SHBG and help weight loss.

Weight loss

Because of excess testosterone and insulin resistance, losing weight can be quite challenging for women with PCOS. These women truly have a metabolic cause for their extra weight and many follow a low-carbohydrate diet designed to lose or maintain weight. However, weight loss achieved through dietary changes and exercise can help women with PCOS in several ways as losing weight reduces a person's risk of cardiovascular disease and type 2 diabetes mellitus, which reduces the ovarian production of testosterone.

REFERENCES

1. Wendelin DS, Pope DN, Mallory SB (2003) Hypertrichosis, *J Am Acad Dermatol* **48:** 161–179.
2. Dawber RPR (2002) Hirsuties, *J Gender Spec Med* **5**: 34–42.
3. Trueb RM (2002) Causes and management of hypertrichosis, *Am J Clin Dermatol* **3(9):** 617–627.
4. Homberg R (2002) What is polycystic ovarian syndrome? A proposal for a consensus on the definition and diagnosis of PCOS, *Human Reprod* **17:** 2495–2499.
5. Simpson NB, Barth JH (1997) Hair patterns: hirsutism and androgenetic alopecia. In: *Diseases of the hair and scalp*, 3rd edn, ed. Dawber RPR (Oxford, Blackwell Science) pp 67–122.
6. Richards RN, Meharg GE (1995) Electrolysis: observations from 13 years and 140 000

hours of experience, *J Am Acad Dermatol* **33:** 662–666.

7. Liew SH (2002) Laser hair removal: guidelines for management, *Am J Clin Dermatol* **3:** 107–115.

8. Barman Balfour JA, McClellan K (2001) Topical eflornithine, *Am J Clin Dermatol* **2:** 197–201.

9. Dawber RPR (1998) Treatment of androgen-related hair disorders: antiandrogens. In: *Dermatologic therapy*, ed. Olsen EA (Copenhagen, Munksgaard) pp 63–67.

10. Wong IL, Morris RS, Chang L (1995) A prospective randomised trial comparing finasteride to spironolactone in the treatment of hirsute women, *J Clin Endocrinol Med* **80:** 233–238.

5 Alopecia areata

AETIOLOGY

Alopecia areata (AA) accounts for up to 2% of new dermatological outpatient attendances in the UK and USA. It is not at present possible to attribute cases of AA to a single cause. Among the many factors that appear to be implicated are the patient's genetic constitution, the atopic state, non-specific immune and organ-specific auto-immune reactions, and possibly emotional stress. The process can be inhibited to a variable extent by several very different therapeutic measures: corticosteroids, local irritants, photochemotherapy, induction of contact dermatitis, or oral ciclosporin. The different chemistries and modes of action of these therapies have opened new channels of research. However, recent studies have done no more than reinforce the generally held belief that both genetic predisposition and the atopic state influence prognosis, but the triggering mechanisms remain obscure.

The incidence of a family history of AA has been reported as from 4.27% up to 9%. The mode of inheritance is thought to be autosomal dominant with variable penetrance. Racial factors may also be important; for example, AA has been found to be common among Japanese in Hawaii. There have been several studies of AA in twins, with some pairs showing concurrence in onset. HLA studies have shown conflicting results, from no increase in class 1 HLA markers in some series to increased HLA-DR4 and DR5 (DRW11) or DQ in others. Various explanations have been proposed for an association between certain HLA haplotypes and AA. Molecular mimicry might erroneously initiate or maintain an immune response directed to autoantigens, and certain haplotypes might present antigens more efficiently to helper T cells. Combinations of some of the already mentioned haplotypes may be associated with a more severe course of AA. Certain haplotypes have been negatively associated with AA, and some appeared to be associated with a better clinical response to immunotherapy.

The association between AA and the atopic state has been confirmed in many studies. AA is significantly associated with Down's syndrome, in which susceptibility to autoimmunity is well known. There is widespread agreement with the hypothesis that AA is an autoimmune disease despite the fact that the evidence is at best circumstantial. It should be recognized that no specific circulating organ-specific autoantibody of any pathogenic relevance has yet been found. Support for an immune mechanism has come from three main areas of research: autoimmune diseases, humoral immunity and cell-mediated immunity.

Thyroid disease is the most frequently described disease in association with AA, but the published figures are contradictory, i.e. from 8% with clinical disease to 24% with abnormal thyroid function tests. Reliable statistics based on the prospective study of a large number of patients are lacking. Other 'autoimmune' associations related to AA include Hashimoto's disease, pernicious anaemia, Addison's disease, testicular atrophy, vitiligo, lupus erythematosus, rheumatoid arthritis, polymyalgia rheumatica, myasthenia gravis, ulcerative colitis, lichen planus and the candida–polyendocrinopathy syndrome.

> **Alopecia areata is probably a specific autoimmune disease, but is not yet confirmed as such**

Studies of organ-specific antibodies in AA have given conflicting results, perhaps due to small groups of patients and controls and differing methodology. Increased circulating thyroid, gastric parietal and smooth muscle cell autoantibodies may be found.

Studies of cell-mediated immunity in AA also yield an inconsistent picture. Again, small studies may have led to conflicting results. Circulating total T-cell numbers have been reported to be reduced or normal, and suppressor T-cell numbers have been variously reported to be reduced, normal or increased. Non-antigen-specific spontaneous and antibody-dependent cell-mediated cytotoxic responses of peripheral blood lymphocytes have also been reported to be increased. This conflict is explainable if one accepts the general statement that a reduction in the numbers of circulating T cells occurs in AA, the level of reduction being related to disease severity or the evolution of the disease over time. Similarly, the impairment of helper T-cell function and the change in suppressor T-cell numbers may also reflect changes in disease activity.

The strongest direct evidence for autoimmunity comes from the consistent findings of a lymphocytic infiltrate in and around hair follicles (Figures 5.1, 5.2) and Langerhans' cells have also been seen in the peribulbar region. Biopsies from scalps of patients treated with the contact allergen diphencyprone and oral and topical minoxidil have shown a reduction in the peribulbar T-cell population in regrowing AA but no change in the absence of regrowth. Direct immunofluorescent examination has demonstrated antibodies to various hair follicle components in AA, but their significance remains controversial. No response of lymphocytes from patients with AA to crude scalp extract in vitro has been demonstrated, but other in vitro studies found ectopic expression of MHC type II antigen HLA-DR by epithelial cells in the presumptive cortex and root sheaths of hair follicles in active lesions of AA. This is thought to represent a mechanism by which cells may present their own specific surface antigens to sensitized MHC-restricted T-inducer cells.

AA therefore appears to belong to the group of organ-specific autoimmune diseases. There is a shared hereditary susceptibility, an increased frequency of organ-specific antibodies and an altered T-cell regulation of the immune response in patients with AA. However, unlike most organ-specific autoimmune diseases, specific, aetiologically important, direct activity against hair follicle components has yet to be demonstrated in a clinically relevant situation. Further research in this area is clearly required. Prospective long-term studies and the relationship between lymphocytes and disease activity are worthy of further attention.

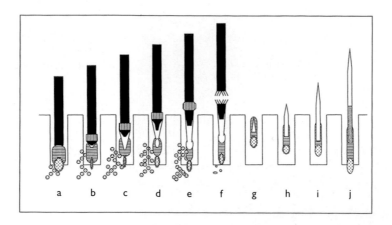

Figure 5.1

Alopecia areata. At any time during anagen the hair follicle can be the centre of an inflammatory process initiated by lymphocytes (a). The consequences of the penetration of invading lymphocytes into the follicular structure and the local delivery of cytotoxic substances are sudden shrinkage of the dermal papilla, arrest of the normal differentiation programme of keratinization and pigmentation, induction of apoptotic bodies in the outer root sheath and narrowing of the hair shaft (b). The density of the infiltrate increases with time and a mixed population of lymphocytes continues to organize toxic conditions for the hair follicle (c). An accelerated telogen stage is initiated (d). When the hair moves upwards, the fragilized segment (a consequence of the sudden arrest of the normal differentiation process) reaches the scalp surface (e), which results in hair breakage (f). When such hairs are examined, they look like exclamation marks: this is a pathognomonic sign of the expanding patch of alopecia. When the inflammation decreases, a new hair cycle starts (g) and the thin, newly synthesized hair shaft merges at the scalp surface (h). If the infiltrate disappears either spontaneously or after treatment, the vellus hairs (h) eventually grow further into terminal-type hairs (i, j) or after a short vellus cycle the hair follicle initiates a terminal-type pigmented hair shaft. The immune process may, however, be able to maintain the follicle in the active process of AA. If so, the hair cycle does not progress beyond anagen stage 3–4 (g). A chronic phase would develop when the infiltrate prevents progression of the root downwards. Very short hair cycles might occur without clinically visible hair production (repeat g–h–g–h . . .).

A wealth of case lore suggests that stress may be an important precipitating factor in some cases of AA. Attempts at objective evaluation using standard psychiatric procedures such as the Rorschach test have shown over 90% of patients with AA to be psychologically abnormal and up to 29% to have psychological factors and family situations that may have affected the onset or course of the disease. Alleged cures by suggestion or sleep therapy have been claimed to support the stress hypothesis. The application of the Bernereuter personality index in AA showed a 'feeling of inferiority, introspection and a need for encouragement', but whether this is associated with induction of AA or is only a behavioural consequence of the disease is still unclear.

There have been many unsuccessful attempts to induce experimentally patches

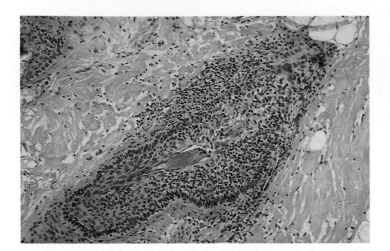

Figure 5.2
Alopecia areata – a catagen hair
follicle surrounded by the
lymphocyte 'swarm'.

of AA. The athymic nude or SCID mouse
might be a useful model in which to study
AA. Especially, transfer of specific human
autologous subsets of T cells into the
system induced AA in donor scalp grafts as
opposed to transfer of serum factors that did
not affect human hair growth in the grafted
scalp samples. Ciclosporin A, a potent modulator of T-cell activity, stimulated hair
growth in nude mice. Hair grafts from
patients with AA and alopecia universalis
have been transplanted successfully on to
athymic nude mice and hair regrowth within
the grafts was stimulated by ciclosporin A.
Both findings are indirect evidence of the
pathogenetic role of the infiltrate. Indeed, as
infiltrating cells in the graft are diluted in the
host, the inhibition of human hair growth is
relaxed. This process is accelerated when
ciclosporin A is applied. Interesting work in
progress includes the alopecia (DEBR) rat,
which loses hair in association with a
marked peri- and intrafollicular infiltrate.
However, each animal model must be evaluated with its own biological specificities; in
the DEBR rats, cell infiltration precedes the
appearance of antibodies, whereas in
C3H/HeJ mice the sequence appears to be
reversed. Interestingly, using these rodent
models, transplantation of AA skin onto

unaffected recipient animals was followed
by disseminated AA in the recipient animal.
The same experiments performed on IL10
knockout recipients also demonstrated that
functionally normal inflammatory pathways
are necessary for the expansion of AA. In
man there is little evidence that a humoral
response would be clinically significant.
Even though not an absolute proof, spread
of AA into hair follicle transplants taken
from a non-affected scalp area and placed
in an AA-affected area documents the
importance of the local infiltrate in this
process.

PATHOLOGY AND PATHODYNAMICS

It is proposed that AA begins with inflammatory infiltration of the deeper parts of the
transient segment of the hair follicle. This
explains why the condition remains reversible. Then AA progresses as a wave
extending centrifugally to the surrounding
follicles, which enter catagen/telogen prematurely, and this has become a widely
accepted view (Figure 5.1). Anagen/telogen
ratios vary considerably with the stage and

duration of the disease process. Biopsy specimens taken early in the course of the disease show the majority of follicles in telogen or late catagen. Some anagen hair bulbs are situated at a higher level in the dermis than normal. A peribulbar lymphocytic infiltrate is seen around follicles, this being more dense in early lesions, consisting predominantly of T cells with increased numbers of Langerhans' cells. The infiltrate disappears during regrowth but the sequence of events is unknown. Established lesions show no decrease in follicle numbers. Anagen development is halted when the inner root sheath has assumed a conical shape with evidence of early cortical differentiation but no cortical keratinization. This stage is equivalent to anagen III, which is equivalent to the embryonic development stage III. Characteristic abnormalities of the hair shaft in AA have been recognized for over a century. Pathognomonic are the exclamation mark hairs, which are, however, not always present. They are club hairs of normal calibre and pigmentation, but the distal ends are ragged and frayed. Below their broken tips they taper towards a small but otherwise normal club. In the areas showing early regrowth, some follicles contain multiple fine hair shafts. The single consistent histological feature is the presence of a dense peribulbar and intrafollicular lymphocytic infiltrate. The upper, permanent portion of the hair follicle may also be involved in the infiltrate either in anagen or telogen. Lesional anagen follicles demonstrate injury which is confined to keratinocytes in the presumptive cortex in the anagen III stage. In an extension of this work, a hypothetical model has been proposed which satisfies the histological evidence and explains the formation of exclamation mark hairs and the non-destructive nature of the disease.

Electron microscopic studies of AA have revealed that lesional anagen follicles have evidence of non-specific injury to matrix cells around the upper pole of the dermal papilla and to cells of the presumptive cortex. Degenerative changes in the suprapapillary matrix are also present, showing aberrant expression of HLA-DR in cells of the precortical matrix and presumptive cortex. This suggests that the presence of HLA-DR antigen in cells of the precortical matrix provides evidence that this site could be of fundamental importance in the pathogenesis of AA and may be the primary target for the disease process.

The concept of fundamental damage occurring in the cells of the precortical matrix and the presumptive cortex does permit explanation of the alterations in the hair cycle. AA affects the follicle in anagen but does not cause an abrupt cessation of mitotic activity in the matrix; why non-pigmented hairs are relatively spared remains an enigma (Figure 5.3). Once in telogen the follicle is thought to be 'safe', but when re-entry into anagen takes place the attack is resumed, anagen development can go no

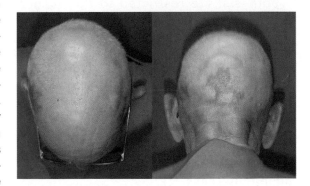

Figure 5.3
Combined androgenetic alopecia and AA. Preservation of pigmented hairy islands in the crown of this man makes the disease more visible. Although balding is associated with less hair cycling, it does not prevent extension of AA . . . it makes AA clinically less visible!

further, and the follicle returns prematurely to telogen. There is therefore a cyclical process, which may explain why follicles are not destroyed permanently. The variations observed in the number of normal telogen hairs, dystrophic hairs and exclamation mark hairs can be interpreted by the postulate that the follicle can respond in three different ways to pathological trauma depending on the severity of the insult. At its most severe the process damages and weakens the hair in the keratogenous zone and at the same time precipitates the follicle into catagen and then telogen. Such hairs break when the keratogenous zone reaches the surface of the scalp; these are later extruded as exclamation mark hairs. Alternatively, a follicle may simply be precipitated into normal catagen and subsequently be shed as a club hair. Such follicles may then produce dystrophic anagen hairs. Finally, it is possible that some follicles are injured just sufficiently to induce dystrophic changes, while they continue to grow in the anagen phase. Attacks, according to the currently available evidence and hypothesis, are restricted to the anagen phase of the growth cycle. Growth is indeed associated with a lot of activities, cell division being the most evident, but also reactivation of pigmentation, modulation of many receptors and secretion of many bioactive substances (e.g. growth factors). This dramatic modification of the local ecosystem associated with growth and pigmentation might be a trigger for immune reactivation of resident or circulating immune cells.

The nature of the infiltrate shows variation according to the course of the disease, but the T4/T8 ratio is positive. The follicular microenvironment is profoundly modified. There is overexpression of HLA class II antigens and ICAM-1, especially in hair matrix and precortical cells, and also in dermal papilla cells. In the microvascular system there is increased expression of various adhesion molecules between endothelial cells or between these cells and other cells such as leucocytes (ICAM-1, ELAM-1, VCAM-1), allowing easier transit into the dermal compartment. As these compartments are interconnected, there is evidence of systemic activity as well (increased numbers and higher proliferative index of activated T cells, and increased circulating IL2 receptors). The definitive and orderly sequence of primary and secondary changes eventually induced by the release of cytokines (IFN-γ or TNF-α induction of HLA class II antigen expression; IFN-γ, TNF-α and TGF-β inhibition of hair bulb proliferation) by the activated T cells is not yet available.

Most authorities regard AA as a clinicopathological entity, but the bewildering variety of its associated diseases and the unpredictability of its course would be more readily explained if AA were a heterogeneous clinical syndrome. Ikeda's classification, which takes into account other clinical features in addition to the alopecia itself, together with observations in Holland and the UK generally supporting Ikeda's hypothesis, suggests that there may be considerable geographical variation in the relative incidence of the various types of AA. Ikeda's classification categorizes AA into the following four types (as recorded in Japan):

- *Type I:* the common type, accounting for 83% of patients. It occurs mainly between the ages of 20 and 40 years, and usually runs a total course of less than 3 years. Individual patches tend to regrow in less than 6 months, and alopecia totalis develops in only 6% of patients.
- *Type II:* the atopic type, accounting for 10% of patients. The onset is usually in childhood and the disease runs a lengthy course in excess of 10 years. Individual patches tend to persist for

1 year and alopecia totalis develops in 75% of patients.

- *Type III:* the prehypertensive type, accounting for 4% of patients. It occurs mainly in young adults and runs a rapid course, with alopecia totalis developing in 39% of patients.
- *Type IV:* the 'combined' type, accounting for 5% of patients. It occurs mainly in patients over 40 years and runs a prolonged course, but results in alopecia totalis in only 10% of patients.

There has been little support for Ikeda's prehypertensive type, but most authors agree that the presence of atopy confers a poor prognosis and slow rate of remission. Almost all the published work on AA regards it as a single entity. The clinical description below follows this convention since Ikeda's approach to the disease has not yet been applied sufficiently widely for its validity to be established. Ikeda's clinical subtypes may at least be useful for clinical, prognostic and therapeutic comparative studies.

The available statistics on age and sex incidence are all based on hospital attendance figures and therefore do not reflect the true incidence of AA. The reported sex incidence has varied widely from males outnumbering females by 3 to 1, through equality to twice as common in females. In Italy, observations confined to children with AA showed less than 1% of 213 cases beginning in the first year (Figure 5.4), and the peak incidence in the fourth and fifth years. Onset before the age of 2 years has been recorded in under 2% of cases in North America.

In summary, if all clinical variants of AA are grouped together, the hospital statistics of most countries show the sexes to be approximately equally affected, and the onset to occur at any age, with the peak incidence lying at some point between the ages of 20 and 50 years.

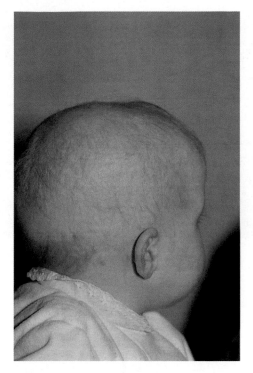

Figure 5.4
Alopecia totalis in an infant.

CLINICAL FEATURES

The characteristic initial lesion of AA is commonly a circumscribed, totally bald, smooth patch. It is often noticed by chance by a parent, hairdresser or friend (Figure 5.5). A very mild inflammation has occasionally been noticed, and the skin may be pinkish and slightly oedematous. The scalp is more elastic, but whether this is specifically associated with inflammation or is secondary to the lack of hair in those areas is not known. Exclamation mark hairs may be present at the margin of the lesion (Figures 5.6, 5.7), where hairs which appear normal may also be very readily extracted. Subsequent progress is very varied. The initial patch may regrow within a few months, or further patches may appear after an interval of several weeks and then in a cyclical fashion

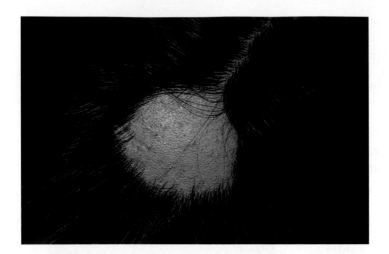

Figure 5.5
Alopecia areata – a single patch.

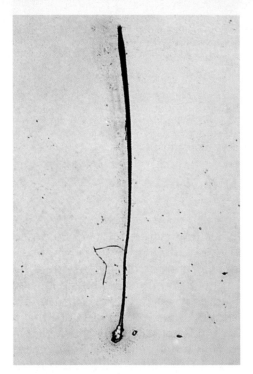

Figure 5.6
Exclamation mark hair from an active area.

the scalp has been reported within 2 days of onset. However, diffuse hair loss may occur over part or all of the scalp without the development of bald areas. Regrowth is often at first fine and unpigmented (Figure 5.19), but usually the hairs gradually resume their normal calibre and colour. Regrowth in one region of the scalp may occur while the alopecia is extending in others.

The scalp is the first affected site in over 60% of cases. In dark-haired men patches in the beard and other sites are conspicuous and in such individuals are often the first to be noticed (Figures 5.9, 5.10). The eyebrows and eyelashes are lost in many cases of AA and may be the only sites affected. The term 'alopecia totalis' is applied to total or almost total loss of scalp hair (Figure 5.4) and alopecia universalis is the loss of all body hair. The extension of alopecia along the scalp margin is known as ophiasis, a 'serpent-like' spread round the scalp edges, starting from the occipital area (Figure 5.16). AA strictly confined to one-half of the body has been reported after a head injury.

(Figure 5.8). A succession of discrete patches may rapidly become confluent by the diffuse loss of remaining hair (Figures 5.9–5.19). In some cases the initial hair loss is diffuse and total denudation of

PROGRESS

The outlook for the sufferer of AA is even more gloomy than is generally recognized.

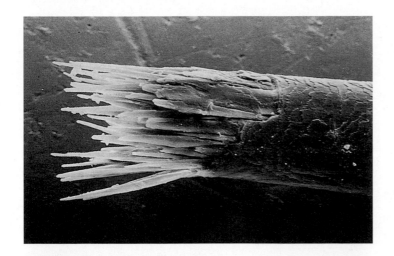

Figure 5.7
Exclamation mark hair from an active area showing the frayed tip (scanning electron micrograph).

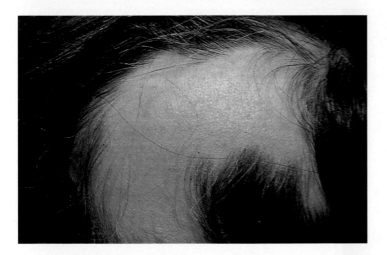

Figure 5.8
Alopecia areata – multiple adjacent patches.

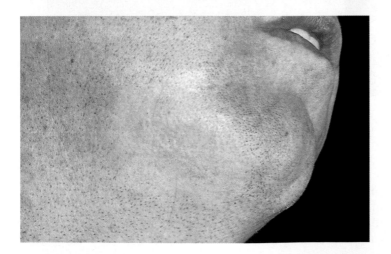

Figure 5.9
Alopecia areata – beard patch.

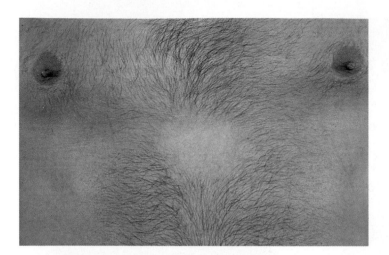

Figure 5.10
Alopecia areata – chest lesion.

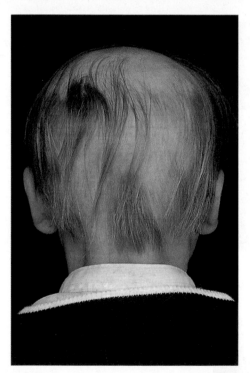

Figure 5.11
Alopecia areata – diffuse pattern.

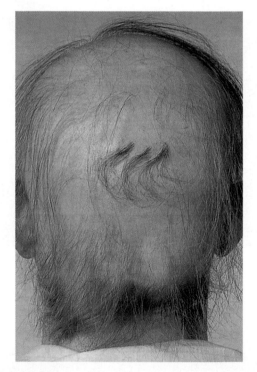

Figure 5.12
Alopecia areata – diffuse pattern.

Further evidence of heterogeneity in AA is provided by the difference in prognosis reported from various countries. In a series in Chicago the duration of the initial attack was less than 6 months in 33% and less than 1 year in 50%, but 33% never recovered from the initial attack. The incidence or relapse in the whole of this series of 230 patients was 86%, but in those followed up for 20 years it was 100%. Of those patients

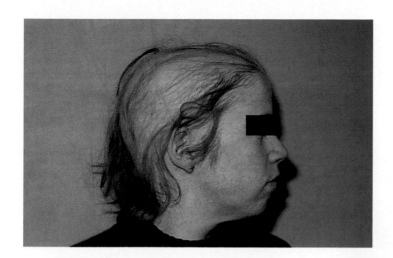

Figure 5.13
Alopecia areata – diffuse pattern.

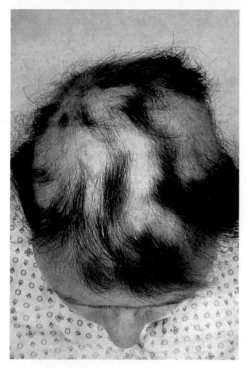

Figure 5.14
Alopecia areata – reticulate pattern.

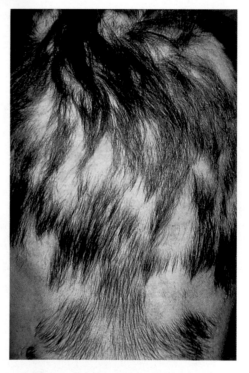

Figure 5.15
Alopecia areata – reticulate pattern.

developing AA before puberty, 50% became totally bald and none recovered. In contrast, only 25% of those developing AA after puberty became totally bald and 5.3% recovered. Workers from the Mayo Clinic reported that only 1% of children and 10% of adults with alopecia totalis showed complete regrowth. In another series complete recovery of alopecia universalis occurred in only 10 of 50 patients, the poorer prognosis

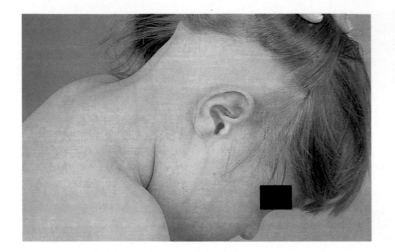

Figure 5.16
Alopecia areata – ophiasis type.

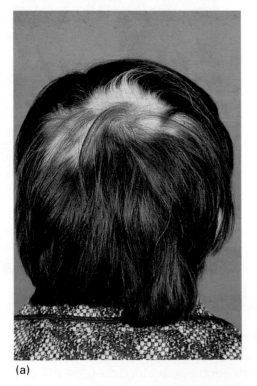

(a)

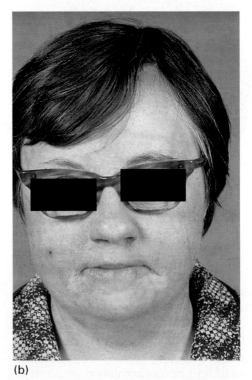

(b)

Figure 5.17
(a, b) Alopecia areata in Down's syndrome patient with hypothyroidism.

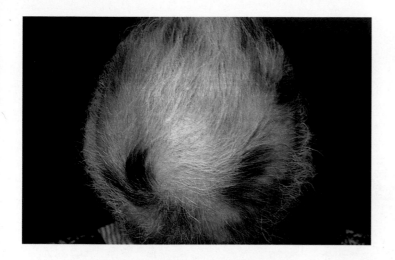

Figure 5.18
Alopecia areata – patchy regrowth of unpigmented hair.

being in cases of prepubertal onset. In no case of AA is a completely confident prognosis justifiable. One woman who lost all her hair at the age of 16 years recovered it almost completely only at the age of 50, despite eight pregnancies.

> **Alopecia areata may selectively attack pigmented hair and cause rapid whitening**

AA in the atopic state undoubtedly has a poor prognosis, and if hair loss is total before puberty it is unlikely to regrow permanently. AA at any age in a non-atopic subject may be given a reasonably good prognosis providing it has remained circumscribed for over 6 months. The ophiasic pattern of AA deserves its bad reputation, particularly if associated with atopy.

White hair in alopecia areata

White hairs may be spared initially by the disease process. Patients with sudden diffuse onset of AA may thus appear to 'go white' over the course of a few days (Figure 5.19). This has been reported in several famous historical personalities. Regrowing hair is often temporarily apigmented (Figures 5.17, 5.18).

ASSOCIATED CLINICAL CHANGES

Nails

The reported incidence of nail dystrophy in AA ranges from 7% to 66%. The nail involvement varies from marked alteration of the nails to diffuse fine pitting (Figure 5.20). It may involve the majority of nails, but solitary nail involvement may also occur. Gross nail dystrophy is said to be proportional to the degree of hair loss. Onychodystrophy may precede or follow resolution of the AA. In some cases the nail dystrophy appears as an isolated feature and affects all the nails (20-nail dystrophy). Surface modifications include ridging with frequent onychorrhexis, cross-fissures, Beau's lines or transverse lines of uniform pits, which may be similar to those seen in psoriasis.

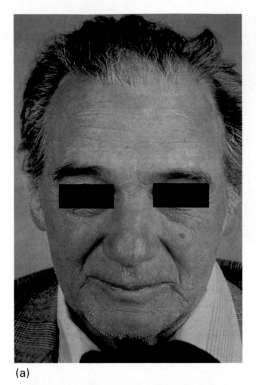

(a)

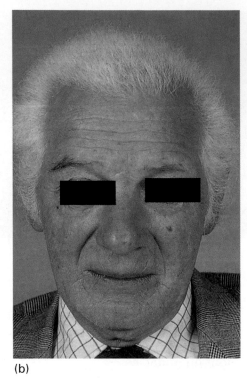

(b)

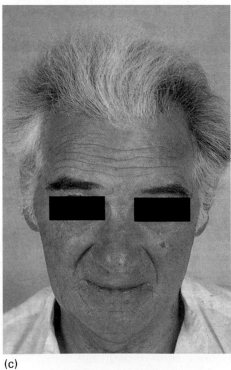

(c)

Figure 5.19
(a) Normal subject. (b) Rapid greying
2 weeks later. (c) Some regrowth.

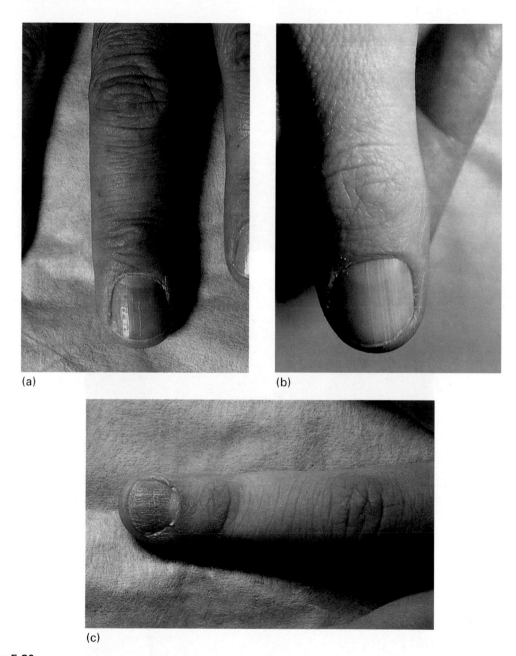

(a)

(b)

(c)

Figure 5.20
(a–h) The spectrum of nail changes associated with AA.

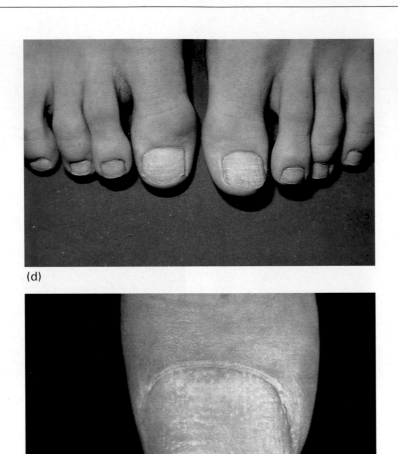

(d)

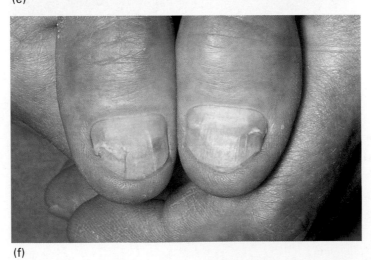

(e)

(f)

Figure 5.20 Continued

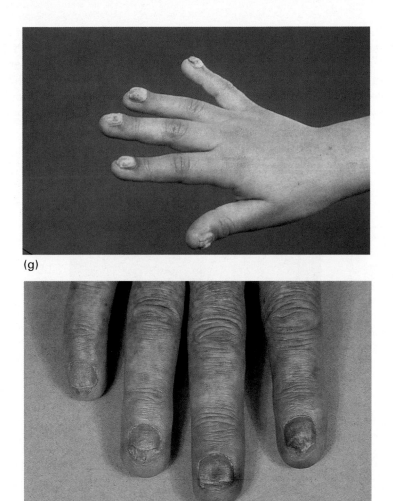

(g)

(h)

Figure 5.20 Continued

Eyes

There are many reports of cataracts in association with alopecia totalis. However, in one study symptomless punctate lens opacities were found with equal frequency in 58 patients with AA and in normal controls. Horner's syndrome, ectopia of the pupil, iris atrophy or tortuosity of the fundal vessels may possibly be linked to AA.

Differential diagnosis

The clinical presentation of a non-scarring alopecia with a clean scalp surface, preserved follicular openings, and a sudden development of a single patch or more extensive alopecia with episodes of spontaneous regrowth is characteristic. Some patients with other diseases may be included by mistake in the AA group. The authors have seen a few patients referred with the diagnosis of AA while the actual disorders were as diverse as triangular alopecia of Sabouraud, atrichia with papules or Marie–Unna hypotrichosis, or an unusual severe symmetrical scarring sebor-rhoea-like dermatitis referred with the diagnosis of AA (Figure 5.21). As will be described later, these disorders have their own characteristics that should help differentiation from AA. In difficult cases a scalp biopsy and discussions between clinician

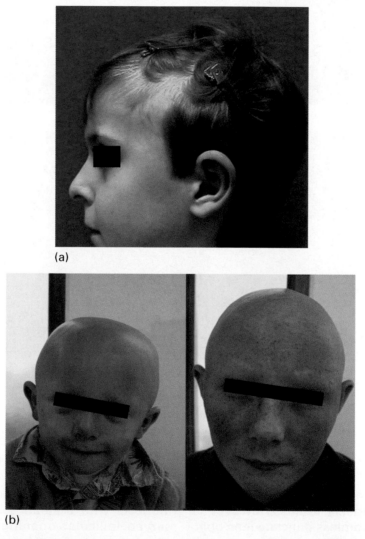

(a)

(b)

Figure 5.21
Patients occasionally referred with the proposed diagnosis of AA. Differential diagnosis includes frequently triangular alopecia of Sabouraud (a) and more exceptional cases of genetic disorders such as atrichia with papules (b) and Marie–Unna hypotrichosis (c) or acquired very unusual severe symmetrical scarring seborrhoea-like dermatitis (d).

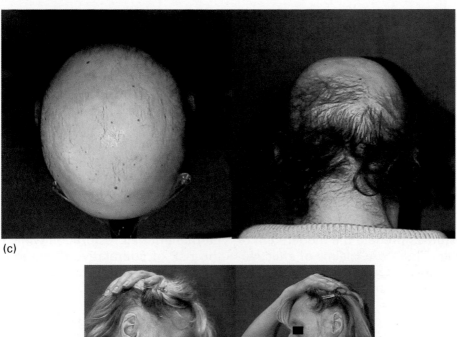

(c)

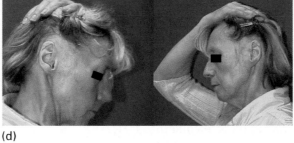

(d)

Figure 5.21 Continued

TREATMENT

The variable and uncertain natural history of AA accounts for the multiplicity of uncritical claims for a large variety of therapeutic procedures. In order to overcome this problem workers have tended to choose patients with alopecia totalis or alopecia universalis because these conditions tend to run a more stable course, and are traditionally more difficult to treat. Although there is an undoubted relationship between AA and alopecia totalis or alopecia universalis, the latter conditions are not necessarily good

and pathologist should help further separation of true AA.

models in which to test for therapeutic efficacy in AA. This approach treats AA as a homogeneous entity, which may not be justified. Ikeda's type I might be expected to run a relatively benign course with a high natural remission and only 6% developing alopecia totalis, whereas Ikeda's original type II (atopic) group are much less fortunate with 75% developing alopecia totalis. It seems reasonable, therefore, that future clinical trial design should, at least, separate the atopic subjects before randomization rather than during analysis.

The sad fact that there is no universally proven treatment for AA is evident from the multiplicity of claims for therapeutic success. The analysable evidence is derived from four main types of therapy:

1. non-specific irritants, e.g. dithranol and phenol
2. immune inhibitors, e.g. systemic steroids and PUVA
3. immune enhancers and inhibitors, e.g. contact dermatitis induction (topical diphencyprone) ciclosporin A and inosiplex
4. drugs of unknown action, e.g. minoxidil.

Counter-irritants

Many irritants have been employed in AA, but most studies predate the modern era of clinical trials. Therefore, claims of effectiveness for phenol, benzoyl benzoate and UVB at erythema doses cannot be substantiated. However, claims for dithranol have some scientific support, a good cosmetic response having been shown to occur in 25% of patients with severe AA. However, all the patients experienced pruritus, local erythema and scaling. The intervention of cytokine release from damaged interfollicular or intrafollicular keratinocytes and/or outer root sheath cells might be of importance for the resolution of the inflammatory process.

Systemic corticosteroids

Systemic corticosteroids restore normal hair growth in many cases of AA. The hairs show abrupt repigmentation and thickening without discontinuity of the shaft. Controversy remains, however, as to the justification for prescribing these potentially hazardous drugs, because most cases relapse at some stage during or after withdrawal of treatment. Very high doses, up to 100 mg prednisolone daily, have been recommended, but the universal side effects of steroids are to be expected. More than two-thirds of patients will experience hair

loss after stopping treatment. These problems have prompted other dermatologists to try mixed regimes of systemic, topical and intralesional steroids. In summary, systemic steroids should not be considered, except in a few specific circumstances at the discretion of the prescriber and after obtaining informed consent from the patient declaring that information has been given as to possible secondary effects. The rule of success announced with pulse therapies (milder disease, shorter duration, younger patient) does not fit with the ethics of medical treatment; it raises false hopes for permanent hair restoration while increasing the risk of cumulative damage associated with high-dose repeat or chronic corticosteroid therapy.

> **The best way to treat alopecia areata is possibly not to start! – no treatment is specifically 'curative'**

Topical and intralesional steroids

Attempts to reduce the hazard of systemic steroids have included both topical and intralesional administration. There have been a number of claims for the effectiveness of topical application using fluocinolone and halcinonide and clobetasol propionate. At best, persistent regrowth occurs in those cases in which it might have been expected to occur spontaneously. In some cases troublesome folliculitis and comedo formation may result.

Intralesional steroids have proved more helpful, but the positive indications for their use remain limited. Intralesional triamcinolone suspension is preferred, administered either by needle injection or by jet injection. Intralesional corticosteroids have

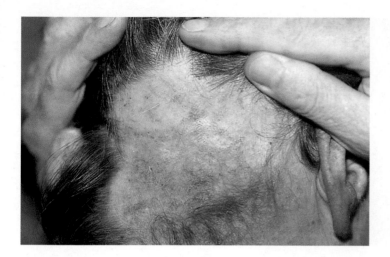

Figure 5.22
Scalp atrophy due to overtreatment of AA with intralesional steroid.

a small but useful role in the management of AA. They can be used to accelerate regrowth in a circumscribed patch of AA which is cosmetically disfiguring or difficult to conceal and can be useful for maintaining regrowth of the eyebrows in alopecia totalis, but great care must be exercised to avoid steroid side effects in the eye. High pressure should also be avoided as loss of vision has been reported, resulting from an infarction caused by crystals in the ophthalmic artery following the use of high pressure in the temporal area. It appears that high pressure pushes fluid containing the crystals of steroids along a line of least resistance, which can alter blood circulation in the territories served by the blood vessels. Atrophy may be an unsightly complication of intralesional corticosteroids and is usually confined to the injection site (Figure 5.22).

Topical immunotherapy

The use of potent sensitizing chemicals to induce and maintain contact dermatitis of the scalp has produced regrowth of hair in some sufferers of AA with both localized and severe forms (Figures 5.23–5.25).

Variable success has been attributed to dinitrochlorobenzene (DNCB), squaric acid dibutyl ester (SADBE) and diphencyprone (DPC) with sporadic reports of success with extracts of the plant *Primula obconica*. Many clinical trials have been carried out with successes from 10% up to 78%, the effect being greatest in localized AA and least in alopecia totalis and alopecia universalis. Patients with a family history of AA, those with a personal or family history of atopy and those who failed to produce a dermatitis reaction all failed to produce good regrowth. Reports of mutagenicity and carcinogenicity of DNCB led to the use of other potent sensitizers free from mutagenic activity which are not likely to be encountered in everyday life or in the workplace. Most recent studies have shown encouraging results with DPC, but many complete failures have also been recorded. It cannot be stated too strongly that such sensitizers are extremely difficult to work with and may cause problems to the pharmacist, to the doctor or nurse applying the treatment, to the patient and to any other individuals who may contact the treated skin!

The mechanism of action of contact sensitization in AA remains speculative. Local immune mechanisms have been suggested.

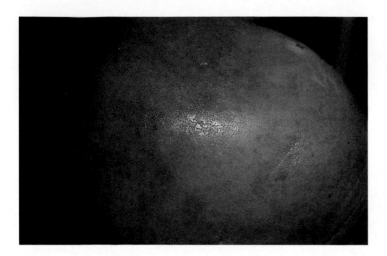

Figure 5.23
Alopecia totalis – no regrowth
following topical DNCB therapy.

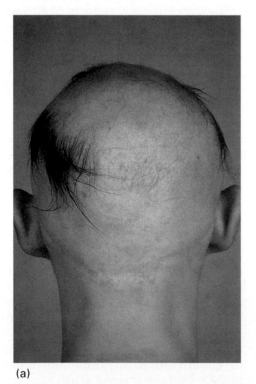

(a)

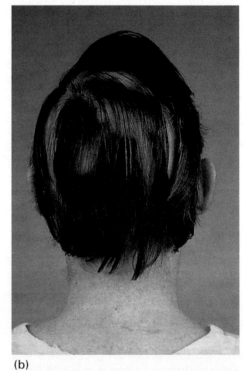

(b)

Figure 5.24
(a) Alopecia areata, almost alopecia totalis, prior to topical diphencyprone (DPC) treatment. (b) Four
months after commencing DPC treatment.

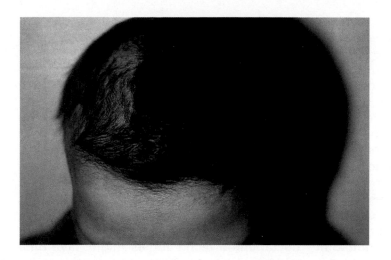

Figure 5.25
DPC treatment – initially to left scalp only and subsequently to right scalp.

It has been proposed that effector T cells are attracted into the area. The occurrence of localized antigen competition has also been suggested, and other workers have extended this theory to claim that repeated application activates non-specific suppressor mechanisms to suppress the effector cells responsible for AA. Once again the effect might be through modulation of epithelial autocrine mechanisms with release of cytokines.

> **It is logical in principle to treat those patients with the best prognosis!**

The role for topical contact sensitization in the treatment of AA is limited. Side effects include pruritus, oedema (especially in the forehead and eyelids), oozing, blistering, secondary infection and urticaria. The rate of response of alopecia totalis seems to be so disappointing that the risks of uncomfortable side effects probably outweigh any benefits, but these methods may be worth trying in patients with tufted, almost total, alopecia and long-standing patchy alopecia.

Photochemotherapy

Hair regrowth may be induced in AA with 8-methoxypsoralen (8-MOP) and sunlight. The use of 8-MOP plus UVA (PUVA) has been claimed to be successful in up to 60% of patients. In a study carried out in France, good responses occurred only when total body irradiation was employed. Up to 30% of patients may respond, but 20–40 treatment exposures may be necessary to achieve benefit. High relapse rates of 50–90% have been reported for all series on stopping therapy. There is a poor response in alopecia totalis. PUVA has many effects on the local immune response within skin, and these may be important in the action of PUVA in AA. Early reports of successful treatment with topical haematoporphyrin plus UVA have yet to be confirmed. Total body PUVA is probably more effective than local irradiation, but since the dose needs to exceed several hundred joules the treatment is rarely justified.

Minoxidil

Minoxidil (2-4-diamino-6-piperidinopyrimidine-3-oxide) is a potent vasodilator used for the treatment of severe hypertension. Its oral use is limited because of a reversible but cosmetically unacceptable hypertrichosis of the face, arms and legs. Preliminary reports of a high success rate with topical minoxidil in AA were followed by double-blind and dose–response studies which were less encouraging – no difference was found between a 3% solution of minoxidil and placebo in moderate, patchy AA. In continuation studies a better response was seen after 64 weeks. The outcome is probably dependent on initial severity. The highest success rate has been obtained by using 5% topical minoxidil solution.

The mechanism of action of minoxidil in AA is also unknown. Evidence points towards an effect on circulating and tissue lymphocytes and hair follicle keratinocytes. Topical minoxidil is yet another therapy whose initial promising reports have not been substantiated.

Immune modulation

Drugs that alter the immune state might be expected to shed some light on the pathogenesis of AA and may also be of therapeutic benefit. Oral ciclosporin A, a powerful modulator of T-cell function, has been shown to produce regrowth in alopecia totalis. However, oral ciclosporin A is potentially both nephro- and hepatotoxic. Topical ciclosporin A has been tried in concentrations from 5% to 10% (w/v) in various oily excipients and produced sporadic patchy regrowth which was little better than placebo. Oral inosiplex has been investigated in uncontrolled studies. It may produce some hair growth but the effect is usually lost within 2–3 weeks of cessation of treatment. Other double-blind, placebo-controlled studies showed a better response than placebo; however, only partial re-growth was seen but growth was maintained in the majority after crossover to placebo.

There is room for properly prepared placebo-controlled clinical trials with new topical immunomodulatory regimes. The challenge is not only in the hands of laboratory researchers and clinicians but also in those of the pharmaceutical companies, who are invited to extend their field of research into an area they are not familiar with. Together with clinical research centres and also patient organizations, cooperation in building up consensus trials and using documented technologies might save time and bring practical therapeutic options for AA sufferers.

SUMMARY

The decision whether or not to treat AA should be made at an early stage. Nothing can justify the prolonged use of expensive placebos. If the prognosis is poor – for example, in a prepubertal atopic with total alopecia – a full explanation and help in adjusting to the problems of wearing a wig will be of far greater value to the child than the unwarranted raising of hopes. However, in the majority of cases in which the prognosis is good, reassurance, aided if necessary by topical or intralesional corticosteroids, can be advised. Systemic corticosteroids are justifiable only in exceptional circumstances. Of the newer therapies, topical DPC currently seems to show the most promise (Figure 5.25) and more sophisticated immune regulatory approaches might lead to proper control of disease activity. It is most logical to treat those patients with an apparently good prognosis in order to lessen the chances of any relapse after response. Reassuring patients with a personal history of severe AA that hair will regrow naturally after

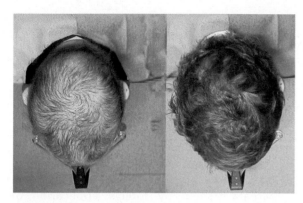

Figure 5.26
Clinically significant initial hair regrowth (left) and almost total (right) restoration in a patient after chemotherapy. In her past history alopecia totalis responded well to topical DPC immunotherapy; chemotherapy-induced hair loss appeared to cause more distress in this 'experienced' AA sufferer than in any other patient!

chemotherapy for cancer is also important (Figure 5.26)

> **Many patients with alopecia areata are enormously encouraged by even transient or partial response to treatment – but medical false optimism may have a negative effect**

FURTHER READING

Barahamani N, de Andrade M, Slusser J, Zhang Q, Duvic M (2002) Interleukin-1 receptor antagonist allele 2 and familial alopecia areata, *J Invest Dermatol* **118:** 335–337.

Freyschmidt-Paul P, McElwee KJ, Happle R, et al (2000) Interleukin-10-deficient mice are less susceptible to the induction of alopecia areata, *J Invest Dermatol* **119:** 980–982.

Freyschmidt-Paul P, Sundberg JP, Happle R, et al (1999) Successful treatment of alopecia areata-like hair loss with the contact sensitizer squaric acid dibutylester (SADBE) in C3H/HeJ mice, *J Invest Dermatol* **113(1):** 61–68.

Friedli A, Salomon D, Saurat JH (2001) High-dose pulse corticosteroid therapy: is it indicated for severe alopecia areata? *Dermatology* **202:** 191–192.

Gilhar A, Landau M, Assy B, et al (2001) Melanocyte-associated T cell epitopes can function as autoantigens for transfer of alopecia areata to human scalp explants on Prkdc(scid) mice, *J Invest Dermatol* **117:** 1357–1362.

Gupta MA, Gupta AK (1998) Depression and suicidal ideation in dermatology patients with acne, alopecia areata, atopic dermatitis and psoriasis, *Br J Dermatol* **139(5):** 846–850.

Happle R (1991) Topical immunotherapy in alopecia areata, *J Invest Dermatol* **96:** 71–72.

Hoting E, Bochm A (1992) Therapy of alopecia areata with diphencyprone, *Br J Dermatol* **127:** 625–629.

Mcdonagh AJ, Tazi-Ahnini R (2002) Epidemiology and genetics of alopecia areata, *Clin Exp Dermatol* **27:** 405–409.

McElwee KJ, Hoffmann R (2002) Alopecia areata – animal models, *Clin Exp Dermatol* **27:** 410–417.

McElwee KJ, Boggess D, King Jr LE, Sundberg JP (1998) Experimental induction of alopecia areata-like hair loss in C3H/HeJ mice using full-thickness skin grafts, *J Invest Dermatol* **111(5):** 797–803.

McElwee KJ, Pickett P, Oliver RF (1996) The DEBR rat, alopecia areata and autoantibodies to the hair follicle, *Br J Dermatol* **134:** 55–63.

Perriard-Wolfensberger J, Pasche-Koo F, Mainetti C, et al (1993), Pulse of methylprednisolone in alopecia areata, *Dermatology* **187:** 282–285.

Seiter S, Ugurel S, Tilgen W, Reinhold U (2001) High-dose pulse corticosteroid therapy in the treatment of severe alopecia areata, *Dermatology* **202:** 230–234.

Shapiro J, Tan J, Ho V, Abbott F, Tron V (1993) Treatment of chronic severe alopecia areata:

a clinical and immunopathologic evaluation, *J Am Acad Dermatol* **29:** 729–735.

Tobin DJ, Fenton DA, Kendall MD (1990) Ultrastructural observations on the hair bulb melanocytes and melanosomes in acute alopecia areata, *J Invest Dermatol* **94:** 803–807.

Tobin DJ, Orentreich N, Fenton DA, Bystryn JC (1994) Antibodies to hair follicles in alopecia areata, *J Invest Dermatol* **102:** 721–724.

Tobin DJ, Sundberg JP, King LE, Boggess D, Bystryn JC (1997) Autoantibodies to hair follicles in C3H/HeJ mice with alopecia areata-like hair loss, *J Invest Dermatol* **109(3):** 329–333.

Tosti A, De Padova MP, Minghetti G, Veronesi S (1986) Therapies versus placebo in the treatment of patchy alopecia areata, *J Am Acad Dermatol* **15:** 209–210.

Tsuboi H, Fujimura T, Katsuoka K (1996) Hair growth in the skin grafts from alopecia areata (AA) grafted onto severe combined immunodeficient (SCID) nude mice, *Hair Research for the Next Millennium*. Editors: D Van Neste, VA Randall, Excerpta Medical International Congress Series 1111. Publ: Elsevier, Amsterdam 265–269.

Van Neste D, de Bruyère M, Breuillard F (1979) Increases of T cell subpopulations in the peripheral blood of patient with alopecia areata treated by topical application of 1-chloro-2:4-dinitrobenzene (DNCB), *Arch Dermatol Res* **266**: 323–325.

Van Neste D, Szapiro E, Breuillard F, Goudemand J (1980) A study of HLA antigens and immune response to DNCB in alopecia areata, *Clin Exp Dermatol* **5**: 389–394.

6 The scaly, sore or itchy scalp

The diseases described in this chapter may seem widely different in pathogenetic terms. They are brought together because their treatment principles frequently overlap and most of them are only controllable: with conditions on the hairy scalp, the aesthetics of treatment must always be carefully considered or compliance may be poor, however good the therapy may seem in purely medical terms. The patient has symptoms to relieve, not (often inexact) disease definitions![1]

PITYRIASIS CAPITIS (DANDRUFF)

The presence of coarse terminal hair on the scalp often makes exact diagnosis of diseases on this site very difficult on clinical judgement alone. Therefore, with inflammatory and infective processes that are easy to diagnose on relatively hairless skin, one should always think in differential diagnostic terms of the hairy scalp. It now seems reasonable to accept pityriasis as near-physiological scaling of the scalp or other hairy regions, which may or may not be fortuitously associated with 'seborrhoea' or with baldness. Pityriasis capitis is popularly known as dandruff (Figure 6.1). Pityriasis is a cosmetic affliction of the newborn, recurring during adolescence and adult life, and is relatively rare and mild in children unless some inflammatory skin disease is present. Its peak incidence and severity are reached at the age of about 20 years and it is quite rare after 50 years. The age incidence suggests that an androgenic influence is important and the level of sebaceous activity may be a factor. However, gross seborrhoea may occur without pityriasis, and, commonly, severe pityriasis may be present without clinically apparent excessive sebaceous activity.

In the normal scalp the horny layer consists of 25–35 fully keratinized and closely coherent cells. In pityriasis there are usually fewer than 10 layers of cells, and these are often parakeratotic and irregularly arranged, with deep crevices resulting in the formation of the flakes visible clinically.

The 'fungal' origin of pityriasis was accepted in the 19th century. *Pityrosporum* yeasts increase in number at puberty. The large numbers of yeasts in pityriasis have been regarded as secondary to the increasing physiological scaling. In other investigations of yeasts in subjects with pityriasis, it was concluded that *Pityrosporum* yeasts were significantly related to pityriasis. It had

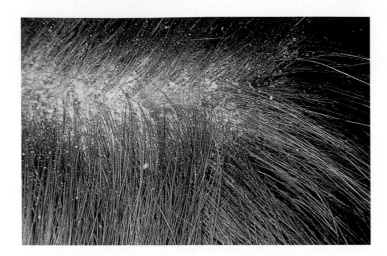

Figure 6.1
Pityriasis capitis.

previously been demonstrated that the application of yeast inhibitors to one-half of the scalp produced a greater reduction in pityriasis than did the application of a bacterial inhibitor to the other half of the same scalp.

Other quantitative studies of the microflora have not finally resolved the problem of their precise role in the production of pityriasis. *Pityrosporum ovale* is more abundant in pityriasis than in the normal scalp, and even more so in seborrhoeic dermatitis.

The balance of evidence suggests that scalp yeasts play no primary role in causing pityriasis capitis but are present in abundance because of the increased availability of scalp 'nutrients'. On historical and scientific grounds, it is possible to present the contrary view, bearing in mind the importance of the good effects of antipityrosporum agents as supporting the infection aetiology.

Clinical features

The clinical appearance is illustrated in Figure 6.1. Small white or grey scales accumulate on the surface of the scalp in localized, more or less segmental, patches, or more diffusely. After removal with an effective shampoo, the scales form again within 4–7 days. The condition first becomes a cos-

metic problem during the second and third decades, but there are long- and short-term variations in its severity. There are also variations in the ease with which the scales become detached and drift 'unaesthetically' among the hair shafts or fall on the collar and shoulders.

In those subjects whose scalp becomes greasy at or after puberty, the seborrhoea binds the scale in a greasy 'paste' and it is no longer shed, but accumulates in small adherent mounds – so-called pityriasis steatoides. The development of clinically evident inflammatory changes in such individuals leads to seborrhoeic dermatitis. Pruritus is not a feature of simple pityriasis. It is very much more common when inflammatory changes develop in the seborrhoeic scalp, and such recurrent episodes may be clearly related to periods of stress, flushing and sweating. Acne necrotica, which may be intensely irritable, can also complicate pityriasis.

Diagnosis

With the notable exception of the greasy scalp of the newborn, the presence of more than very mild pityriasis in a young child throws doubt on the diagnosis. Extreme and persistent scaling, even though it lacks the characteristic features of psoriasis, is always suspect, particularly if there is a family history of this disease. Widespread scaling, sometimes with scarring, may occur in some forms of ichthyosis. At any age, if pruritus is troublesome, pediculosis capitis must be carefully excluded and differentiated from irritant dermatitis with peripilar keratin casts.

Small areas of scaling with dull, broken hair shafts are typical of *Microsporum* ringworm. Localized scaling in children is therefore an indication for examination of the scalp under Wood's light, and of the broken hairs under the microscope. A nervous hairpulling tic may result in twisted and broken hairs of normal texture in a patch of postinflammatory scaling, i.e. trichotillomania. Profuse, sticky, silvery scale suggests pityriasis amiantacea.

Treatment

Pityriasis in its milder forms is a physiological process. The object of treatment is to control it at the lowest possible cost and inconvenience to the patient, appreciating that any procedure found to be effective will need to be repeated at regular intervals.

The evidence presented for *Pityrosporum* yeasts being aetiologically important has converted many clinicians to specific antipityrosporum therapy with imidazole compounds, e.g. Nizoral shampoo (ketoconazole).

In the average case, one of the many proprietary shampoos may be found effective. Preparations containing zinc pyrithione or zinc omadine, which reduce the yeast populations, are generally very easy to use in the cosmetic sense.

PITYRIASIS AMIANTACEA

Pityriasis amiantacea is a reaction of the scalp, often without evident cause, in which thick 'asbestos-like' scales accumulate. It may complicate seborrhoeic dermatitis, psoriasis or lichen simplex. Cases which some dermatologists would accept as early psoriasis are labelled pityriasis amiantacea by others. If such cases are excluded there is no definite association between pityriasis amiantacea and psoriasis. Pityriasis amiantacea may occur at any age, but the average age at which it occurs is 25 (range 5–40) years.

Pathology

The most consistent findings are spongiosis, parakeratosis, migration of lymphocytes into the epidermis, and a variable degree of acanthosis. In cases with severe inflammation, there is synchronization of the hair cycles. Hairs in telogen are, however, fixed in the thick scales and retained for a longer period of time than usual. New cycles are initiated and regrowing hairs can be found in patches which are synchronized, underneath the compact parakeratotic scales. The essential features responsible for the asbestos-like scaling are diffuse hyperkeratosis and parakeratosis together with follicular keratosis, which surrounds each hair with a sheath of horn.

Clinical features

The clinical appearance is illustrated in Figures 6.2–6.5. Masses of sticky, silvery scales, overlapping like the tiles on a roof, adhere to the scalp and are attached in layers to the shafts of the hairs which they surround. The underlying scalp may be red and moist or may show simple erythema and scaling, or the features of psoriasis, seborrhoeic dermatitis or lichen simplex.

A relatively common form seen mainly in young girls complicates recurrent or chronic fissuring behind one or both ears. The scales

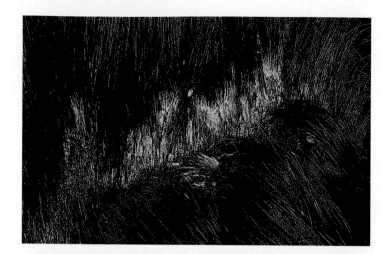

Figure 6.2
Pityriasis amiantacea.

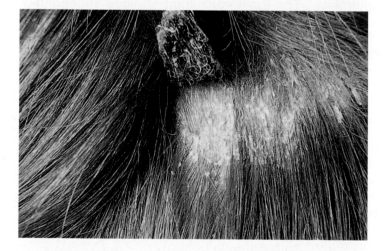

Figure 6.3
Another example of pityriasis amiantacea.

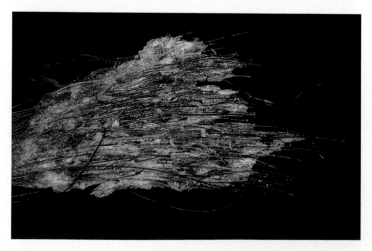

Figure 6.4
Pityriasis amiantacea – close-up of sticky, silvery scales.

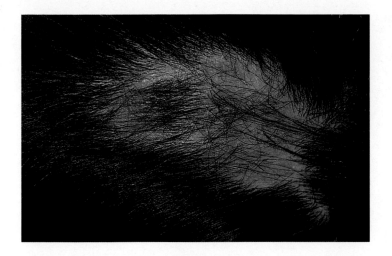

Figure 6.5
Hair loss after pityriasis amiantacea.

extend some distance into the neighbouring scalp. Another form extends upwards from patches of lichen simplex in the occipital site and is seen mainly in middle-aged women. The disease is usually confined to small areas of the scalp, but may be very extensive, either involving a large area diffusely, or affecting a number of small patches. The latter form in children often proves to be psoriasis by its subsequent course. The majority of patients notice some hair loss in areas of severe scaling. The hair regrows when the scaling is effectively treated. Tufts of thin, newly regrowing hairs can be seen when the scales are tilted. If scarring alopecia occurs, it may well be related to secondary bacterial infection and intense inflammation (Figure 6.5).

Usually, the distinctive appearance makes the diagnosis easy, but the identification of the underlying disease may not be easy.

Treatment

Where pityriasis complicates lichen simplex or psoriasis, the underlying condition must be treated, but it may be useful initially to eliminate the abundant scale by the use of oil of cade ointment or a topical tar/salicylic acid ointment, which is effective also in many cases in which no preceding disease of the scalp is discovered. Either preparation should be washed out of the scalp after 4–5 hours with a suitable shampoo, e.g. tar shampoo. Even then the condition sometimes tends to recur. The alternative application of antibacterial and steroid products in a gel or hydrophobic base helps in clearing the condition.

If psoriasis is associated, then the same local or systemic treatment principles used in general may be effective in treating the scalp. Potent topical corticosteroid scalp liquids may be beneficial in some cases.

SEBORRHOEA

Seborrhoea (Figure 6.6) may be defined as the production of a quantity of sebum which is excessive for the age and sex of the individual, but this definition is inadequate in clinical practice since many patients in whom the level of sebum excretion is not abnormal seek advice because they find the greasiness of their hair cosmetically unacceptable. Seborrhoea in practice is that level of sebum production which the patient considers to be excessive! There is a subtle

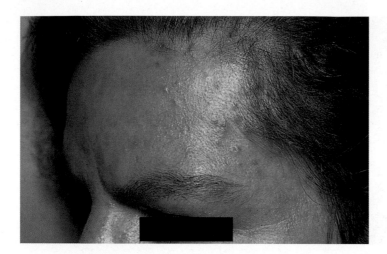

Figure 6.6
Seborrhoea and greasy hair.

interaction between the feeling of greasiness due to the level of sebum production and physical factors independent of sebum production, such as the oiliness due to heating (melting point of lipids and waxes) or due to sweating (presence of emulsifiers).

Aetiology

Sebaceous glands are present over the entire surface of the skin except the palms and the soles and the dorsa of the feet. The largest glands are on the face and scalp and on the scrotum. The glands in the central area of the chest and back are larger than those elsewhere on the trunk. Sebaceous glands in the skin all open into hair follicles, but the pilary component of the pilosebaceous unit may be only a very small vellus hair.

The sebaceous glands are functional at birth, and in early infancy under the influence of maternal androgens, but throughout childhood they remain tiny and inactive. With the approach of puberty, at which androgen levels begin to rise, usually at about the age of 9 or 10 years, the sebaceous glands enlarge and the production of sebum begins. Between 13 and 16 years of age the production of sebum is equal between males and females, but the level increases in males to reach a peak at the age of about 20. In males it remains high into extreme old age; in females there is a marked decrease after the menopause. Oestrogen decreases the size of sebaceous glands and thus the production of sebum.

There is considerable variation in the normal level of sebum production in sexually normal males, and those with abundant sebum may complain about it. In those genetically predisposed to acne this may accompany the seborrhoea. Men with common baldness may complain of the conspicuous greasiness of the scalp, but in such patients greasiness is merely more evident and the level of sebum production is no greater than in non-bald control subjects. It appears that the same amount of sebum is dispersed on fewer hairs, which results in a relative increase in greasiness.

For the same reasons, and in combination with different hairstyles in women, seborrhoea may have far greater significance. Seborrhoea (and acne in those predisposed), together with hirsutism and baldness, is one of the triad of cutaneous parameters of androgenetic activity.

Clinical features

The patient complains that the scalp and hair are excessively greasy and therefore unmanageable.

Management

Symptomatic treatment without any attempt to evaluate the significance of the symptom is difficult to justify. Admittedly, the seborrhoea may be a physiological variant in an otherwise entirely normal patient. However, in a significant proportion of women, the seborrhoea is a manifestation of increased androgenetic activity, which has consequences other than purely cosmetic ones.

The association of hirsutism or of androgenetic alopecia should be noted. The menstrual history should be recorded. If the association of hirsutism, or of alopecia of androgenetic pattern, or of menstrual irregularity, suggests the possibility of an abnormality in systemic androgen metabolism, this should be investigated and treated. If the seborrhoea is an isolated symptom, topical means to control it are recommended. The aims of topical treatment are (1) inhibition of sebaceous glands, (2) inhibition of lipid synthesis in the glands and (3) inhibition of microbial lipolysis of triglycerides. The use of isopropyl alcohol as a vehicle reduces sebum depletion, tar or oestrogens and/or antiandrogens reduce lipid synthesis, and lipolysis is reduced by isopropyl alcohol, colloidal sulphur or selenium disulphide. The use of lotions containing oestrogens is often advocated in some European countries and their thorough investigation and evaluation is clearly desirable. It is usual in cases in which there is no indication for systemic treatment to suggest the use of proprietary, cosmetically acceptable shampoos marketed for the condition, leaving the patient to establish empirically the choice of preparation and the frequency of application to provide the greatest symptomatic relief and 'aesthetic' satisfaction.

SEBORRHOEIC DERMATITIS

The prevalence of seborrhoeic dermatitis shows wide geographical variation, but the extent to which this is climatic or racial is still uncertain. In the UK, seborrhoeic dermatitis appears to be significantly more frequent among the Celts than in other ethnic groups. International comparisons are still more difficult to make as differences in diagnostic criteria and in nomenclature are so frequent.

> **Seborrhoeic dermatitis may occur with androgenetic alopecia and it exaggerates the hair loss**

Aetiology

The cause of seborrhoeic dermatitis is unknown, but a genetic factor is almost certainly implicated. Clinically different syndromes with some features in common occur in the infant when sebaceous activity has been re-established by endogenous androgen production. The sebum excretion rate, however, is not increased in seborrhoeic dermatitis, but the sebum contains less than the normal proportion of free fatty acids, squalene and wax esters and relatively increased quantities of triglycerides and cholesterol.

Attempts to relate seborrhoeic dermatitis to the activities of *Pityrosporum* yeasts have recently been more successful than in previous centuries. It is therefore often considered to be an inflammatory variant of pityriasis capitis.

Pathology

The histological changes combine features of chronic eczema with features of psoriasis. The ultramicroscopic appearance is not specific and resembles that seen in discoid eczema. Yeast forms are usually present in excess.

Clinical features

The clinical appearance is illustrated in Figures 6.7–6.10. Pityriasis capitis is usually regarded as the precursor or the mildest form of seborrhoeic dermatitis of the scalp.

'Greasy' scales, often yellow in colour, combine with exudate to form crusts, beneath which the scalp is red and moist. The eyebrows and the nasolabial folds are often also involved. As the condition deteriorates, perifollicular erythema and scaling gradually extend to form sharply marginated patches, dull red in colour and covered by greasy scales. There may be only a few discrete patches, or the scalp may be diffusely affected with extension of the dermatitis beyond the frontal margin. Scratching and secondary infection may enhance eczematization with much exudation and crusting. Secondary bacterial infection may cause an increase in these inflammatory changes or the development of pustulation. Often associated with seborrhoeic dermatitis of the scalp is blepharitis. Small crusts form along the eyelid margins with increased population of *Demodex folliculorum*, and occasionally eyelashes may be destroyed. The retroauricular region is commonly affected by seborrhoeic dermatitis, either alone or in association with scalp lesions. There may be a crusted retroauricular fissure from which dull red scaling extends into the scalp and to the back of the pinna. The concha and the external auditory canal may be similarly affected (Figure 6.9). The popularity of beards has led to an increase of seborrhoeic dermatitis at this site (Figure 6.10). Erythema and greasy scaling are most severe on the cheeks. On the shaven chin a superficial folliculitis of the beard is common. Less often, a deep follicular infection occurs, which may leave permanent scars. Seborrhoeic dermatitis of other hairy regions of the body may accompany dermatitis of the scalp.

Diagnosis

There is a tendency to diagnose seborrhoeic dermatitis too freely. Many other skin condi-

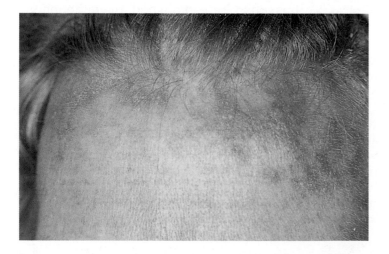

Figure 6.7
Seborrhoeic dermatitis – scalp and forehead.

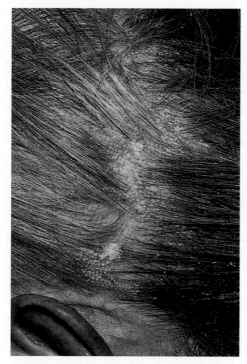

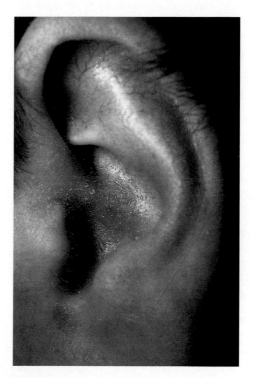

Figure 6.8
Seborrhoeic dermatitis – scalp.

Figure 6.9
Seborrhoeic dermatitis – otitis externa.

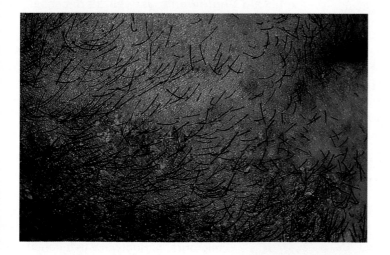

Figure 6.10
Seborrhoeic dermatitis – beard.

tions may occur in grossly seborrhoeic subjects and the diagnostic criteria should therefore be strict.

The heavy scales of psoriasis are usually easy to differentiate, particularly if psoriatic skin lesions or nail involvement can be found. Occasionally the existence of a hybrid condition may be suspected, particularly on the face. In cases of doubt, a biopsy may be helpful.

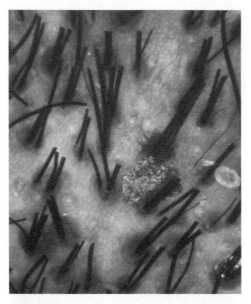

Figure 6.11
Demodex – clinical view of scalp. Chronic itchy sensations were associated with diffuse hair loss (African subject; close-up photograph). A scalp biopsy showed mixed superficial infiltration with mast cells in regard to infested sebaceous gland openings in the infundibulum (red dot showing scalp surface sampling (Fig. 6.12) and biopsy site [histology not shown]).

Tinea capitis may readily be confused with seborrhoeic dermatitis, particularly those forms of tinea caused by anthropophilic *Trichophyton* species. Wood's light examination and fungal culture should always be carried out in doubtful cases.

The study of whether the chronic itching with diffuse hair and follicular *Demodex*

colonization is a variant of seborrhoeic dermatitis is inconclusive (Figures 6.11, 6.12).

Lichen simplex of the nape of the neck, a relatively common condition particularly in women, can be confused with seborrhoeic dermatitis, but the characteristic site and the severity and persistence of the itching suggest the correct diagnosis. Less commonly, lichen simplex may occur at the side of the scalp about the ear.

Treatment

Seborrhoeic dermatitis of the scalp may respond to the same measures as pityriasis capitis, but if it is extensive or severe, daily application of a corticosteroid lotion is helpful. The scalp should be shampooed twice or more each week until the dermatitis is under control. The range of shampoos available has expanded enormously in recent years, and most are now cosmetically acceptable and easy to comply with. They contain anti-inflammatory, antiseptic, antifungal or 'antiscale' ingredients as well as necessary cosmetic substances. The choice of shampoo can often be left to the patient's aesthetic judgement as the agents in these particular vehicles have not been evaluated in depth pharmacologically in proper comparative clinical trials. Leaving a therapeutic component (gel or washable ointment) in contact during the night before a shampoo might be a reasonable approach twice weekly.

If secondary infection is present, a topical antibiotic–corticosteroid combination or, if

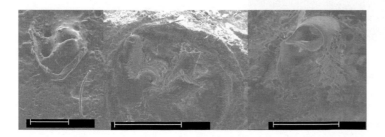

Figure 6.12
Demodex–scanning electron micrograph. Root view (left panel) with tiny exogen hair suggests androgenetic alopecia. Surface view (middle panel) shows follicular opening filled with hair and bottom of *Demodex* at larger magnification (right panel).

the secondary infection is severe and extensive, systemic antibiotics should be prescribed.

Severe and extensive seborrhoeic dermatitis may tend to relapse. Some patients therefore prefer to continue to use a treatment shampoo (e.g. zinc pyrithione or ketoconazole) prophylactically. Hence, much remains to be done in the area of 'cosmeceuticals' to maximize the drug and aesthetic functions of therapeutic shampoos.

SEBORRHOEIC DERMATITIS OF INFANCY

The relationship of this distinctive syndrome to seborrhoeic dermatitis of adults is problematical. During the early days or weeks of life, grey, greasy crusts form on the scalp (Figure 6.13), particularly on the frontal and parietal regions. A pink, scaly erythema may develop in the neck folds and in other skin flexures. Many authorities now state that seborrhoeic dermatitis of infancy is a manifestation of the atopic state, but even if this is part of the truth, it is still important to preserve it as a distinct clinical entity, because this specific type of dermatitis has a good prognosis, usually resolving spontaneously within a few months.

> **Seborrhoeic dermatitis of infancy is probably an atopic state with a fairly good prognosis**

PSORIASIS OF THE SCALP

Psoriasis is a genetically determined disorder of the skin. There is some racial variation in its prevalence, but few large-scale and reliable surveys have been reported. The prevalence in adults in north-west Europe is about 1.5–2%. The mode of inheritance of psoriasis is not known and there may indeed be more than one genotype. In the genetically predisposed individual, the first attack may develop at any age, but the mean age of onset is in the third decade, and psoriasis is uncommon in the first 2 or 3 years of life. The initial attack and subsequent recurrences may be provoked by streptococcal infection, and perhaps by stress, but may also occur for no obvious reason.

Pathology

The distinctive histological features of psoriasis are acanthosis with elongation of the

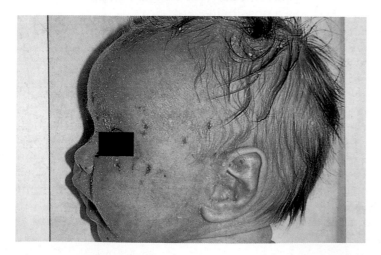

Figure 6.13
Seborrhoeic dermatitis of infancy – probably a type of atopy.

rete ridges and absence or reduction of the granular layer, especially over the rete pegs. The horny layer is parakeratotic and there are collections of polymorphonuclear leucocytes in the upper dermis. The dermal papillae are oedematous. The criteria for the histological differential diagnosis of psoriasis from seborrhoeic dermatitis of the scalp are well established. Features favouring psoriasis are condensed hyperkeratosis with focal parakeratosis, PAS-positive serum inclusions, polymorphonuclear leucocyte abscesses within the horny layer, and spongiform pustules and polymorphonuclear leucocytes within the epidermis. The criteria for seborrhoeic dermatitis are irregular acanthosis with relatively thin ortho- or parakeratotic horny layer, spongiosis and spongiotic vesicles, and exocytosis of lymphocytes and many yeast elements.

> **Psoriasis of the scalp usually has very 'sharp' margins and heavy scaling – but the scalp should always be viewed under Wood's light to exclude a fungal cause**

Clinical features

The scalp is frequently involved in psoriasis, and is often said to be a classical site for the disease (Figure 6.14). In children and young adults, it is sometimes the first site to be affected, and in some patients it remains the only one. In the majority of cases, however, other sites are sooner or later involved. Often the scalp remains constantly affected to some degree over many years, whereas lesions elsewhere may come and go.

The classical feature of psoriasis is a palpable, bright pink plaque covered in silvery scale. However, the earliest change, particularly in children, may be less distinctive.

There may be patchy or diffuse scaling without any special features or there may be asbestos-like scale in layers (pityriasis amiantacea appearance). The correct diagnosis may be suspected if there is a family history of psoriasis or if the patient has lesions elsewhere.

Although extensive loss of hair occurs only in the erythrodermic forms of psoriasis, some increased shedding of telogen hairs and some reduction in hair density is common in plaques of psoriasis.[2]

In severe psoriasis of the scalp, masses of heaped up scale form a solid cap which may extend just beyond the hair margin.

Diagnosis

The diagnosis of typical psoriasis is usually easy. Atypical lesions suggestive of psoriasis should lead to examination of the commonly affected sites, including the nails, for traces of psoriasis, even if the patient denies their presence. Small patches on knees or elbows are easily overlooked by the patient.

A very persistent scaly plaque on the bald scalp should be histologically examined to exclude Bowen's disease. Small psoriasiform plaques (even in the hairy scalp) remaining largely unchanged over many years should also suggest Bowen's disease as a possibility.

Treatment

A detailed explanation of the problem of psoriasis should always be given and the patient should be reassured that although the tendency to psoriasis cannot be eradicated, the attacks can be controlled and very long remissions may occur.

The commonest causes of treatment failure, particularly in scalp lesions, is the patient's inability to carry out the treatment

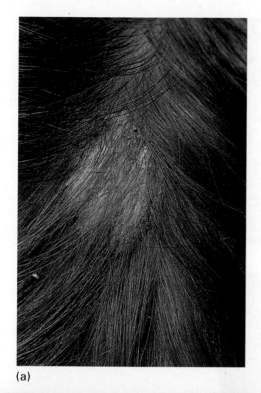

(a)

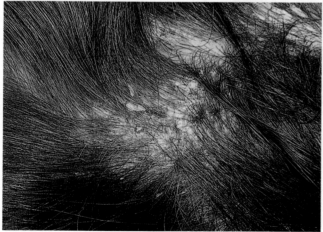

(b)

Figure 6.14
(a–e) The spectrum of scalp psoriasis.

thoroughly and the lack of nursing or help. Treatment of scalp psoriasis poses problems to the patient. Many of the oily, tar-containing or dithranol-based products used on other body sites successfully are impractical for the hairy scalp. Corticosteroid scalp liquids used daily and tar-containing shampoos are the commonest treatments in clinical practice. Most recently, salicylic acid has again become available in shampoo formulations, usually combined with tar. These modern products are much easier to comply

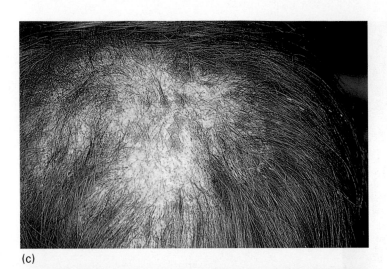

(c)

Figure 6.14 Continued

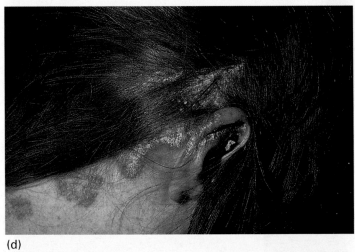

(d)

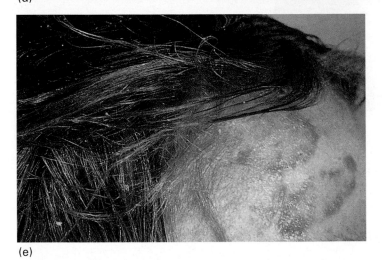

(e)

with on a regular basis. Many patients comply better if treatment shampoo alternates with a good cosmetic shampoo, which may have the same surfactants to cleanse and condition hair.

Patients with psoriasis require careful supervision. The disease itself can be a cause of severe stress, and full discussion of the problems arising as a result forms an important part of treatment.

Where routine topical treatments prove inadequate, many of the general antipsoriatic measures should be considered, such as antimitotic agents and even X-radiation (Grenz ray).

HAIR CASTS

Hair casts (peripilar keratin casts or 'pseudonits') are firm, yellowish, white accretions ensheathing, but not attached to, scalp hairs and freely movable up and down the affected shafts. Such lesions are often found in scaly and seborrhoeic disorders of the scalp (Figures 6.15–6.18).

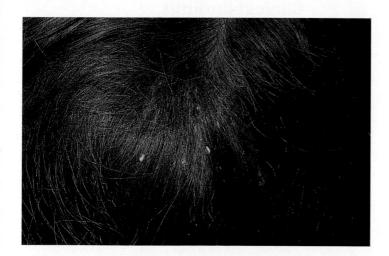

Figure 6.15
Hair (peripilar) casts.

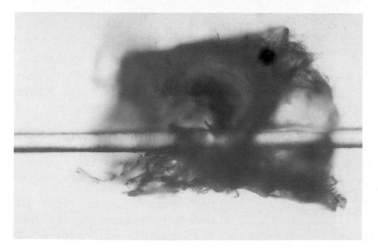

Figure 6.16
Hair cast – infundibular type.

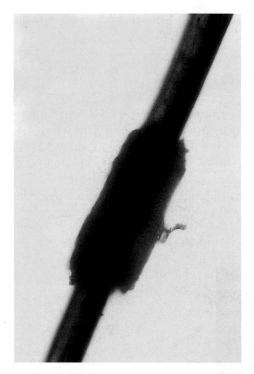

Figure 6.17
Hair cast – root sheath type.

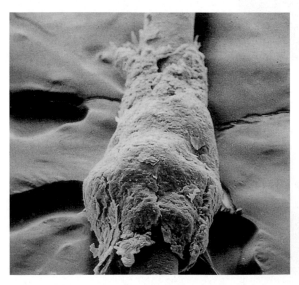

Figure 6.18
Hair cast (scanning electron micrograph).

In cross-section, casts are composed of a central layer of retained internal root sheath and an outer, thick keratinous layer. Scalp histology shows the follicular openings to be packed with parakeratotic squames, which break off at intervals to form hair casts.

Casts are found quite commonly in scaly, mainly parakeratotic conditions of the scalp such as psoriasis, pityriasis capitis, seborrhoeic dermatitis and pityriasis amiantacea. Casts may be associated with traction hairstyles and hairsprays.

Clinical findings

Hair casts may occur as an isolated abnormality unrelated to any overt scalp disease; such cases may mimic pediculosis capitis (Figure 6.15). Girls and young women are most commonly affected.

Hundreds of casts may develop within a few days. It is possible that this type may represent an unusual manifestation of psoriasis.

In patients with scaly parakeratotic diseases of the scalp, persistent dandruff which resists apparently adequate treatment is likely to be due to multiple hair casts.

Diagnosis

In the absence of associated scalp disease, casts may be mistaken for pediculosis capitis, trichorrhexis nodosa or hair knots. Of these nodal shaft abnormalities, only hair casts are freely movable along the hair.

Treatment

Any causative scalp disease must be treated. Keratolytic preparations and shampoos that readily improve scalp scaling frequently fail to remove casts. Prolonged brushing and combing is necessary to slide casts off the affected hairs. Retinoids might help through regulation of keratinization.

TINEA CAPITIS

Tinea capitis[3,4] is a fungal infection of the scalp in which the basic feature is invasion of hair shafts by a dermatophyte fungus (Figures 6.19–6.30). In this section are also included infections on other parts of the head and neck.

Most species of dermatophyte are capable of invading hair, but some species, such as *Microsporum audouinii, Trichophyton schoenleinii* and *T. violaceum*, have a particular predilection for the hair shaft. *Epidermophyton floccosum, T. concentricum* and *T. interdigitale* are exceptional in apparently never causing tinea capitis. All dermatophytes causing scalp fungal infection can invade glabrous skin and many attack nails as well. The species of dermatophyte fungus most likely to cause tinea capitis vary from country to country and often from region to region. Moreover, in any given location the species may change with time, particularly as new organisms are introduced by immigration. It is of interest that in tinea capitis, anthropophilic species predominate.

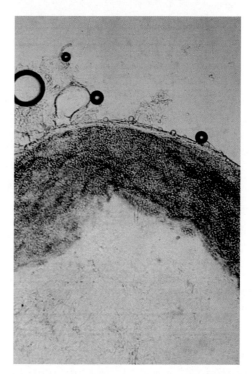

Figure 6.20
Dermatomycosis – endothrix hair infection.

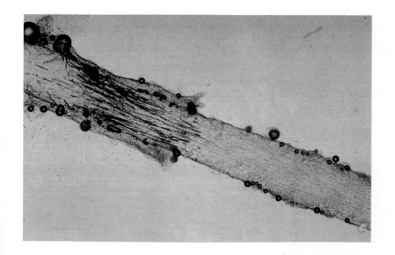

Figure 6.19
Dermatomycosis – ectothrix hair infection.

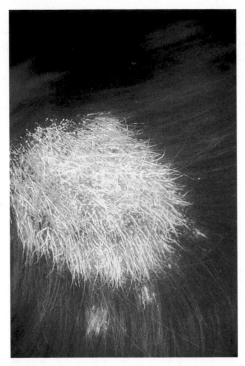

Figure 6.21
Tinea capitis – Wood's light fluorescence in
Microsporum canis type.

In recent years, there has been an
increase in *M. canis* as the dominant organism in infections in Europe and a spread of

T. tonsurans in urban communities in the
USA.

> **Patchy hair loss of fungal cause is
> much more common in children**

Pathogenesis

The spores of fungi causing tinea capitis can
be demonstrated in the atmosphere close to
the scalp of patients with the condition. It is
highly likely that scalp hair acts as a trapping
device, possibly enhanced by electrostatic
forces. It is known that contamination of hair
without any clinical findings may occur
among classmates of children with tinea
capitis. It is proven that, if actual hair infection is to occur, invasion of the stratum
corneum of the scalp skin must first develop.
Trauma assists inoculation, which is followed
after approximately 3 weeks by overt hair-
shaft infection. Spread to other adjacent follicles proceeds for a period during which there
is often a period of regression with or
without an inflammatory phase.

There are several types of hair invasion
which are worthy of note (Figures 6.19, 6.20).

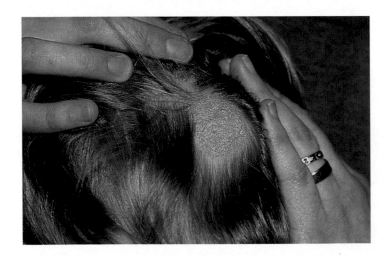

Figure 6.22
Tinea capitis – similar patch to that
shown in Figure 6.21.

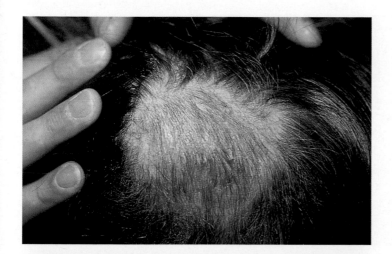

Figure 6.23
Tinea capitis – hair breakage and some inflammation.

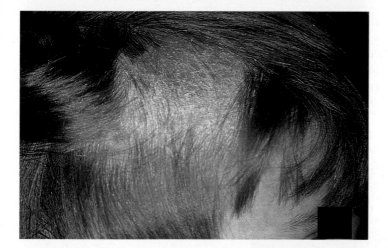

Figure 6.24
Tinea capitis – more severe inflammation.

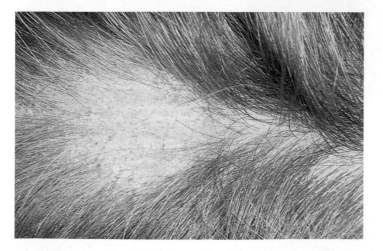

Figure 6.25
Tinea capitis – *Trichophyton violaceum* infection.

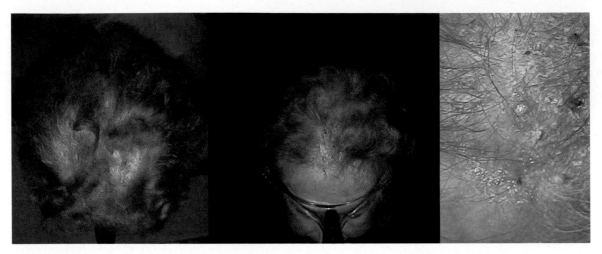

Figure 6.26
Tinea capitis incognita. Adult patient, with paraproteinaemia but not immunocompromised,
showing a diffuse scaly and inflamed scalp. The chronic course, the repeatedly erroneous diagnosis
of scalp eczema or psoriasis, the prolonged application of topical steroids without cure and the
presence of a diffuse scaling, and in some places crusts and pus formation, the relative resistance to
treatment (cure after 3 months of Lamisil®) suggests a scalp equivalent of tinea incognita
(*Microsporum canis* after contact with infected cat).

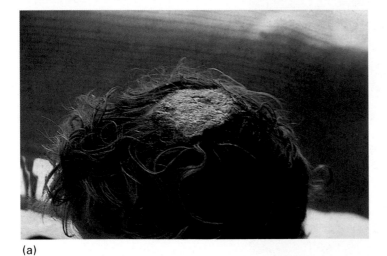

(a)

Figure 6.27
(a–h) The spectrum of kerion
infection on the head and neck due
to *Trichophyton verrucosum* of
bovine origin.

Microsporum type

In small-spored ectothrix (e.g. *M. canis*), the
hair shaft is invaded in mid-follicle. The
intrafollicular hyphae continue to grow
inwards towards the bulb of the hair.
Secondary extrapilary hyphae burst out and
grow in a tortuous manner over the surface
of the hair shaft, which is of course growing
outwards continuously. These secondary
extrapilary hyphae segment to produce a
mass of small (2–3 μm diameter) arthrospores, each one of which becomes rounded
off and eventually spherical. The size of

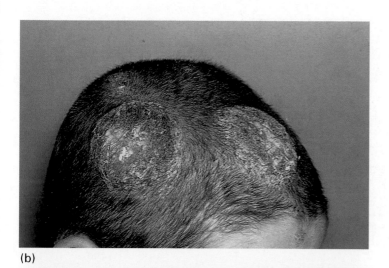

(b)

Figure 6.27 Continued

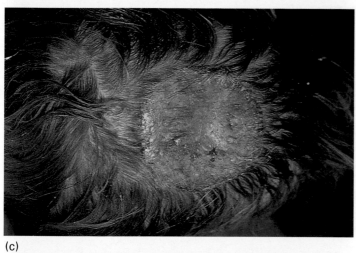

(c)

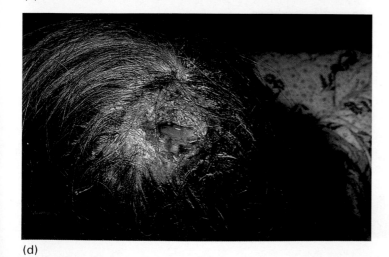

(d)

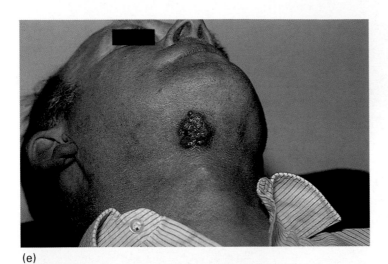

(e)

Figure 6.27 Continued

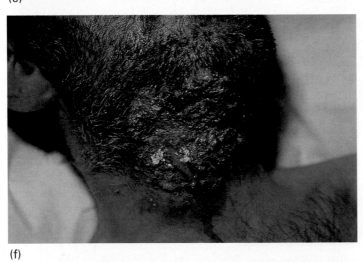

(f)

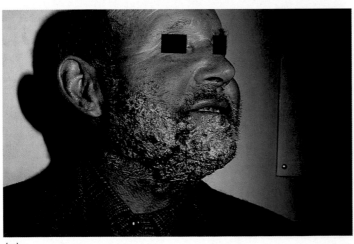

(g)

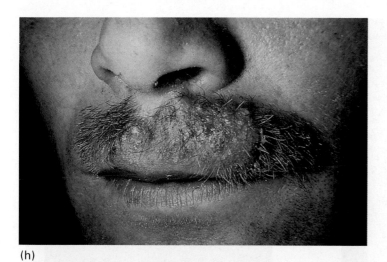

(h)

Figure 6.27 Continued

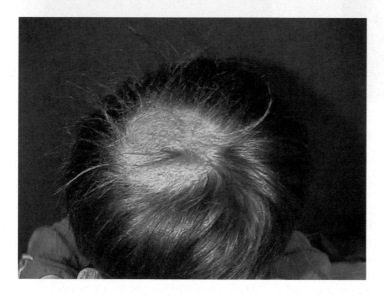

Figure 6.28
Kerion. When taken at the most acute stage, recovery of hair growth in a kerion is possible if oral steroids are given to prevent follicular destruction. Kerion is a trichological emergency!

After many weeks of infection as in this case (*T. verrucosum*), albeit treated with topical and oral antimycotics, permanent hair loss becomes inevitable. Some remnant follicular subunits may recombine, as in this patient after 1 year, but fuzzy hair is not cosmetically significant.

these spores is such that they cannot easily be distinguished as separate structures under the low power of the light microscope. With Wood's light, bluish green fluorescence is characteristically present in this type of hair invasion (Figures 6.19, 6.21).

A similar type of hair invasion occurs with other *Microsporum* spp., e.g. *M. gypseum*. The spores, although similarly arranged, are larger, in this case about 5–8 μm. Fluorescence has been reported in some cases.

Trichophyton types

In large-spored ectothrix (in chains) (e.g. *T. verrucosum*) the arthrospores are spherical, arranged in straight chains and again confined to the outer surface of the hair shaft. They apparently arise from straight primary extrapilary hyphae and, although the size varies with species, they are distinctly visible under the low power of the light microscope. There is no fluorescence.

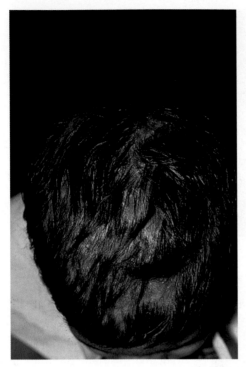

Figure 6.29
Trichophyton schoenleinii infection – favus, late
stages with scarring.

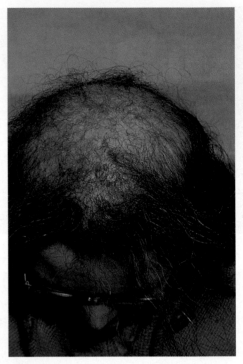

Figure 6.30
Another example of *T. schoenleinii* infection –
favus, late stages with scarring.

In endothrix (e.g. *T. tonsurans*) intra-pilary hyphae fragment into arthrospores which are entirely within the hair shaft (Figure 6.20). Hair thus affected is especially fragile and breaks off close to the scalp surface. This type is non-fluorescent.

In the favic type (e.g. *T. schoenleinii*) broad hyphae and air spaces are seen in the hair shaft, but arthrospores are always absent. The affected hair is less damaged than in other types and may continue to grow to considerable lengths. Greenish grey fluorescence is present. Air spaces probably represent sites in which intrapilary fungal hyphae have regressed. The clinical picture usually left by this infection is one of cicatricial alopecia (Figures 6.29, 6.30).

Clinical features

The clinical appearance of fungal infection of the scalp is quite variable, depending on the type of hair invasion, the level of host resistance and the degree of inflammatory host response. The appearance, therefore, may vary from a few dull grey, broken-off hairs with a little scaling, detectable only on careful inspection (Figures 6.22–6.26), to a severe, painful, inflammatory mass covering most of the scalp. In all types the main features are partial hair loss with inflammation of some degree. It is useful to recognize several basic clinical pictures.

Small-spored ectothrix infections

In *M. audouinii* and *M. ferrugineum* infections, the basic lesions are patches of partial alopecia often circular in shape, but showing broken-off hairs, dull grey from their coating of arthrospores. Inflammation is of minor degree, but fine scaling is characteristic, usually with a fairly distinct margin. There may be several or many such patches arranged more or less randomly. In *M. canis* infection the picture is similar, but there are more inflammatory changes. In infection caused by all these species, green fluorescence under Wood's lamp is usual, but non-fluorescent cases have been reported. Children are affected more frequently than adults, although the occasional case of tinea capitis in older patients must not be forgotten. The attack rate for epidemic infections caused by anthropophilic species may be as high as 30% within a school class. In the past, infection rates of both *M. audouinii* and *M. canis* were much higher.

Kerion

The most severe pattern of reaction is known as a kerion (Figure 6.27). It is a painful, inflammatory mass in which such hairs as remain are loose. Follicles may be seen discharging pus, there may be sinus formation and on rare occasions mycetoma-like grains may be found. Thick crusting with matting of adjacent hairs is common. The area affected may be limited, but multiple plaques are not rare and occasionally a large confluent lesion may involve much of the scalp. Regional lymphadenopathy is common. Although this violent reaction is usually caused by one of the zoophilic species, typically *T. verrucosum* or *T. mentagrophytes*, occasionally a geophilic organism is isolated and anthropophilic infections

which have been relatively inactive for weeks may suddenly become inflammatory and develop into kerions if a high degree of hypersensitivity develops. The possibility that secondary bacterial infection may be playing some part should not be ignored. In such cases a swab should be sent to the bacterial laboratory in addition to the plucking of hairs for mycology. Generally, however, pustule formation represents an inflammatory response to the fungus itself, and/or to the perforating folliculitis.

Agminate folliculitis

A somewhat less severe inflammatory fungal infection of the scalp consisting of sharply defined, dull red plaques studded with follicular pustules is also seen in zoophilic infections.

Endothrix infections

In *T. tonsurans* and *T. violaceum* infections, a relatively non-inflammatory type of patchy baldness occurs. Formation of black dots (swollen hair shafts) as the affected hair breaks at the surface of the scalp is a classical sign in this condition, but such findings may not be very conspicuous. The patches, which are usually multiple, may show minimal scaling, sometimes mimicking discoid lupus erythematosus or seborrhoeic dermatitis. They are commonly angular in outline rather than round. A low-grade folliculitis is often seen, and sometimes a frank kerion may develop.

Favus

Infection with *T. schoenleinii* is seen sporadically in many countries including South Africa, those of the Middle East, Pakistan, the USA, the UK and Australia. The classical picture of tinea capitis due to this organism is characterized by the presence of yellowish, cup-shaped crusts known as scutula. Each scutulum develops round a hair, which pierces it centrally. Adjacent crusts enlarge to become confluent, forming a mass of yellow crusting. Many patients may show less distinctive changes, in early cases perhaps amounting to no more than perifollicular redness and some matting of the hair. Extensive patchy hair loss with cicatricial alopecia and atrophy among patches of normal hair may be found in long-standing cases where much of the hair loss is irreversible due to the destruction of the bulge area of the hair follicle (Figures 6.29, 6.30). In these patients the glabrous skin is commonly affected by the development of similar yellowish crusts. Some nail involvement is found in 2–3% of patients. Although the initial infection probably occurs in childhood in nearly all cases, it shows little if any tendency to clear spontaneously at puberty, particularly in women. Families with several generations affected are well recognized.

Differential diagnosis

The differential diagnosis of tinea capitis includes all conditions capable of causing patchy baldness with inflammatory changes of the scalp. Alopecia areata may show erythema, and although it is itself not a scaly condition, it may coexist with seborrhoeic dermatitis. Such cases can be confusing, though careful examination usually shows that the scaling and the hair loss are not coextensive. Exclamation mark hair must be distinguished from the broken hairs of tinea capitis. Traumatic alopecia from hairdressing procedures and trichotillomania may also be confused. Seborrhoeic dermatitis is usually more diffuse than tinea capitis, but in pityriasis ('tinea') amiantacea, the

changes are often localized. In this condition the scaling is adherent to the hair, but breakage of the hair shaft does not normally occur. In psoriasis, hair loss is found only occasionally and again broken-off hairs are not usually present.

In impetigo, which may be secondary to pediculosis capitis, loosening of the hair is not normally present, but matting and crusting may cause confusion with inflammatory ringworm. An abscess of the scalp is much more acutely painful, typically causing systemic upset and fever, and shedding of loosened hair is much less evident than in kerion. Discoid lupus erythematosus, lichen planus and other causes of cicatricial alopecia may sometimes have to be considered.

Control

It is of considerable importance with scalp fungal infection to discover the species involved. Some information may be obtained from the clinical picture or the presence or absence of fluorescence, but culture is required for a diagnosis to be accurately established. Where animal species are concerned the source should be proved mycologically: it is not always the expected one. The course of action to be taken depends upon the situation and the value placed upon the animal. A small, much-loved domestic pet can often be treated successfully and economically with griseofulvin. Cattle ringworm in calves will normally settle spontaneously. A group of highly infected laboratory mice should probably be destroyed.

With anthropophilic infections, careful investigation of the outbreak or epidemic is recommended, and exclusion of children from school is probably necessary. Apart from the risk of spreading infection, there is often a sound sociological basis for keeping an infected child at home. It demonstrates social awareness and responsibility by the family and avoids a situation in which the family may be accused of spreading infection. With zoophilic infections such as *M. canis* ringworm, children can normally be allowed to remain at school as infectivity from human to human is low.

Treatment

The mainstay of treatment in all these conditions is oral griseofulvin, though trials of the newer antifungals have shown very promising results.[3,4] Topical therapy has little place, except as an adjunct to oral therapy; it is sensible to remove matted crusts and to carry out routine frequent shampooing. Although massive, single-dose griseofulvin therapy and intermittent dose schedules (25 mg/kg twice a week) have had some success, in general, conventional continuous daily or twice-daily griseofulvin treatment is advisable. In small-spore ectothrix infections, griseofulvin for 4–6 weeks is usually adequate. Where possible, infected hair should be clipped away to reduce the infectivity of the patient and careful monitoring is recommended. In chronic *T. tonsurans* and *T. schoenleinii* infections, much longer therapy may be needed.

In a study of griseofulvin versus the new oral antifungals, mycological or clinical cure was reported in over 80% treated.[3] Monotherapy with oral terbinafine, itraconazole and fluconazole all showed similar efficacy in tinea capitis over a 2–3 week period with fewer side effects than a 6 week course of griseofulvin. For *M. canis* infections a longer course than 3 weeks is advised.

With scalp kerions, removal of crusts using wet compresses should not be neglected, and the possibility of coexisting bacterial infection should be considered. If confirmed by culture, systemic antibacterial chemotherapy should be instituted. In general, the kerions are less painful than their inflammatory appearance suggests, but analgesics may be needed. Occasionally, in children with extensive kerions, admission to hospital or frequent attendance at the outpatient clinic, where skilled nursing is available, may be of great value, and is much appreciated by the worried parents. Permanent hair loss from scarring is usually less than would be expected. Ketoconazole shampoo may be used to prevent spread in the early phases of therapy. In severe inflammatory forms there is a case for using oral prednisolone to inhibit the inflammatory response, and, indeed, a short period of oral corticosteroids also helps by resolving the oedema and oozing and by preventing secondary scarring.

> **Oral antifungal therapy is the rule in scalp infection**

PRURITIC SYNDROMES

Pruritus of the scalp may occur as an isolated symptom in the absence of any objective changes. The patient is often middle-aged, the pruritus is spasmodic and may be intense, and exacerbations are frequently related to periods of stress or fatigue. Such patients are often extremely demanding.

Pruritus is also the predominant manifestation of acne necrotica, in which scattered vesicles followed by small crusts are a source of severe discomfort. Dermatitis herpetiformis may involve the scalp. Grouped papules and vesicles in recurrent crops may be associated with similar lesions of the trunk and limbs.

Lichen simplex is a frequent cause of pruritus of the nape and occipital region in women, and may also be localized above one or both ears. In the affected region, the scalp is thickened and scaly.

Reactions to hair dyes and other hair cosmetics more commonly involve the ears, neck, forehead or face than the scalp itself. However, intense irritation of the scalp is sometimes the initial symptom of a sensitization reaction and, rarely, eczematous changes may affect the whole or part of the scalp. In such cases there is associated reversible hair loss. Apart from hair cosmetics and medicaments, the wearing of a hat may also cause a scalp reaction.

Seborrhoeic and atopic dermatitis and other inflammatory disorders, such as Norwegian scabies (Figures 6.31, 6.32), may be pruritic, but pruritus is seldom a presenting symptom. Psoriasis is not usually pruritic.

In children and in women of any age, pediculosis should be excluded, no matter what the social status or the age of the patient. Multiple insect bites are sometimes a puzzling source of irritation in children, and are usually rapidly complicated by bacterial infection as a result of excoriation. In infants, in the elderly and in the immunosuppressed, scabies may cause scalp irritation. In the immunosuppressed, itch may be paradoxically absent.

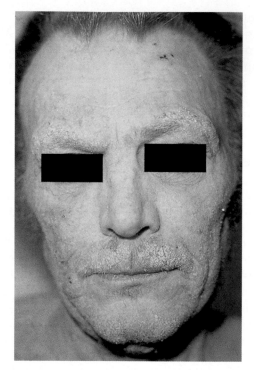

Figure 6.31
Norwegian scabies.

Overuse or abuse of antiparasitic shampoos may complicate the clinical picture in scalp irritation syndromes and possibly promote secondary hair loss.

Figure 6.32
Norwegian scabies – biopsy showing follicular *Acarus* organisms.

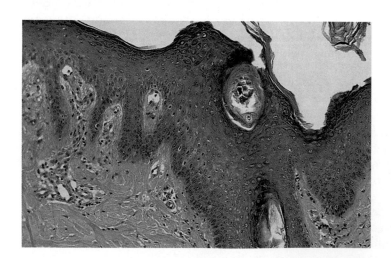

> **The scalp is a common site for parasitophobia**

LICHENIFICATION AND LICHEN SIMPLEX

Lichenification is a 'leathery' thickening of skin resulting from repeated rubbing and scratching (Figures 6.33, 6.34). The surface skin lines and creases are exaggerated within the abnormal area. Lichenification may occur secondary to many pruritic dermatoses or develop as a localized abnormality without any predisposing diseases, the so-called lichen simplex or primary lichenification (Figure 6.35).

The pathological changes vary from site to site. Typical findings include hyperkeratosis and acanthosis; localized areas of spongiosis and parakeratosis may also be present. All components of the epidermis are hyperplastic. The dermal changes vary according to the primary cause and the duration of the lesion. A mixed chronic inflammatory cell infiltrate is usually present

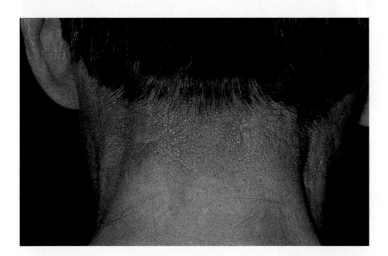

Figure 6.33
Lichenification – nape of neck.

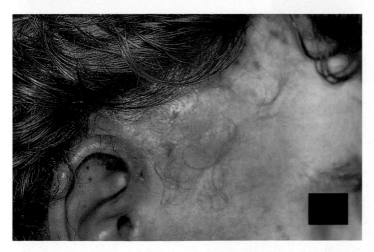

Figure 6.34
Lichenification – temporoparietal lesion.

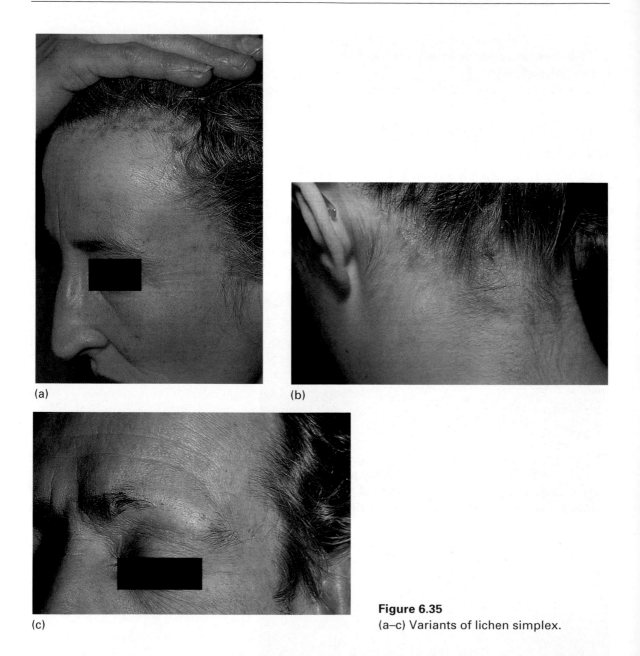

(a)

(b)

(c)

Figure 6.35
(a–c) Variants of lichen simplex.

in the upper dermis, often associated with fibrosis and Schwann cell proliferation.

Emotional tensions play an important part in the development and persistence of lichenification, which may indeed persist long after the primary disease has remitted. The fact is the basis of the often-used synonym 'neurodermatitis'. Not all individu-als produce lichenified skin on rubbing and scratching; atopic subjects are particularly prone. In many subjects, the same disease and chronic rubbing and scratching produce nodules – nodular prurigo or nodular lichenification. Afro-American subjects fre-quently produce papular and follicular lichenification.

The main symptom is pruritus, which may be very severe despite minimal signs. The most common diseases predisposing to secondary lichenification are atopic dermatitis, nummular eczema, lichen planus, seborrhoeic dermatitis, asteatotic eczema and, rarely, psoriasis. Chronic photodermatoses and psoriasis may cause a lichenified appearance in areas where little scratching and rubbing occur. Lichenified patches may occur on any pruritic area that is amenable to rubbing and scratching.

Lichen simplex (Figure 6.35) is defined as localized lichenification due to rubbing and scratching of skin previously apparently normal, i.e. primary lichenification. In general, the local physical signs and histopathological changes are the same as in secondary lichenification. Lichen simplex is rare before puberty, the peak incidence being between 30 and 50 years of age. Women are more frequently affected than men. In lichen simplex, only a few lesions are present, and in 50% of cases only one lesion occurs. The commonest area affected is the nape of the neck.

Lichen nuchae occurs as a single plaque on the nape of the neck. It may be very scaly and mimic psoriasis, and attacks of secondary bacterial infection are common (Figures 6.33, 6.35b). On other parts of the scalp the presenting signs may be localized breaking of hair associated with underlying pruritus (trichoteiromania).

This pattern is particularly likely to affect the temporal and parietal areas of the scalp. Allergic or irritant reactions to hair cosmetics must be carefully excluded.

Treatment

Primary lichenification requires careful psychological assessment and treatment; the patient should be given insight into the underlying stresses and an understanding of the need to break the scratching habit.

Topical treatment needs to be anti-inflammatory, occlusive in sites where this is possible; topical steroid liquids or creams are most commonly used, whereas intralesional triamcinolone may be effective in recalcitrant cases. Superficial X-radiation may be helpful in the most recalcitrant cases.

CONTACT DERMATITIS

Contact dermatitis (contact eczema) may be conveniently defined, for the present purposes, as an inflammatory condition of the skin caused by an external agent. If photodermatitis is excluded, two broad divisions are recognized: irritant and allergic dermatitis.

Irritant dermatitis

A skin irritant is defined as a substance that is capable of causing cell damage in most people if it is applied for a sufficient length of time, with sufficient frequency and in sufficient concentrations. The scalp is generally considered to be resistant to irritant damage, possibly because of a relatively thick epidermis and horny layer, and a rapid epidermal 'turnover time'; i.e. it replaces its natural barrier layer relatively quickly both spontaneously and after any cell damage. It should be noted, however, that substances that are recognized as highly irritant on other sites are rarely applied to the scalp with sufficient frequency for a sufficient time or in sufficient concentrations. For example, hairdressers frequently develop irritant contact dermatitis of the hands from contact with shampoos, but the dilute shampoo solution applied to the scalp does not cause dermatitis because it is soon rinsed off. Shampoos may rarely irritate the skin of the forehead and scalp margins in susceptible individuals, such as those with atopic eczema, and inflame the conjunctival surface of the eye.

In practice, thioglycollates, bleaching preparations and heat are the commonest causes of irritant dermatitis of the scalp. It is important to remember that irritant dermatitis affects only skin that has been in direct contact with the offending agent.

Allergic dermatitis

Allergic dermatitis implies dermatitis due to the development of allergy to a substance previously applied to the skin. Most substances causing dermatitis of this type are of small molecular mass, less than 10 kDa, and act only as partial antigens or haptens. To form complete antigens, they must combine with epidermal protein. The immunological response requires the presence of epidermal Langerhans' cells to recognize the allergen and normal regional lymph glands for the cell-mediated antibody response to occur in the epidermis. The dermatitis developing in this way may spread away from the site of contact, particularly if the allergen is applied repeatedly. The scalp is relatively resistant to allergens. As with irritants, this resistance may be due to the thick horny layer, but this cannot be the only factor, since eczematous contact allergy is not entirely dose related.

Less well defined is the occurrence of immediate-type hypersensitivity with or without concurrent eczematous allergy. This type I reactivity is most commonly seen with hair dyes of paraphenylenediamine type.

Clinical appearance

Irritant dermatitis affecting the scalp may commence with burning or soreness and tightness of the scalp within a short time of contact with the irritant. Liquid irritants most typically cause these symptoms at the scalp margins. The signs vary from slight erythema to marked oedema and exudation.

Complete resolution usually takes no more than a few days. Hair breakage may occur from certain substances, e.g. thioglycollates. If the scalp inflammation is severe enough, diffuse hair loss may occur days to weeks after the insult, due to local inflammatory telogen effluvium.

In *allergic dermatitis* the clinical picture varies considerably. Irritation of the scalp or scalp margins with little visible change, and occipital lichenification due to chronic scratching, may be the only signs. More severe cases present with acute, subacute or chronic eczema, either localized to the scalp and adjacent areas or spreading to affect other parts of the head and neck. Acute signs may mimic angio-oedema (Figure 6.36), bilateral erysipelas or dermatomyositis if periorbital oedema occurs. Many weeks, rarely months, may elapse between the onset and the spontaneous cure of allergic

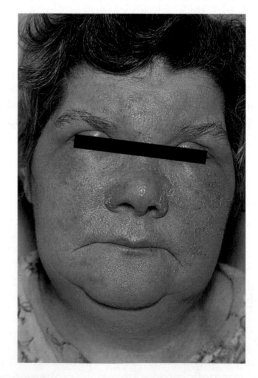

Figure 6.36
Allergic contact dermatitis due to hair dye.

dermatitis. Rarely, telogen effluvium may occur after contact dermatitis.[5] Occasionally, allergic contact dermatitis to hair products occurs at remote sites (back, feet) because of the habit of shampooing in the shower. Such non-typical locations must be remembered when the cause of allergic dermatitis is due to haircare products.

> **Allergic contact dermatitis due to scalp products may only affect the scalp margins**

Agents causing contact dermatitis

Hair dyes

Approximately 40% of women in the USA use some form of hair dye. Vegetable dyes are still used, though less commonly than in the past. Henna does not cause eczematous allergy, but may precipitate contact urticaria and more frequently allergic rhinitis and asthma. Camomile is still present in some shampoos and rinses; it contains the dye apigenin (trihydroxyflavone), which is a potent sensitizer in those handling the plant, but not when used cosmetically.

Metallic dyes are now only rarely used. Some contain nickel and chromium, but these are securely chelated into complex molecules.

Temporary dyes (colour rinses) and semi-permanent dyes are generally safe products though the latter are often marketed as shampoos and may give rise to an irritant reaction in susceptible individuals or allergic dermatitis due to o-nitroparaphenylene-diamine (ONPPD).

Permanent dyes are more likely to cause allergic sensitization than any other hair cosmetic preparations. Paraphenylene-diamine (PPD) may cause acute eczematous dermatitis of the head and neck, but hand dermatitis in those handling PPD is the commonest pattern. PPD is a potent sensitizer. Such is the notoriety of PPD that it has been banned as a hair dye in many countries, but this ban may soon be relaxed since the European Community has decreed that hair dyes may contain up to 6% PPD. Cases of PPD allergy are now less common because of better education of hairdressers and users and improved purity of the PPD (contaminants could act as potential irritants or cosensitizers), and also because the chemical reaction during the dyeing process is more accurately controlled and completed, leaving little or no free PPD. Fully polymerized PPD is harmless and inert so that reactions to dyes in wig hair do not therefore occur. In practice, hair dyeing by individuals at home is more likely to produce allergy in the user, or in those afterwards in contact with the hair, due to residual free dye remaining on the hair because of inadequate care during the dyeing process. Paratoluenediamine (PTD) is 50% less likely to cause allergy than PPD.

If allergy to a hair dye is suspected, patch testing should be carried out using 1% ONPPD, 1% PPD and 1% PTD. Cross-reactivity may be a problem: for example, para-dye dermatitis may be potentiated by certain antihistamines and rubber antioxidants.

> **Hand eczema in hairdressers due to hair dyes is much more common than eczema in the client**

Hair bleaches

These are commonly sold as twin packs containing hydrogen peroxide and ammonium persulphate. The latter is potentially both an irritant and a sensitizer. It is a histamine releaser causing facial swelling and scalp itching – this is more likely in dermographic subjects. If excessive concentrations are applied for too long, an acute irritant reaction may occur with hair breakage. For patch testing, 1% aqueous ammonium persulphate should be used.

Permanent wave solutions

Sensitivity reactions to thioglycollates are extremely rare, though mild transient irritant dermatitis is not uncommon. Necrosis of the scalp has been described from incorrect use of a thioglycollate solution, compounded by attempted reversal of the reaction with a borate neutralizer. Necrosis may be due to the heat generated.

Hair straighteners (relaxers) and depilatories

These often contain thioglycollates but are less likely to cause significant reactions than permanent wave solutions.

Setting lotions

The main ingredient is usually polyvinyl-pyrrolidone, which seems to have no allergic potential. If a reaction to such lotions occurs, it is more likely to be due to added dyes.

Hair tonics, stimulants and restorers

Such preparations are generally innocuous. Burning and exudation of the scalp may occur due to a stimulant containing century plant extract, which is rarely used on the scalp in common baldness.

Shampoos

Since they are applied in dilute solution for a short time, irritant reactions are rare, though shampoos are an infrequent cause of hand dermatitis in hairdressers.

Men's hair creams

Allergy to perfume, lanolin or preservatives may occur.

Hairnets

These are no longer popular, but may still be worn by some older women. The eruption affects the neck, ears and frontal hairline, simulating seborrhoeic dermatitis and lichen simplex. All the cases described have shown positive patch tests, either to the net or to its marginal elastic. Azo- and anthroquinone dyes, PPD and certain disperse dyes are the commonest specific allergens.

Hatband dermatitis

The site affected by the dermatitis varies, though most cases involve the forehead. Leather used to be the most frequent allergen, but fabric and plastic are now the more likely offenders. Dermatitis has been described from laurel oil used to add lustre to felt hats. Some hatbands have a varnish finish containing colophony.

Wig reactions

Ill-fitting wigs may cause friction and irritant damage to localized parts of the scalp, typically under the adhesion band. Allergic dermatitis may be caused by adhesive substances. Allergy cannot develop against completely polymerized hair dye in wigs.

ACNE NECROTICA

This descriptive clinical syndrome has been regarded as a folliculitis compounded by focal scratching and 'picking'. It may occur at any age past puberty, but teenaged girls and middle-aged men seem to suffer most. Itching is often profound, particularly at the frontal scalp margin, and the patients become very demanding.

The histological changes are not pathognomonic. There is usually folliculitis complicated in the more severe lesions by necrosis destroying the follicle and the neighbouring dermis. Some lesions submitted to biopsy show only infected excoriations. Differential diagnosis includes pemphigus foliaceus.

Clinical features

Acne necrotica and its variant, acne frontalis, present as indolent papulopustules with central necrosis, healing slowly to leave varioliform scars (Figures 6.37, 6.38).

They may be slightly painful and are pruritic. They occur most characteristically along the frontal hairs, but also involve the scalp, where they may leave small patches of cicatricial alopecia. Less often they occur on the cheeks and neck or on the chest and back. Untreated, the condition in all its variants runs a long course, although there may be only a small number of active lesions present at any one time.

A severe form may coexist with the forms just described, but much more commonly occurs alone. Pruritus, which may be distressingly severe, leads the patients to seek medical advice. The primary lesions are small papulopustules, but these are rapidly excoriated.

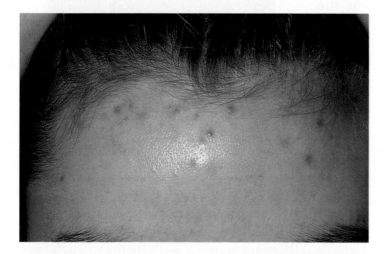

Figure 6.37
Acne necrotica.

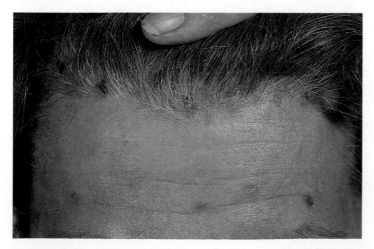

Figure 6.38
Another example of acne necrotica.

New lesions continue to develop at irregular intervals, but the pruritus seems often to be disproportionately severe in relation to the objective change (Figure 6.38).

Diagnosis

In acne necrotica the distribution of the lesions and their morphology serve to differentiate such diseases, now uncommon in temperate regions, as papulonecrotic tuberculides, tertiary syphilis and pemphigus foliaceus.

The severely pruritic form should never be diagnosed unless pediculosis and dermatitis herpetiformis have been excluded, the former by searching for the lice (Figures 6.39–6.41), and the latter by the presence of lesions elsewhere.

Treatment

All forms show a temporary response to broad-spectrum antibiotics and such treatment is useful in severe cases. Many patients find it necessary to take a small maintenance dose, e.g. oxytetracycline 250 mg twice daily, as in acne vulgaris. Topical corticosteroid antibiotic preparations are of some value, but provide only temporary benefit.

PEDICULOSIS CAPITIS

Pediculosis capitis is due to the head louse *Pediculus humanus capitis*. The female head louse is 3–4 mm long, slightly larger than the male. During 40 days of life she lays a total of approximately 300 eggs, 8 per day. The eggs are firmly attached to the hair shaft close to the swarm scalp end (Figures 6.39–6.41). After 1 week, the eggs hatch, producing larvae similar to small adults – they begin feeding on the

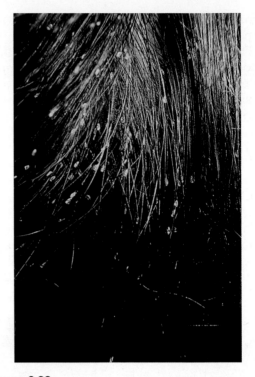

Figure 6.39
Pediculosis capitis – ova capsules on scalp hair.

blood of the host almost immediately. The louse begins to mate within 10 days after 3 moults.

Clinical features

There are typically no more than 10 adult lice alive on the scalp at the peak of the infection, though empty oval capsules attached to the hairs may add up to thousands (Figure 6.39). Itching is usually severe and persistent. Scratching and secondary bacterial infection may lead to matting of hair.

Treatment

Malathion and carbaryl have been the principal treatment agents since resistance to the organochlorides emerged. The liquid

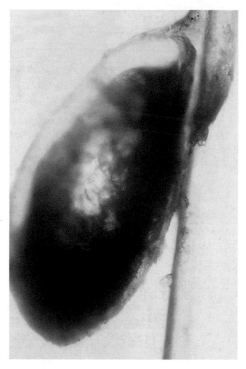

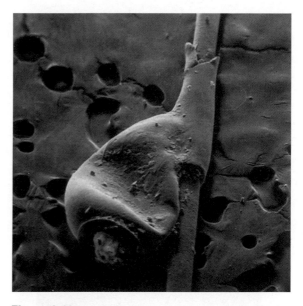

Figure 6.41
Pediculosis capitis – ova capsule (scanning electron micrograph).

Figure 6.40
Pediculosis capitis – ova capsule (light micrograph).

treatment is left on the scalp for 12 hours before washing off. A repeat treatment may be required 7–10 days later. Physical removal of the lice is an important adjunct with a 'louse comb' and brushing. Since resistant strains are appearing, an 'old' drug is regaining popularity – ivermectin, which has been mainly used for onchocerciasis. It is only required to give a single oral dose.[6]

FOLLICULAR KELOIDALIS NUCHAE (ACNE CHELOIDALIS)

This chronic inflammatory folliculitis of the nape of the neck occurs almost exclusively in males, and is certainly more severe and also much more frequent in Afro-Americans[7] than in Caucasians. It may begin at any time after puberty, usually between the ages of 14 and 25 years. Many of those affected suffer or have suffered from acne vulgaris; many others have no other skin lesions. The cause of the condition is unknown, but a genetic factor is probably implicated. Histologically, chronic folliculitis and foreign body granulomata surrounding fragments of hair are the main features.

Follicular papules and pustules develop in irregularly linear clusters on the nape just below the hairline and extend in further crops at long or short intervals towards the occiput (Figure 6.42). Firm 'keloid' papules follow the folliculitis and become confluent to form horizontal bands or plaques (Figure 6.43). These may coexist with new follicular papules and discharging sinuses.

Treatment with topical antibacterial agents and with systemic antibiotics may possibly restrain the progress of the inflammatory changes, but not reliably or completely. The keloids may be successfully excised by plastic surgery. Oral retinoids

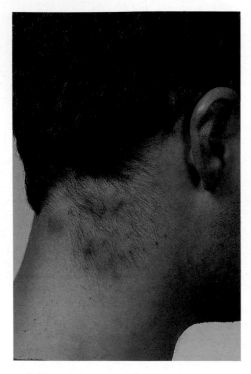

Figure 6.42
Acne cheloidalis.

have failed to give any consistent benefit but may temporarily arrest the progress of the early follicular inflammatory phase. Oral antiandrogen therapy may give some benefit when the disorder occurs in women.

REFERENCES

1. Dawber RPR, Wojnarowska F (1997) Scalp disorders. In: *Textbook of dermatology*, 6th edn, eds Champion RH, Burton JL, Ebling RJG, Burns A (Oxford, Blackwell Scientific Publications), pp 2634–2638.
2. Runne U, Kroneisen-Wiersma P (1992) Psoriatic alopecia: acute and chronic hair loss in 47 patients with scalp psoriasis, *Dermatology* **185:** 82–87.
3. Gupta AK, Adams P, Diova N (2001) Therapeutic options for the treatment of tinea capitis: griseofulvin versus the new oral antifungal agents, terbinafine, itraconazole and fluconazole, *Paediatr Dermatol* **18:** 433–438.
4. Rainer SS (2000) New and emerging therapies in paediatric dermatology, *Dermatol Clin* **18:** 73–78.
5. Tosti A, Piraccini BM, Van Neste DJJ (2001) Telogen effluvium after allergic contact dermatitis of the scalp, *Arch Dermatol* **137:** 187–190.
6. De Berker D, Sinclair R (2000) Getting ahead of head lice, *Aust J Dermatol* **41:** 209–212.
7. Perkins W (2002) Acne keloidalis nuchae. In: *Treatment of skin disease*, eds Lebwohl MG, Heymann WR, Berth-Jones J, Coulson I (London, Mosby), pp 4–5.

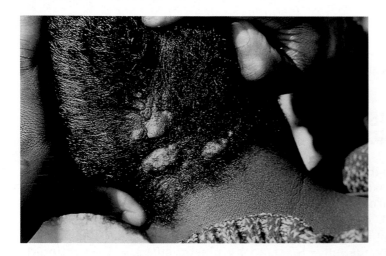

Figure 6.43
Acne cheloidalis with severe nodular scarring.

7 Hair colour

Although melanin is by definition a black pigment, scientists have long used the term to describe a range of pigments from yellow to black. Biologists usually define melanin as the pigment derived from the melanophore in the human, the melanocyte. The superficial structures of vertebrates contain such melanin pigments – skin, hair, scales and feathers.

To understand and study the nature of the basic mechanisms that regulate pigmentation in humans, one must consider the process in sequence. Four classes of factors regulate mammalian melanin pigmentation:

1. Those regulating the number and position of melanocytes in the hair and skin.
2. Those regulating tyrosinase and melanin synthesis. Melanin synthesis is an enzyme-mediated process that changes tyrosine into eumelanin and phaeomelanin. Several enzymes mediate this reaction, including tyrosinase, TRP-1 (tyrosinase-related protein-1), and TRP-2 (tyrosinase-related protein-2).
3. Those governing the morphology and distribution of melanosomes in melanocytes.
4. Those controlling the transfer of melanosomes from melanocytes to ker- atinocytes and the distribution of melanosomes in the latter cells.

Many of the disease states to be described later show examples of specific defects within this overall scheme.[1]

Human hair pigmentation depends entirely on the presence of melanin from melanocytes, but the actual colour perceived depends also on physical phenomena. The range of colours produced by melanins is limited to shades of grey, yellow, brown, red and black. In contrast, many lower animals display colours due to such pigments as porphyrins and carotenoids in addition to melanins.

Much of the research done on melanogenesis and its cellular control is in relation to cells in other epithelial surfaces, mainly the epidermis. Despite this, there is no reason to believe that the biochemical events in hair bulb melanocytes are different, and the work that has been carried out clearly suggests that they are indeed similar.

Hair colour is partly due to physical factors as well as melanin

MELANIN CHEMISTRY[1]

Many problems remain to be resolved regarding the structure of natural melanins. The whole range of human hair colour is due to two types of melanin: eumelanins, which give mainly black and brown hair; and phaeomelanins, which give predominantly red, auburn and blond hair (Figure 7.1). In general one can say that though individuals have one of these pigments for their hair colour, they are both present – dark hair is mainly from eumelanins and red hair from phaeomelanins. Auburn hair is a mixture of both. Whatever the hair colour seen by the eye, isolated eumelanins are brown to black in colour and are insoluble, whereas phaeomelanins are reddish brown and alkali soluble.

Hair bulb tyrosinase activity does not decline linearly with age but tends to be maximal in middle age. The possible relationship of specific tyrosinases to human hair colours is still ill-defined. There seems little doubt that the hair bulb produces eumelanin similar to that found in other sites.

It has been traditional to believe that each individual produces the same melanins throughout life. This is probably untrue; for example, cases have been described in which red scalp hair began to turn dark brown in later life, suggesting a change in 'balance' from phaeomelanogenesis to eumelanogenesis. Many other natural hair colour changes may reflect similar biochemical changes.

MELANOCYTES AND MELANOGENESIS

The melanocyte is the site of pigment production in the hair bulb. Functional melanocytes are situated in the bulb at the apex of the dermal papilla among the germinative cells of the hair matrix; hair bulb melanocytes are only active during the phases of hair production (anagen II–VI), whereas tyrosinase synthesis occurs during the early anagen stage. The main body of the cells is in contact with the basement membrane (Figures 7.2–7.6). Amelanotic melanocytes are also present in the external root sheath and other parts of the follicle.

In black hair follicles, deposition of melanin within melanosomes continues until the whole unit is uniformly dense.

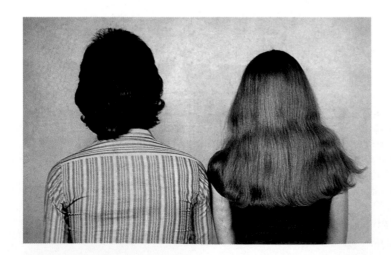

Figure 7.1
Black (eumelanin) and red (phaeomelanin) hair colours.

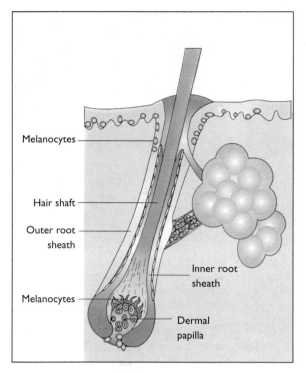

Figure 7.2
Diagram showing main sites of functionally active follicular melanocytes.

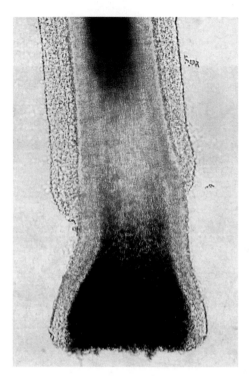

Figure 7.3
Plucked anagen hair stained to show intense melanin pigment in the bulb (lower third).

Lighter-coloured hair shows less melanin deposition and blond hair follicles show melanosomes with a 'moth-eaten' appearance. Red and blond hair follicles have spherical melanosomes; those in brown and black hair are ellipsoidal.

Melanocytes in the hair bulb (and epidermis) differ from those found in internal structures in donating pigment to receptor cells, i.e. the hair matrix cells (keratinocytes) that ultimately differentiate to produce the hair cortex. No pigment is donated to presumptive cuticular and internal root sheath cells, though pigment granules are detectable in the cuticle of human nostril hair and in the coat of many animals (Figure 7.7). In the epidermis each melanocyte has a relationship with a defined pool of adjacent keratinocytes to which,

under suitable conditions, it donates melanosomes usually via dendritic processes. Under certain circumstances, melanocytes may transfer pigment. At present, there is no definite evidence to show whether a similar defined pool of receptor cells exists for each melanocyte in the hair follicle; it remains a probability.

Melanocytes are functionally active only during the anagen phase of the hair cycle (stages II–VI). They were formerly thought to disappear during telogen, but it is now known that they remain at the surface of the papilla in a shrunken, adendritic form. It is possible that the full complement of melanocytes present during successive anagen phases is the result not only of reactivation of 'dormant' cells but also of new cells due to melanocyte replication.

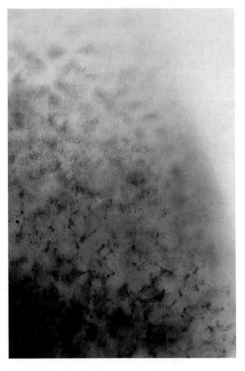

Figure 7.4
Melanin pigment in the melanocytes and matrix cells of the hair bulb – cortex precursor compartment.

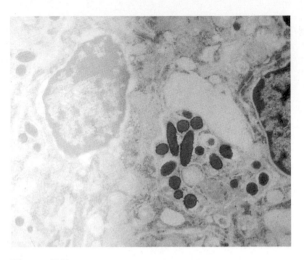

Figure 7.5
Pigmented melanosomes in a hair bulb melanocyte (electron micrograph).

Melanin granules are distributed throughout the hair cortex (Figure 7.8) but in greater concentration towards the periphery. Paracortex is thought to contain more granules than the less dense orthocortex. The pigment granules of black and brunette hair have oval pigment grains with a more

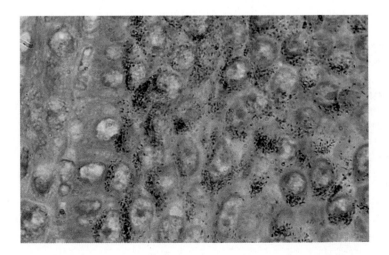

Figure 7.6
Melanin 'capping' in hair bulb matrix cells.

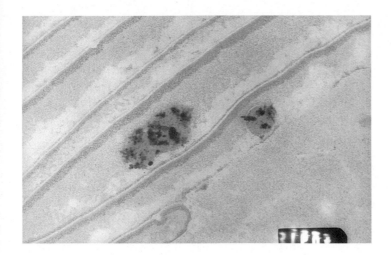

Figure 7.7
Melanin granules (unusually) seen in the hair cuticle (electron histomicrograph, silver methenamine stain).

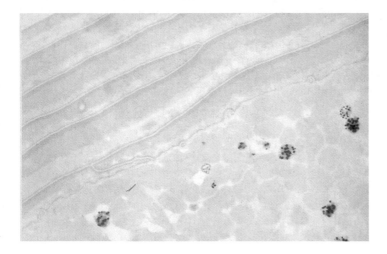

Figure 7.8
Melanin granules in the hair cortex (electron histomicrograph, silver methenamine stain).

or less homogeneous inner structure and sharp boundaries. Their surface is finely grained with a thin, surrounding, membrane-like layer of osmophilic material. Black hair granules are also relatively hard as judged from ultramicrotome sectioning, and have a high refractive index. A greater number of such granules are present in dark hair than in lighter shades. Blond hair granules are smaller, partly ellipsoid and rod-shaped in longitudinal section. They also frequently have a rough, irregular and pitted surface.

HAIR COLOUR DUE TO PHYSICAL PHENOMENA

The white colour of hair seen when melanin is absent is an optical effect due to reflection and refraction of incident light from various interfaces at which zones of different refractive index are in contact (Figure 7.9). Thus, in general, non-pigmented hair with a broad medulla appears paler than non-medullated hair. Normal 'weathering' of hair along its length

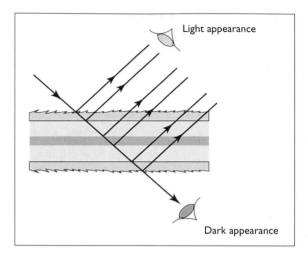

Light appearance

Dark appearance

Figure 7.9
Diagrammatic view of the main hair structure interfaces that reflect and refract light.

may lead to the terminal part appearing lighter than the rest due to a similar mechanism – the cortex and cuticle become disrupted and form numerous interfaces for internal reflection and refraction of light. This also applies in excessive 'weathering', in which patients often note a lightening in colour of the brittle hair. A similar phenomenon is responsible for the whitish bands of pili annulati. Since these optical whitening effects are due to reflection and refraction of incident light, when such hairs are viewed by transmitted light microscopy, they appear dark. Newly formed unpigmented hair with no medulla appears yellowish rather than white. This is probably the intrinsic colour of dense keratin as orientated in hair fibres. However, the perceived colour is affected by the physical characteristics of the hair shaft and may bear little relationship to the true chromaticity of the shaft.

Hair colour in humans is probably only decorative, having no essential biological function. The racial and genetic colour differences that have evolved are probably related to the UV radiation-protective colours seen in the skin; i.e. dark-skinned races have dark hair. Hair pigment, however, is not important in protection against the effects of sunlight, though there is evidence to suggest that hair bleached by sunlight and hair with less natural melanin 'weathers' less well; i.e. the structure of hair colour appears to be a matter of serendipity.

Lanugo hair present in utero is unpigmented. Vellus hair is also typically unpigmented in white-skinned individuals, but, in men in particular, some vellus fibres may pigment slightly after puberty. Hair colour varies according to body site in most people. Eyelashes are usually the darkest. Scalp hair is generally lighter than genital hair, which often has a reddish tint even in subjects having essentially brown hair, and hair on the lower and lateral scrotal surfaces is lighter than on the pubes. Apart from individuals with red scalp hair, a red tint to axillary hair is commonest in brown-haired individuals.

Hair on exposed parts may be bleached by sunlight. Very dark hair first lightens to a brownish red colour but rarely becomes blond even after strong sunlight exposure; brown hair, however, may be bleached white.

> **'Weathering' and exposure to UV radiation can both give rise to 'paling' of hair – an optical (pallor) effect**

CONTROL OF HAIR COLOUR

Hair colour is under close genetic control; however, the exact hormonal and cellular mechanisms controlling melanocyte function are not clearly worked out. An intimate relationship must exist between the factors controlling melanocyte and matrix cell activity since melanocyte mitosis and melanosome production and transfer occur only during the anagen phase of the hair cycle. A negative feedback system has been postulated. Enzyme degradation products of melanosomes within matrix cells may cross cell membranes to melanocytes and control further melanin production or transfer. A melanocyte-specific 'chalone' acting within a negative feedback system may well exist for follicular melanocytes.

Follicular melanocytes are known to respond like epidermal melanocytes to melanocyte-stimulating hormone (MSH), which can darken light-coloured hair. Three forms of MSH have been described: these are small peptide hormones consisting of 12–18 amino acids. In vertebrates they are produced from the intermediate lobe of the pituitary gland. All three melanotrophins are cleavage products of a common precursor peptide, pro-opiomelanocortin. Corticotropin (adrenocorticotrophic hormone, ACTH) and α-MSH contain homologous internal sequences. Thus, the hyperpigmentation that occurs in Addison's disease, Nelson's syndrome and ectopic ACTH syndrome may be the result of ACTH, α-MSH and even other peptides with common sequences. The effects of hormones other than MSH on hair pigmentation have yet to be elucidated. Oestrogens and progestogens may increase hair colour in view of their effect on the epidermis during pregnancy.

VARIATIONS IN HAIR COLOUR

Genetic and racial aspects

Mammalian hair colour has long been a subject of considerable interest to geneticists, and in a variety of species, including humans, a number of genetic variants have been described. Genetic studies of hair colour not only provide us with knowledge of gene function but also give us an insight into the mechanism of hair pigmentation. From laboratory and animal studies a general conformity has been shown in the complement of genes affecting hair colour. It is reasonable to assume that an essentially similar complex of genes may be involved in humans. Human hair colour is influenced by at least four gene loci which are probably allelic. The chief obstacle to more detailed studies of hair colour inheritance in humans is the absence of clear data on 'crosses' between individuals with 'pure' Caucasoid, Negroid and Mongoloid skin. Ethnic differences in hair colour are very conspicuous, as are the differences in hair morphology, though colour and hair form are inherited separately. Dark hair predominates in the world. Among Caucasoids there is wide variation in colour within geographical regions. Blond hair is most frequent in northern Europe and black hair in southern and eastern Europe. Foci of blondness are to be found even in North Africa, the Middle East and in some Australoids. Congoid, Capoid, Mongoloid and Australoid hair is mainly black.

Red hair

Red hair (rutilism) has attracted more attention than other colours because it is less common and because it is distinctive and relatively rare. The melanocyte-stimulating hormone receptor gene (MC1R) is associated with red hair; this gene is located on chromosome 16.[2] The melanin pigment is predominantly phaeomelanin. In Italy and in the UK, excluding East Anglia, the distribution of red hair is similar to that of blood group O. The incidence of red hair varies from 0.3% in northern Germany, to 1.9% in Copenhagen, to as high as 11% in parts of

Scotland. Like hair of many other colours, red hair often darkens with age from red through brown to sandy or auburn in the adult. The skin of red-heads is generally pale, burns easily in sunlight and pigments very little even after prolonged and frequent sun exposure. Enquiries in Continental Europe revealed that red hair was thought to be associated with the idea of being less serious!

Bright red hair in childhood often darkens with age

Heterochromia

This is defined as the growth of hair of two distinct colours in the same individual. A colour difference between scalp and moustache is not uncommon. In fair-haired individuals, pubic and axillary hair, eyebrows and eyelashes are much darker than scalp hair. In humans, eyelashes are generally the most darkly pigmented hairs. Black- and brown-haired subjects commonly have red or auburn sideburns. In other than the fair-haired, genital hair is usually lighter-coloured than scalp hair and may have a reddish tint even in those with brown pubic hair. Of a series of South African whites, 33% had red axillary hair while this was only occasionally seen in coloureds; also hair on the lower and lateral aspect of the scrotum was lighter than on the pubes. In brown-haired individuals a reddish tint is more common in axillary hair than on the scalp.

Scalp hair generally darkens with age. Rarely, a circumscribed patch of hair of different colour occurs. This usually has a genetic basis, though the mode of inheritance is not known in humans. Patchy differences of hair colour are of five main types:

1. tufts of very dark, coarse hair growing from a melanocytic naevus
2. hereditary, typically autosomal dominant heterochromia, e.g. tufts of red hair at the temples in a black-haired subject or a single black patch in a blond
3. partial asymmetry of hair and eye colour may occur sporadically – perhaps as a result of somatic mosaicism
4. the white forelock of piebaldism
5. the 'flag' sign in kwashiorkor.

GREYING OF HAIR

Greying of hair (canities) is usually a manifestation of the ageing process and is due to a progressive reduction in melanocyte function (Figures 7.10, 7.11). This may be genetically programmed to occur as early as adolescence, reflecting the intense biological activity in the hair bulb, which may in some follicles produce melanocyte 'senescence' by the second decade of life. The larger medullary spaces of older people may contribute to the process.

There is a gradual dilution of pigment in greying hairs; i.e. the full range of colour from normal to white can be seen both along individual hairs and from hair to hair. Loss of hair shaft colour is associated with a decrease and eventual cessation of tyrosinase activity in the lower bulb. In white hairs, melanocytes are infrequent or absent, or possibly dormant. It has been suggested that autoimmunity plays a part in the pathogenesis of greying. Grey hair certainly has an association with the autoimmune disease pernicious anaemia. The age of onset of grey hair is primarily dependent on the genotype of the individual, although acquired factors may play a part. The visual impression of greyness is more obvious (seen earlier) in the fair-haired. In Caucasoid races, white hair first appears at the age of 34.2 ± 9.6 years, and by the age of 50 years,

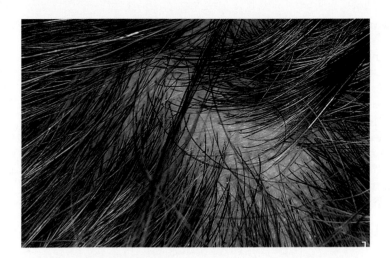

Figure 7.10
Irregular greying of hair.

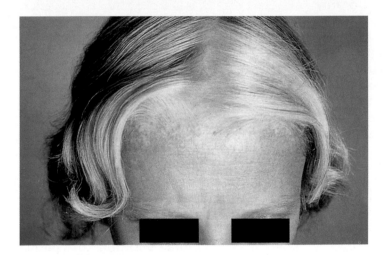

Figure 7.11
Prominent greying of hair – in this case it was premature and associated with early onset pernicious anaemia.

50% of the population have at least 50% grey hairs. The onset in black Africans is 43.9 ± 10.3 years, and in Japanese between 30 and 34 years in men and 35 and 39 years in women. The beard and moustache areas commonly become grey before scalp or body hair. On the scalp, the temples usually show greying first, followed by a wave of greyness spreading to the crown and later to the occipital area.

Rapid onset, allegedly 'overnight' greying of hair, has excited the literary, medical and anthropological worlds for centuries. Many reports have been overdramatized, but it does certainly occur. Historical examples often quoted include Sir Thomas More and Marie Antoinette, whose hair apparently became grey over the night preceding their execution. The mechanism for rapid greying is thought to be the selective shedding of pigmented hairs in diffuse alopecia areata, the non-pigmented hairs being retained.

Despite occasional reports to the contrary, in general greying of hair is progressive and permanent, although melanogenesis during anagen may be intermittent for a time before finally stopping. Most of the reports of the return of normal hair colour from grey are examples of pigmented regrowth following alopecia areata, which eventually repigments in many cases. The reported repigmentation of grey hair in association with addisonian hypoadrenalism may result from a mechanism similar to that in alopecia areata or vitiligo, in view of the known association between these diseases. Darkening of grey hair may occur following large doses of *p*-aminobenzoic acid.

Premature greying of hair

Premature greying of hair is arbitrarily defined as onset of greying before 20 years of age in Caucasoids and 30 years of age in Negroids. It probably has a genetic basis and occasionally occurs as an isolated auto-somal dominant condition. The association between premature greying and certain organ-specific autoimmune diseases is well documented. The relationship is probably not one of common pathogenesis but of genetic linkage. It is often stated that prema-ture greying may be an early sign of pernicious anaemia, hyperthyroidism and, less commonly, hypothyroidism, all auto-immune diseases which individually have a genetic predisposition (Figure 7.11). In a controlled study of the integumentary associations of pernicious anaemia, 11% of patients had premature greying. In Böök's syndrome, an autosomal dominant trait, premature greying, is associated with premolar hypodontia and palmoplantar hyperhidrosis.

The premature ageing syndromes, proge-ria and Werner's syndrome (pangeria) (chromosome site 8p12-p11.2), may have very early greying as a prominent feature. It does not occur in metageria, acrogeria, or total lipodystrophy. In progeria it is associ-ated with marked loss of scalp hair at as early as 2 years of age.

In dystrophic myotonica, the onset of grey hair may precede the myotonia and muscle wasting.

Premature canities is an inconstant feature of the Rothmund–Thomson syn-drome; when present, it typically com-mences in adolescence.

One-third of patients with chromosome 5p-syndrome (cri-du-chat syndrome) have prematurely grey hair.

> **Premature hair greying may be associated with autoimmunity, e.g. pernicious anaemia**

Localized white hair (poliosis)

Poliosis is defined as the presence of a localized patch of white hair due to the absence or deficiency of melanin in a group of neighbouring follicles. The changes in melanogenesis are the same in the hair folli-cle as in the affected epidermis.

Hereditary defects

Piebaldism[3] (white spotting or partial albinism) is an autosomal dominant abnor-mality with patches of skin totally devoid of pigment, which remain unchanged through-out life. It is due to several mutations at the W locus, the gene encoding *C-kit* receptor. Most commonly a frontal white patch (Figure 7.12) occurs – the white forelock – which may be the only sign. Melanocytes are decreased in number, but are mor-phologically abnormal and contain normal non-melanized premelanosomes, and also premelanosomes and melanosomes of abnormal appearance. Similar pathological changes are seen in Tietze's syndrome of generalized 'white spot' loss of skin and

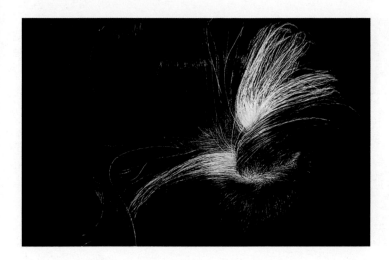

Figure 7.12
Poliosis.

hair pigment, complete deaf-mutism and eyebrow hypoplasia. Whether or not melanocytes are present in the affected areas remains controversial.

Waardenburg syndrome shows skin changes so similar to piebaldism that they are presumed to have a similar pathogenesis (chromosome site 2q35). Symptoms and signs are present from birth and include dystopia cantharum with lateral displacement of the medial canthi, hypertrophy of the nasal root and hyperplasia of the inner third of the eyebrows with confluent brows. Total or partial iridal heterochromia may occur as may perceptive deafness. The white forelock is present in 20% of cases. Premature greying may develop with or without the white forelock. Piebaldism and congenital nerve deafness may occur in the absence of other overt signs of Waardenburg syndrome, suggesting that this association may be genetically distinct.

In vitiligo, the white patches of skin frequently have white hairs within them (Figure 7.13). The histological changes are consistent with an 'autoimmune injury' to the melanocytes, but without hair shedding.

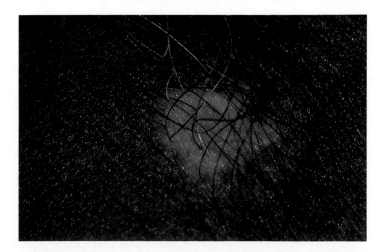

Figure 7.13
Grey hairs in a patch of vitiligo.

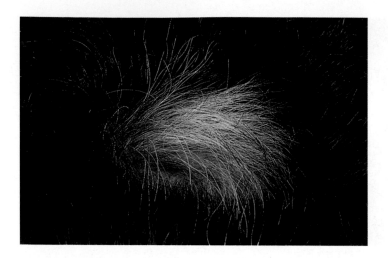

Figure 7.14
Alopecia areata – regrowing hair, some apigmented.

The Vogt–Koyanagi–Harada syndrome consists of a post-febrile illness comprising bilateral uveitis, labyrinthine deafness, tinnitus, vitiligo, poliosis, alopecia areata and meningitis. Alezzandrini's syndrome combines unilateral facial vitiligo, retinitis and poliosis of eyebrows and eyelashes; perceptive deafness is rarely associated.

In alopecia areata, regrowing hair is frequently white (Figure 7.14). It may remain so, particularly in cases of late onset. Though absent hair pigment is only evident at this stage of resolution, melanocytes are lost from the hair bulb quite early and migrate to the dermal papilla. Poliosis occurs in 60% of cases of tuberous sclerosis. Depigmented hair may be the earliest sign.

The pathognomonic signs of Recklinghausen's multiple neurofibromatosis relate to hyperpigmented areas – café-au-lait macules and axillary and perineal freckling. Scalp neurofibromas may have a patch of poliosis overlying them; this must not be mistaken for vitiliginous changes.

Acquired defects

Permanent pigmentary loss may be induced by inflammatory processes which damage melanocytes, e.g. herpes zoster. X-radiation often causes permanent hair loss, but less intense treatment leads to hypopigmented and, rarely, hyperpigmented hair. Patchy white hair may develop on the beard area after dental treatment.

Albinism[3]

In autosomal recessive oculocutaneous albinism (complete, perfect or generalized albinism; chromosome site 15q11.2-q.12), similar changes are found in the hair bulb melanocytes as in the epidermis. This applies to tyrosine-positive and tyrosine-negative types. Melanocytes are structurally normal and active in producing melanosomes of grades I and II. They are, however, enzymically inactive. The melanocyte system is never completely devoid of melanin. In Caucasoids the hair is typically yellowish white (Figure 7.15), though it may be cream, yellow, yellowish red or vibrant red. This range of colour parallels that seen in normal blond Caucasoids. In Negroid albinos the hair colour is white or yellowish brown.

In complete albinism, the hair may be yellow or white

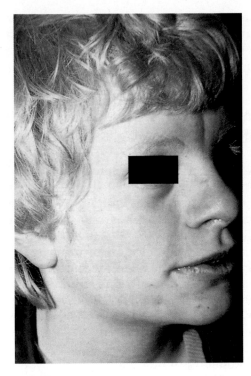

Figure 7.15
Albinism – yellow hair.

Chédiak–Higashi syndrome

This syndrome is an autosomal recessive defect of the membrane-bound organelles of several cell types. Mutations of the LYST locus cause defects in the Chédiak–Higashi syndrome (CHS) protein to occur. It combines oculocutaneous hypopigmentation with a lethal defect of leucocytes. The hair is silvery grey or light blond and may be sparse.

COLOUR CHANGES INDUCED BY CHEMICALS AND PHARMACOLOGICAL AGENTS

Some topical agents temporarily change hair colour. Dithranol and chrysarobin stain light-coloured or grey hair mahogany brown. Resorcin, formerly used a great deal in a variety of skin diseases, colours black or white hair, yellow or yellowish brown.

Some systemic agents alter hair colour by interfering with the eumelanin or phaeomelanin pathway. In other drugs the mechanism is not known. Chloroquine and hydroxychloroquine interfere with phaeomelanin synthesis; i.e. they only affect blond and red haired individuals. After 3–4 months of treatment, the hair becomes increasingly silvery or white. The colour change is usually patchy and first affects the temples or eyebrows. The changes are completely reversible. Mephenesin, a glycerol ester used extensively in the past for diseases with muscle spasms, causes pigmentary loss in dark-haired people. Triparamol, an anticholesterolaemic drug, and fluorobutyrophenone, an antipsychotic drug, both interfere with keratinization and cause hypopigmented and sparse hair. Minoxidil and diazoxide, two potent antihypertensive agents, both cause hypertrichosis and darkening of hair. The colour produced by diazoxide is reddish, whereas minoxidil darkens hair mainly by converting vellus hair to terminal hair, i.e. enhancing normal melanogenesis. Hydroquinone and phenylthiourea interfere with tyrosine activity, causing hypopigmentation of skin and hair.

The scalp hair may have a distinctive silvery colour in argyria (Figure 7.16).

Darkening of white hair has been shown to occur in a patient with Parkinson's disease following the addition of carbidopa and bromocriptine therapy. There is anecdotal evidence that a variety of non-steroidal anti-inflammatory agents can temporarily produce pigment in grey hairs.

COLOUR CHANGES DUE TO NUTRITIONAL DEFICIENCIES

Because specific dietary deficiencies are rare in humans, most clinical knowledge of

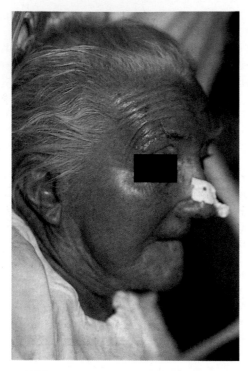

Figure 7.16
Silvery grey hair in argyria.

their effects is derived from laboratory and animal studies. Copper deficiency in cattle causes achromotrichia since it is the prosthetic group of tyrosinase. Loss of hair colour due to this mechanism occurs in humans as Menkes' kinky-hair syndrome, but why the hair twists remains unknown. In protein malnutrition, exemplified by kwashiorkor, hair colour changes are a prominent feature. Normal black hair becomes brown or reddish, and brown hair becomes blond. Intermittent protein malnutrition leads to the 'flag' sign of kwashiorkor (*signe de la bandera*) – alternating white (abnormal) and dark bands occur along individual hairs. Similar changes to kwashiorkor have been described in severe ulcerative colitis and after extensive bowel resection. The lightening of hair colour

from black to brown described in severe iron-deficiency anaemia may be an effect on keratinization rather than melanocytic function.

HAIR COLOUR IN METABOLIC DISORDERS

Phenylketonuria is an autosomal recessive disorder in which the tissues are unable to metabolize phenylalanine to tyrosine because of phenylalanine hydroxylase deficiency. Mental retardation, fits and decreased pigmentation of skin, eyes and hair occur with eczema and dermographism. Black hair may become brown while older, 'institutionalized' phenylketonurias may have pale blond or grey hair. Tyrosine treatment causes darkening towards normal colour within 1–2 months.

The paling of hair seen in homocystinuria is probably due to keratinization changes in view of the error in methionine metabolism. In Menkes' syndrome and chronic iron deficiency pale hair is seen.

Light, almost white, hair and recurrent oedema are the surface manifestations of the hair condition, 'oast-house' disease. Methionine concentration in the blood is raised in this condition.

ACCIDENTAL HAIR DISCOLORATION

Hair avidly binds many inorganic elements and thus hair colour changes are occasionally seen after exposure to such substances (Figure 7.17). Exposure to high concentrations of copper in industrial processes or in tap water or swimming pools may cause green hair, particularly visible in blond subjects. Cobalt workers get bright blue hair,

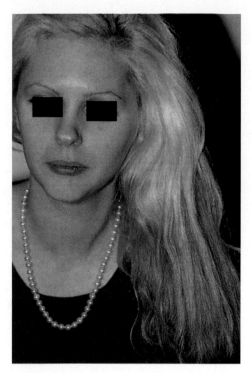

Figure 7.17
Bleached hair – inorganic stain (reddish brown)
from bathing in 'thermal' water; abnormal
colour seen on the distal parts of the hair shafts.

whereas a deep blue tint may be seen in handlers of indigo. A yellowish hair colour is not uncommon in white- or grey-haired heavy smokers due to tar in cigarette smoke; yellow staining may also occur from picric acid and dithranol. Trinitrotoluene (TNT) workers sometimes develop yellow skin and reddish brown hair.

REFERENCES

1. Castanet J, Ortonne JP (2000) Hair pigmentation. In: *Hair and its disorders*, eds Camacho FM, Randall VA, Price VH (London, Martin Dunitz), pp 49–63.
2. Ha T, Rees JL (2001) The melanocortin 1 receptor. What's red hair got to do with it? *J Am Acad Dermatol* **45:** 961–964.
3. Tomita Y (1994) The molecular genetics of albinism and piebaldism, *Arch Dermatol* **130:** 355–358.

8 Psychosociology of hair

The effective diagnosis, assessment and management of many disorders of the hair are impossible without some appreciation of the special psychological significance of the hair. Diseases that produce patterns of hair growth which deviate even slightly from that which the patient regards as normal may in extreme cases cause emotional stress of such a degree as to perpetuate the abnormality, whether or not stress played a role in initiating it.

Perception may appear excessive if it relates to a moderate change; if so, dysmorphophobia should be considered. Furthermore, the insidious chronic evolution of a moderate imbalance of the steady state of hair shedding and regrowth may lead to a depressive status: no one believes that the patient is losing her hair as 'so many are still remaining'. The patient feels totally isolated in the absence of appropriate diagnosis and identification of the kinetic dimensions of what is going on, even subclinically.

Nowadays, it is not possible to reassure a patient without functional exploration and appropriate documentation; stress-related disorders have been a grey zone where patients were all too easily classified. In the present era of increased communication of information, one must have the opportunity to state whether or not a pathological process is taking place and appropriate management, including psychological support, must be initiated.

THE UNCONSCIOUS SIGNIFICANCE OF HAIR

Grooming has recently been shown to be under genetic control in mice. In the social organizations of other mammals, hair, especially on the head (crown, mane), is a significant signal between individual members of the group. Hair mass and colour may be significant factors that regulate the distance that younger members will maintain between themselves and group leaders. Care of the hair coat is a well-known socializing modality in monkeys related to age and sex; haircare and body heat are under certain circumstances more rewarding than food.

The importance of hair in many rituals in a variety of primitive peoples has long been recognized in the anthropological and psychiatric literature, and is associated with the concept of power and physical strength and attractiveness. In modern humans, hair has

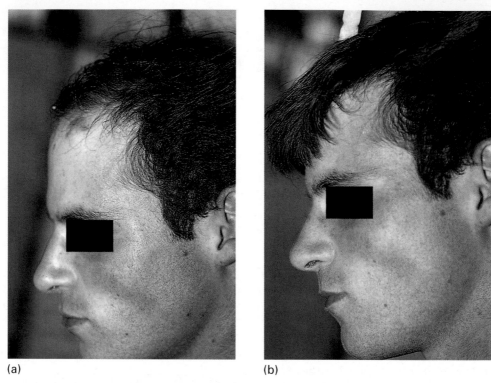

(a)   (b)

Figure 8.1
Minimal androgenetic alopecia without (a) and with (b) hair prosthesis in position.

practically no other significance than as a sexual symbol. A friend psychologist involved in a number of enquiries concluded that hair problems are related to dating and mating, and it has been claimed that there is no normal person without some degree of hair fetishism. Subjects with alopecia may assert that they would prefer to be without an arm or a leg than minus head hair. Even minimal facial hair in a woman may cause great distress. These effects are frequently not based upon reality value, but, like all the effects connected with hair, have their source in profound unconscious 'constellation'. Some men with quite mild androgenetic alopecia will go to great lengths to improve their appearance by prosthetic or surgical means (Figures 8.1, 8.2). Surgical interventions should at least improve the appearance in the long term.

We advocate that decisions on hair transplantation should be taken after proper diagnosis and definition of the kinetics of the hair disorder. Transplanting in a subject with alopecia areata will inevitably lead to hair loss in the grafts and is a medical fault. Similarly, lack of provision of proper information to the patient on the long-term evolution of male pattern balding is not acceptable (Figure 8.3).

Charles Berg, a psychoanalyst of the Freudian school, believed that the normal concern about the hair becoming thin, falling out or becoming greyish, was a displacement of castration anxiety and that shaving the head was symbolic castration! This explanation may seem extreme, but in some societies and religions, shaving the head is associated with celibacy or chastity, as is, to a lesser extent, covering the hair in

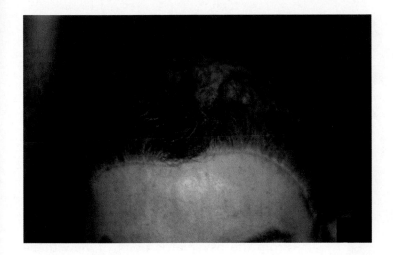

Figure 8.2
Androgenetic alopecia – very poor aesthetic result after scalp flap surgery.

Muslim and Orthodox Jewish society. The Christian wedding veil similarly represents modesty and chastity.

Changing the hairstyle is also a marker of a change in the social status: the braid of younger children in ancient Egyptian culture, for example, or a haircut in a child separating from the child group to enter the world of adults (Jewish society, Amazonian tribes).

The association of hair with sexual attractiveness is clear from even the most superficial survey of the visual arts, books and the output of the advertising industry. The cliché 'a woman's crowning glory' exemplifies the attitude, and the anguish at the loss of head hair and thus of sexual attractiveness is well described and illustrated in the self-help book *Coping with Sudden Hair Loss* by Elizabeth Steele, the founder of the UK Alopecia Society.

This heavy weight of symbolism pertaining to head hair is outweighed by that of body hair, the presence and depiction of which is hedged with taboos. In the French *'culture des salons'*, a specific word was created to name those hairs that would not be looked at or talked about in public – *'poils'*; 'head hairs', in contrast, were of social significance and talking about them was acceptable, so they were specifically called *'cheveux'*. Classical paintings from the 15th to the 19th centuries do not show body hair on female nudes. This omission led the art critic and historian John Ruskin to consider his wife abnormal because of her body hair, which prevented the consummation of their marriage and resulted in its annulment. Pubic hair is often considered a forbidden subject, and may be an object of fetishism. Axillary hair is more likely to be considered normal, acceptable or even attractive in Continental Europe, but is regarded as abhorrent in women or sometimes as a sign of rampant feminism in the UK and the USA. Hairiness of the head, face and body of men is often equated with barbarism, violence and rape.

There can be no doubt that some disorders of hair give rise to anxieties more profound than their objective severity would appear to justify. This may reflect the symbolic significance of hair.

DISTURBANCE OF THE BODY IMAGE

Some 30 years ago, the concept of 'non-disease' was coined and it was pointed out that the absence of diagnostic signs and

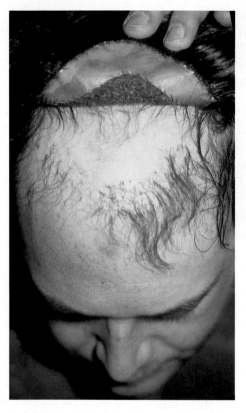

Figure 8.3
Donor dominance in grafts for androgenetic alopecia. Hair follicles contained in grafts taken from an androgen-sensitive area will miniaturize at the same pace in the recipient area (right frontal hair line) as in the androgen-sensitive donor area (lower vertex, not shown here). The transplants on the left frontal line, were taken from an appropriate donor site; i.e. less sensitive to androgen.

symptoms need not imply an absence of significant symptomatology. Of the patients studied, the symptoms are confined to the scalp, the face, and the perineum in the majority. Most affected individuals are adult females. The scalp symptoms are more common in women and are chiefly of excess hair loss; a minority also have irritation and burning. None of these patients have objective signs of hair loss, and are

therefore suffering from the delusion of dysmorphophobia. Many of these patients have depressive illness. Some of these female patients are preoccupied with excess facial hair that is not clinically apparent. Suicidal symptoms must be taken seriously. The present authors have seen similar patients whose principal scalp complaint apart from hair loss was extreme tenderness. In all these patients the objective changes, if indeed there are any, are so slight as to seem trivial even to the most sympathetic observer, yet the patients insist that the symptoms are ruining their life.

From the psychiatric point of view these patients are not a uniform group. Most have a disturbed body image and the majority are depressed. They require most careful management and the more severely affected, who are potential suicide risks, should be referred to a psychiatrist.

Diffuse shedding of hair can occur in patients under very severe stress, but diffuse alopecia should not be glibly attributed to the minor stresses that can be elicited in the history of most individuals. Diffuse shedding of hair beginning some 3 or 4 months after a well-defined major stressful episode may, however, be accepted as provoked by that episode and as potentially reversible in the same way as post-partum or post-febrile alopecia. This may be due to the stress itself or to the profound anorexia and consequent weight loss that often occur with a major life crisis or stress. Hair loss may accompany other 'losses'.

However, chronic or severe acute 'stress' may occasionally develop along with the 'androgenetic' syndrome. Besides psychological support, early investigation and treatment should be undertaken in order to prevent further hair loss. The first symptom of androgenetic alopecia is often profuse but predominantly frontovertical shedding of telogen hairs. This symptom is very easily confused with true diffuse telogen shedding as mentioned above. Whatever the distinction, both reflect shortening of the hair cycle and more shedding. In the case of androgen sensitivity, shortening will lead to the next steps: delayed replacement and more thinning and final atrophy without production of clinically visible hair. In the case of telogen effluvium, chronic shedding and rapid regrowth of short-lived thick anagen hair will not end in balding, but the maximal length of uncut hair will be shorter: a new dynamic equilibrium has been reached ... but with continuous shedding of more hair than earlier in life.

Depressive illness in young women may be accompanied by androgenetic cutaneous changes. Although the patient may herself tend to blame her alopecia, hirsutism or acne for her depression, a detailed history often establishes that the emotional and cutaneous changes developed in parallel. There are controversy and doubt as to the relationship between depression, stress and androgenetic syndromes. Some clinicians have argued that antiandrogen therapy even worsens the depressive status.

In the cutaneous androgenetic syndromes the distress caused by the skin changes can contribute to their perpetuation. Acne and/or hirsutism can seriously impair a sensitive adolescent's capacity to establish normal social relationships with his contemporaries and, if severe, may retard his psychosocial development. The evidence that a self-perpetuating vicious circle can become established has not yet been proven biochemically, but clinical experience suggests that it may occur and that it may indeed be of common occurrence.

The role of stress in precipitating alopecia areata is well known, although the time interval between the alleged precipitating stress and loss of hair has varied from a few days to several months. It follows that if stress can indeed precipitate an attack of alopecia areata, it must do so by more than one mechanism. Some writers have suggested that alopecia may be an auto-immune disorder. Should this prove to be the case, it does not preclude the possible precipitation of an attack by stress, as the science of psychoimmunology is still in its infancy, but can already suggest possible mechanisms. The evidence incriminating stress remains controversial, but it is probable that no dermatologist of experience would exclude its possible role in certain cases.

Alopecia areata can be extremely disfiguring. Whether or not stress plays a part in provoking it, it is certain that the alopecia is often itself a source of severe stress. This relationship is certainly perceived by sufferers. It is not proven that this stress perpetuates the condition, but the possibility should be borne in mind in the management of these patients. Psychological approaches do not significantly modify the course of the disease but do help patients cope with hair loss.

Alopecia in males and females

In studies in Continental Europe, even though bald males were considered more intelligent than their non-bald colleagues, some balding males suffered a loss of self-esteem and some degree of psychological maladjustment that was improved when hair regrowth was initiated with a topical agent. Balding in females resulted in a gradual but in-depth change in social and private behaviour. They had more psychosocial problems, which they attributed to the hair loss, than men with androgenetic alopecia or women without visible dermatological conditions. During such psychosocial enquiries, the women with androgenetic alopecia were rated higher for self-sufficiency and social inadequacy, rigidity and general psychological maladjustment, but had lower scores for injuredness, self-evaluation and self-esteem than men. Globally, men are afraid of looking older, whereas women feel less feminine. If the importance of hair is as described, the fact that smoking might aggravate the problem should be taken as another opportunity to modify human behaviour and diminish the positive images associated with smoking, seeing it rather as a personal and social nuisance.

ARTEFACTS

Artefacts are self-inflicted lesions, but the term as usually employed excludes such lesions produced accidentally through the abuse of mechanical or chemical cosmetic procedures. The most frequent form of deliberate artefact of the scalp consists of plucking the hair, so-called trichotillomania (see pp 97–101). In children, the partially bald patches so produced are seldom of serious psychiatric significance, but the plucking systematically of almost all the head hair in an adult usually indicates a very serious personality disorder, as does extensive self-mutilation of the skin in any region of the body. This tonsure trichotillomania is very rare in men (Figure 8.4), mostly occurring in women from 15 to 35 years of age.

Deliberate physical or chemical production of other injuries of the scalp is very unusual, but it is possible that some cases are undiagnosed. Trichoteiromania due to excess rubbing of scalp has recently been identified as a new variant of hair mania. These subjects are more open to talk about their habit than those affected by true trichotillomania. Trichoklepto-

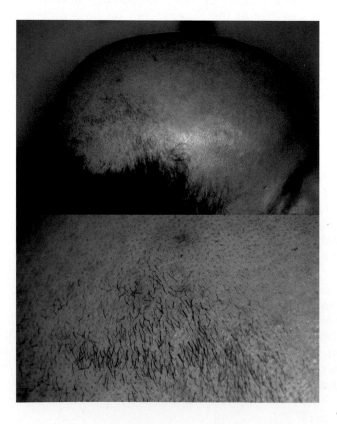

Figure 8.4
Trichotillomania associated with severe male pattern baldness.

mania might describe pulling and taking away hair from another individual (see Figure 3.82).

THE RELIGIOUS SIGNIFICANCE OF HAIR

Hair has two perceived symbolic meanings in a religious context. Shaven or shorn hair, or even total scalp epilation by plucking, is a symbol of bodily – including sexual – dedication to the gods, i.e. celibacy and chastity. Monks and nuns, both Buddhist and Christian, have shaven heads, as do Hindu priests and widows. Hair sacrifice and offering to the gods was widespread in many ancient religions. The hair was offered for fertility, for victory, in fulfilment of a vow, and in place of human sacrifice. The practice continues today. The temple of Tirupati in southern India is a renowned pilgrimage site for such offerings, which, it is said, also contribute to the temple revenues. In contrast, matted, uncut hair is seen as withdrawal from worldly concerns and vanities in the Hindu sadhu (Figure 8.5). Sometimes long hair is a religious requirement, as in the Sikh religion and for the Rastafarians, although in both groups it has now also become a symbol of identity as well as a religious tenet.

In patriarchal religious societies, married females cut their hair as a submission to male authority; wigs are used for appearances in public while natural hair is shown in privacy, once again illustrating the fears of the seductive power of female hair!

HAIR CUTTING AS PUNISHMENT

Many peoples have practised cutting off or shaving the hair as a punishment. The Ainu of Hokkaido, the northernmost island of

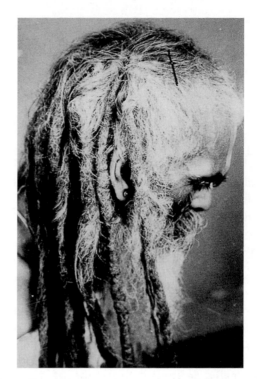

Figure 8.5
Uncut and matted head and face hair – religious sign of withdrawal from worldly concerns and vanities.

Japan, have a long-established reputation for hirsutism: they are in fact a proto-Caucasoid stock who are no more hirsute than many other Caucasoids, although very hairy compared with their Japanese neighbours. Among the Ainu, great emphasis is placed on the possession of a very full beard and abundant head hair and the enforced cutting of hair is regarded as a severe punishment associated with loss of honour. Women's hair is cut as punishment for adultery. The same punishment was used in Europe after the Second World War on women who had associated with soldiers of occupying armies.

The importance placed on short hair by the armed forces of many countries reinforces the popular association between short hair and authority and discipline.

Conversely, Japanese troops imposed the wearing of long hair on Chinese males in order for them to look like females, which was considered injurious.

HAIRSTYLE

The importance of hair as a component of the body image has been mentioned, and vast amounts of money are expended on styling hair. The length, the colour and the style in which it is worn must conform to an accepted stereotype. Some knowledge of recent research on such stereotypes is helpful in increasing a dermatologist's understanding of some of his patients who appear to be endeavouring perversely to demand from their hair qualities with which nature failed to endow it.

Long hair in males in the USA is said by some to be a reflection of group attitudes culturally defined rather than of personal feelings of sexual identity. The finding of some investigators on male students classified as 'deviant' in hair length were not unexpected; the deviants with hair reaching below their shoulders assigned more value to independence and less value to recognition and conformity than the non-deviant students. The stereotypes accepted among students have been found to vary from one university to another even during the same period, being influenced by the conservatism or liberalism of the community in which the university is situated. Long hair has been seen as a protest, but the increasing number of hairstylists for young men seems to indicate that many of them need an artificial aid to win or to retain a desired self-esteem.

In the 1980s short hair was again the norm, and long hair was often a badge of defiance, e.g. the Rastafarian style. Short hair can also be a symbol of defiance, as in the skinheads and punks. The 1920s passion for the 'bob' was seen as such by parents and authority figures. Differentiation of those 'group-associated hairstyles' may be difficult, as many balding males, any age, shave their hair in order to make hair loss less visible, following a trend launched by many sportsmen.

HAIR COLOUR

As with other stereotypes, those concerning hair colour apply to the communities studied and to the period of the study. Nevertheless, they throw considerable light on deeply rooted concepts and prejudices.

Yellow hair or a yellow wig was the trademark of a prostitute in ancient Rome. Blond hair is associated with both innocence, as in so many fairy tales, and, conversely, with sexual allure, as exemplified by Marilyn Monroe and other screen goddesses. Dark hair has connotations of night and mystery and is essential for the 'vamp'. Enquiries in Continental Europe revealed that red hair was associated with the idea of being less serious. Strangely, red hair has been associated with bad odours, indicating deeply rooted unconscious belief in some cultures.

BEARDS

Ancient Egyptian Pharaohs, male or female, associated power with wearing a fake beard. Numerous psychological studies carried out on the subject of beards show a generally positive correlation between the amount of hair on the subject's face and high ratings for masculinity, maturity, good looks, dominance, self-confidence and other desirable traits. Similar findings have been reported from the University of Chicago. However, at the rural and more conservative University of Wyoming, only 12.8% of females preferred men with a very full beard, whereas 40% preferred no facial hair and 42% preferred a moustache but no beard.

MOUSTACHES

Few investigations have been made of the correlation of moustaches with personality traits or of observer reactions to them. In studies of British Army personnel in the years 1950–1960, moustaches were divided into four types:

1. trimmed, flatly covering most of the lip
2. clipped, 'toothbrush'
3. line
4. bushy.

Those with trimmed moustaches did not differ in their assessments from clean-shaven candidates. All those with clipped moustaches failed to pass the selection board (but not of course on account of their moustaches). They were limited in imagination with little appreciation of the opinions of others and they tended to create rather than to decrease interpersonal tensions. Men with line moustaches passed the board at only half the normal rate; those that failed showed obsessive health consciousness. Men with bushy moustaches passed at the normal rate; those that failed tended to self-indulgence and self-display. Australian observations over 20 years ago suggested an association between moustaches and sexual pathology, but did not allow any firm conclusions to be drawn.

Hair and politics have not been studied thoroughly: this subject definitely should be a potential source of information on the perpetuation of hair icons. Think only of the scalp hairstyle of US and USSR presidents during the second half of the 20th century: a sharp contrast between youthful-looking USA and the balding USSR. Whatever the merit of the individuals, images of success and failure were reinforced at the end! Think of the more recent preparation for the 2003 war between the USA and Iraq. Everyone probably remembers the hands of an anonymous hairdresser bringing the last touch on the hair of the president of the USA. This scene was shown on almost all TV screens worldwide – in our opinion during an exceedingly long period of time in view of the gravity of the situation – as the first military actions against Iraq were to be announced officially. On the other side, the Iraqi president conveyed the identification power of the moustaches on his troops. Indeed, as it appeared in magazines, 20 out of 20 military staff surrounding the then ruling Iraqi leader wore similar types of moustaches.

FURTHER READING

Barth JH, Catalan J, Cherry CA, Day A (1993) Psychological morbidity in women referred for treatment of hirsutism, *J Psychosom Res* **37**: 615–619.

Cash TF (1996) Body image and cosmetic surgery: the psychology of physical appearance, *Am J Cosmet Surg* **13(4)**: 345–351.

Cash TF, Price VH, Savin RC (1993) Psychological effects of androgenetic alopecia on women: comparisons with balding men and with female control subjects, *J Am Acad Dermatol* **29**: 568–575.

Freyschmidt-Paul P, Hoffmann R, Happle R (2001) Trichoteiromania, *Eur J Dermatol* **11**: 369–371.

Girman CJ, Rhodes T, Lilly FRW, et al (1998) Effects of self-perceived hair loss in a community sample of men, *Dermatology* **197**: 223–229.

Pomey-Rey D (1986) Hair and psychology. In: *The science of hair care*, ed Zviak C (New York, Marcel Dekker), pp 571–586.

Trueb RM (2003) Association between smoking and hair loss: another opportunity for health education against smoking? *Dermatology* **206:** 189–191.

Index

Page numbers in *italics* indicate figures or tables.